Pharmacy Calculations
for Technicians

Fifth Edition

Don A. Ballington, MS
Tova Wiegand-Green, MS

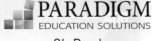

PARADIGM
EDUCATION SOLUTIONS

St. Paul

Managing Editor	Brenda M. Palo
Developmental Editor	Nancy Papsin
Production Editor	Lori Michelle Ryan
Assistant Production Editor	Katherine Lee
Editor/Proofreader	Thomas McNellis
Copy Editor	Kristin Melendez
Director of Production	Timothy W. Larson
Cover and Text Designer	Jaana Bykonich
Permissions Coordinator	Tari Cliff
Illustrator	S4Carlisle Publishing Services
Indexer	Terry Casey
Cover Images	iStockphoto/BahadirTanriover (top left), George Brainard (top right), Shutterstock/Ragne Kabanova (bottom left)

Care has been taken to verify the accuracy of information presented in this book. However, the authors, editors, and publisher cannot accept responsibility for Web, e-mail, newsgroup, or chat room subject matter or content, or for consequences from application of the information in this book, and make no warranty, expressed or implied, with respect to its content.

Trademarks: Some of the product names and company names included in this book have been used for identification purposes only and may be trademarks or registered trade names of their respective manufacturers and sellers. The authors, editors, and publisher disclaim any affiliation, association, or connection with, or sponsorship or endorsement by, such owners.

Art and Photo Credits: Following the index.

We have made every effort to trace the ownership of all copyrighted material and to secure permission from copyright holders. In the event of any question arising as to the use of any material, we will be pleased to make the necessary corrections in future printings. Thanks are due to the aforementioned authors, publishers, and agents for permission to use the materials indicated.

ISBN 978-0-76385-221-4 (text and Study Partner CD)
ISBN 978-0-76385-218-4 (text)
ISBN 978-0-76385-225-2 (eBook)

© 2014 by Paradigm Publishing, Inc.
875 Montreal Way
St. Paul, MN 55102
E-mail: educate@emcp.com
Website: www.emcp.com

Printed in the United States of America

22 21 20 19 18 17 16 15 14   3 4 5 6 7 8 9 10 11

Brief Contents

Contents

Pharmacy Calculations for Technicians, Fifth Edition provides students with the essential mathematics concepts and calculations skills that pharmacy technicians need to assist in the filling of drug doses in both community and institutional pharmacy practices as well as to prepare for the certification exams. Guided by clear, complete examples and practice problems, students begin by reviewing basic mathematical concepts such as fractions, decimals, percents, ratios, and number systems. Students are then introduced to different calculation methods such as ratio and proportion, dimensional analysis, and alligation. The text provides students with plenty of practice in pharmacy math calculations, conversions, measurements, and equations, including calculations required for the preparation of doses, parenteral solutions, and compounded products. These skills are taught using authentic medication labels and real-world applications. In addition, the text teaches business terms and supports calculations related to pharmacy operations. Students learn how to perform calculations for inventory applications, purchasing needs, profit margins, and insurance reimbursements. Lastly, the text offers important chapter features that provide students with the knowledge, skills, and confidence to provide safe and effective care for the patients they serve.

Chapter Features: A Visual Walk-Through

Chapter features are designed to help students learn calculation skills used in current pharmacy practice, including knowledge of basic mathematical concepts, an understanding of pharmacy calculation methods used in the preparation and dispensing of medications, and an insight into effective communication with patients and other healthcare team members.

1

LEARNING OBJECTIVES establish clear goals for pharmacy technician students as they begin their chapter study.

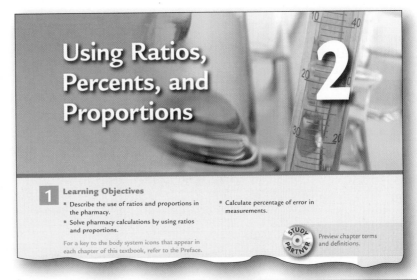

Using Ratios, Percents, and Proportions

2

1 **Learning Objectives**

- Describe the use of ratios and proportions in the pharmacy.
- Solve pharmacy calculations by using ratios and proportions.

- Calculate percentage of error in measurements.

For a key to the body system icons that appear in each chapter of this textbook, refer to the Preface.

STUDY PARTNER Preview chapter terms and definitions.

2 KEY TERMS are high-
lighted using boldfaced
type and are defined both
in context as well as in a
separate Key Terms section
at the end of each chapter.
Students are encouraged
to preview the chapter's
key terms on the Study
Partner CD before begin-
ning their chapter study.

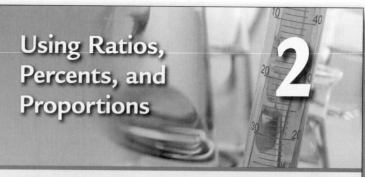

Using Ratios, Percents, and Proportions

2

Learning Objectives

- Describe the use of ratios and proportions in the pharmacy.
- Solve pharmacy calculations by using ratios and proportions.
- Calculate percentage of error in measurements.

For a key to the body system icons that appear in each chapter of this textbook, refer to the Preface.

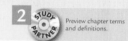 Preview chapter terms and definitions.

2.1 Numerical Ratios

2 A **ratio** is a numerical representation of the relationship between two parts of a whole or of the relationship of one part to the whole. Ratios are written with a colon (:) between the numbers, which may be read as *per, of, to,* or *in*. The ratio 1:2 could mean that the second part has twice the value (e.g., size, number, weight, ~~of the first~~ ~~would mean that~~ ~~something within a total~~

Pages 51–52
Page 53

Key Terms

conversion factor an equivalency equal to 1 that can be used when converting units of measure using the ratio-proportion method

percent the number of parts per 100; can be written as a fraction, a decimal, or a ratio

percentage of error the percentage by which a measurement is inaccurate

proportion an expression of equality between two ratios

ratio a numerical representation of the rela-tionship between two parts of the whole or between one part and the whole

ratio-proportion method a conversion method based on comparing a complete ratio to a ratio with a missing component

3 TIMELY TOPICS in
pharmacy practice are
introduced in this revised
edition, including days'
supply, time conversion,
IV calculations, and insurance reimbursements, to
name a few.

New!

3 ### Calculating Days' Supply

As each prescription is received in the pharmacy, personnel scan the prescription for completeness and validity, interpret the order, and then enter the information into the computer system. The electronic information becomes a part of the patient's perma-nent health record. Some information that must be entered into the computer is not always written on the prescription but must be calculated by the pharmacy technician or pharmacist. The pharmacist must verify the accuracy of the calculations and the data that is entered into the computer. Any calculation that the technician performs that requires written work should be available to the pharmacist when he or she veri-fies the accuracy of the prescription entry and calculations.

Prescriptions are often written for a specified number of doses or a specified dura-tion of time. In either case, the technician will need to calculate the "**days' supply.**" A prescription that is written for a specified number of doses such as #30 and with a dosing schedule of TID (or three times daily), will last 10 days. Another prescription may be written for a patient to use a medication TID for 10 days, and the physician has indicated the quantity as QS (or a sufficient quantity). You would calculate that the patient needs 30 doses to complete the therapy prescribed by the physician.

The most common information that requires a calculation is verifying that the days' supply and the quantity dispensed will meet the needs of the patient according to what the prescriber has indicated.

Example 3.1.6

Calculate the days' supply for the following prescription.

> ℞ **Ibuprofen 800 mg**
>
> take one tablet by mouth two times daily with food
>
> dispense 60 tablets

$$\frac{x \text{ days}}{60 \text{ tablets}} = \frac{1 \text{ day}}{2 \text{ tablets}}$$

$$\frac{(60 \text{ tablets}) \, x \text{ days}}{60 \text{ tablets}} = \frac{1 \text{ day} \, (60 \text{ tablets})}{2 \text{ tablets}}$$

$$x = 30 \text{ days' supply}$$

4

EXAMPLES provide realistic problem statements and show clear, step-by-step solutions. Many of these problems are accompanied by AUTHENTIC MEDICATION LABELS so that students can gain confidence in reading and accurately interpreting these labels before performing pharmacy calculations.

Example 2.3.3

4 The label shown below is the stock your pharmacy has available for gentamicin. How many milliliters will need to be prepared if the patient is prescribed 50 mg?

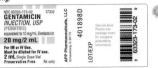

NDC 63323-173-02   17302
GENTAMICIN
INJECTION, USP
(PEDIATRIC)
equivalent to 10 mg/mL Gentamicin
20 mg/2 mL
For IM or IV Use.
Must be diluted for IV use.
2 mL Single Dose Vial
Preservative Free   Rx only

APP Pharmaceuticals, LLC
Schaumburg, IL 60173

401898D

LOT/EXP

63323-173-02

$$\frac{x\,\text{mL}}{50\,\text{mg}} = \frac{2\,\text{mL}}{20\,\text{mg}}$$

$$\frac{(50\text{-mg})\,x\,\text{mL}}{50\text{-mg}} = \frac{(50\,\text{mg})\,2\,\text{mL}}{20\,\text{mg}}$$

$$x\,\text{mL} = \frac{100\,\text{mL}}{20}$$

$$x\,\text{mL} = 5\,\text{mL}$$

Check that the product of the means equals the product of the extremes.

5 mL:50 mg = 2 mL:20 mg
$50 \times 2 = 5 \times 20$
$100 = 100$

2.3 Proportions

Because 2.5% is larger than the acceptable percentage of error, the target range was not met.

5

PROBLEM SETS reinforce chapter content and provide opportunities for students to practice their skills and gain confidence in their abilities. Answers to the Problem Sets can be found in Appendix A.

5

2.4 Problem Set

Calculate the percentage of error for the following measurements; then round to the nearest hundredths place. Assume that the measured amount is equal to the quantity desired.

1. The measured weight was 185 mg, but the actual weight is 189 mg.

2. The measured weight was 500 mg, but the actual weight is 476 mg.

3. The measured weight was 1200 mg, but the actual weight is 1507 mg.

4. The measured weight was 15 mg, but the actual weight is 12.5 mg.

5. The measured weight was 400 mcg, but the actual weight is 415 mcg.

6. The measured volume was 5 mL, but the actual volume is 6.3 mL.

Express the following ratios as fractions and reduce to the lowest terms.

1. 3:7

2. 8:6

3. 3:4

4. 4:6

5. 1:7

Reduce the following fractions to the lowest terms and express each as a ratio.

6. $\frac{2}{3}$

7. $\frac{6}{8}$

8. $\frac{5}{10}$

9. $\frac{1}{9}$

10. $\frac{1}{10,000}$

Applications

State the ratio for the following doses.

11. 30 mg capsule Cymbalta

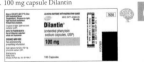

6

12. 100 mg capsule Dilantin

Dilantin
(extended phenytoin
sodium capsules, USP)
100 mg
100 Capsules

6

13. 5 mL dose of oral suspension containing 250 mg amoxicillin

00000-0000-00   reconstitute
w/ 105 mL water
Amoxicillin for Oral
Suspension, USP
250 mg per 5 mL
when reconstituted according to directions
Caution: Federal law prohibits
dispensing without prescription.
150 mL bottle

6

6

BODY SYSTEM ICONS have been placed by the names of all generic and brand name medications discussed in the chapter. These icons help students make connections between certain medications and the body systems that they are prescribed to treat. For a key that explains the meanings of the body system icons, see page xvi.

New!

7

SAFETY IN NUMBERS

are placed in the page margins and alert students to important safety reminders that must be heeded to provide safe and effective patient care.

8

FOR GOOD MEASURE

tips appear in the page margins and offer hints and rules to remember when performing pharmacy calculations.

9

MATH MORSELS

provide general math reminders and tips as they apply to pharmacy calculations.

10

PUT DOWN ROOTS

analyzes the root words of certain math terms so that students can understand how the definitions of these terms emerged from their word parts.

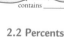

7 Safety in Numbers

For a decimal value less than 1, use a leading zero to prevent errors.

Reading and Writing Decimals

A decimal is read by first reading the whole number, if there is one, to the left of the decimal point, then the decimal point (say "and" or "point"), and then the decimal fraction, to the right of the decimal point.

A decimal is written as a whole number or a zero, then the decimal point (indicating the value of the number to the right of the decimal), and then the fractional portion. The values to the right of the decimal point are multiples of one-tenth: tenths, hundredths, thousandths, ten thousandths, and so on. Figure 1.4 illustrates this relationship in terms of medication.

To further emphasize the value of the calculation when there is no whole number, a zero should be placed to the left of the decimal point. This zero is called a **leading zero**. Using a leading zero will help prevent errors by ensuring a correct reading of the value.

Adding and Subtracting Decimals

When adding or subtracting decimals, place the numbers in columns so that the decimal points are aligned directly under each other. Add or subtract from the far-right column to the left column.

...conversion pr... the unknown a... ...ne value that is to be converted on the left side of the proportion. On the right side of the proportion, put the conversion factor. The **conversion factor** is an equivalency equal to 1. For example, since 1 g = 1000 mg, an example of a conversion factor is 1 g/1000 mg or 1000 mg/1 g. Additional conversion factors are presented in Appendix D.

Example 2.3.5

How many milligrams are equivalent to 3 g?

Begin the solution by setting up a ratio and solving for x, using the conversion factor 1000 mg = 1 g.

$$x \text{ mg}:3 \text{ g} = 1000 \text{ mg}:1 \text{ g}$$

$$\frac{x \text{ mg}}{3 \text{ g}} = \frac{1000 \text{ mg}}{1 \text{ g}}$$

The unit of measurement in the numerators is the same (both are milligrams), and the unit of measurement in the denominators is the same (both are grams). Multiply both sides by 3 g to cancel the grams and isolate the unknown.

8 For Good Measure

When setting up a proportion to solve a conversion, the units in the numerators must match, and the units in the denominators must match.

---

56   Chapter 2 _Using Ratios, Percents, and Proportions_

9 Math Morsels

Moving the decimal point three spaces to the right is the same as multiplying by 1000. Moving the decimal point three places to the left is the same as dividing by 1000.

yields 17,000,000 microliters. (Move the decimal point six places to the right.) Conversely, changing to a larger unit requires division. So, to convert 25 meters to kilometers, divide by 1000 to get 0.025 kilometers. (Move the decimal point three places to the left.) Similarly, 3 microliters divided by 1000 yields 0.003 milliliters, and 22 milliliters divided by 1000 yields 0.022 liters. In each case, move the decimal point three places to the left.

The key to understanding the relationships in the metric system is to remember that the decimal point must be moved three places when converting from one unit to the next. Moving the decimal point three places is essentially equivalent to multiplying or dividing the number by 1000. The three "places" are representative of the three zeros in 1000.

$$1 \text{ kg} = 1000 \text{ g}$$
$$1 \text{ g} = 1000 \text{ mg}$$
$$1 \text{ mg} = 1000 \text{ mcg}$$
$$1 \text{ L} = 1000 \text{ mL}$$

...ve...   ...of that s... converting ...   ...a larger u...

contains _____ g.

2.2 Percents

10 Put Down Roots

The word _percent_ comes from the Latin term _per centum_, meaning "by the hundred." Therefore, _percent_ literally means "per 100."

Percent expresses the number of parts compared with a total of 100 parts. The word _percent_ means "per 100" or "hundredths" and is the same as a fraction in which the denominator is 100. Percent is represented by the symbol %. Percents can be visualized by comparing a stack of 100 pennies (equivalent to $1) next to smaller stacks of pennies (see Figure 2.2). A stack of 5 pennies equals 5 cents and represents 5% of a dollar. Similarly, a stack of 40 pennies equals 40 cents and represents 40% of a dollar.

A percent can be written as a ratio, a fraction, or a decimal. For example, 30% means there are 30 parts in a total of 100 parts.

$$30:100, \quad \frac{30}{100}, \text{ or } 0.30$$

FIGURE 2.2   **Comparison of Percents**

100% of a dollar	40% of a dollar	5% of a dollar
100 pennies	40 pennies	5 pennies

2.2 _Percents_   47

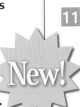

11

NAME EXCHANGE tips remind students that they must be familiar with both the generic name and the brand name of frequently prescribed medications.

New!

12

PHOTOGRAPHS reinforce the text and help students to recognize pharmacy supplies and equipment used for measurement.

13

ILLUSTRATIONS and their accompanying captions and callouts simplify important concepts that technicians need to understand to meet the needs of patients in a pharmacy setting.

14

FIGURES provide additional details and visual reinforcement of chapter topics.

Roman numerals.

Example 1.2.2

11

➤ Name Exchange

Diphenhydramine is generic for Benadryl. It is an over-the-counter medication but will still need a prescription written in some cases.

The following prescription is received in the pharmacy. How many milligrams are in a dose and how many tablets are to be dispensed?

> ℞ diphenhydramine XXV mg
> Sig: take II tab each night
> Disp: XXXII tablets

To calculate the number of milligrams in a dose, start by calculating the amount of milligrams in a tablet. Add the Roman numerals on the prescription.

$$\frac{\text{XXV mg}}{\text{1 tablet}} = 10 + 10 + 5 = \frac{25 \text{ mg}}{\text{1 tablet}}$$

Then, determine the number of tablets taken each night.

2.4 Percentage of Error

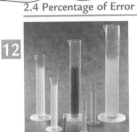

Graduated cylinders are used to accurately measure liquids in the pharmacy.

Percentages are used in a variety of ways when preparing medication doses. In the compounding pharmacy, percentages are used to determine the possible percentage of error and the least weighable quantity of a substance for safe preparation. Percentages are also used when doing the business of the pharmacy, such as calculating the percentage of sales, percentage of discount, and percentage of markup. These applications will be covered in Chapter 9, "Using Business Math in the Pharmacy."

When measuring a liquid or weighing a solid ingredient in the pharmacy, a certain amount of error is expected. Not all graduated cylinders used in the pharmacy are equally accurate, although they are usually much more accurate than the measuring devices found in patients' homes. Graduated cylinders used in pharmacies may be conical or cylindrical, with the cylindrical shape being more accurate. Similarly, pharmacy balances, though generally very accurate when compared with

2.4 Percentage of Error   **61**

---

working know... the volumes of o... ...dications that are commonly prescribed. Most frequently, the dosage amount is between 2 mL and 60 mL, or roughly ½ tsp to 2 fl oz. Oral doses are often verified in the pharmacy by means of reference and established protocols.

13

FIGURE 5.3
Oral Syringe

This oral syringe is marked with both household and metric units of measure.

Example 5.2.3

The pharmacy receives a prescription for 100 mg of amoxicillin to be taken three times daily for 10 days. The

Amoxicillin for Oral Suspension, USP

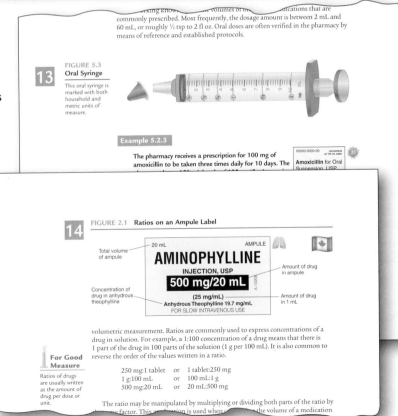

14

FIGURE 2.1   **Ratios on an Ampule Label**

Total volume of ampule — 20 mL

20 mL   AMPULE

AMINOPHYLLINE
INJECTION, USP
500 mg/20 mL
(25 mg/mL)
Anhydrous Theophylline 19.7 mg/mL
FOR SLOW INTRAVENOUS USE

Amount of drug in ampule
Amount of drug in 1 mL
Concentration of drug in anhydrous theophylline

For Good Measure

Ratios of drugs are usually written as the amount of drug per dose or unit.

volumetric measurement. Ratios are commonly used to express concentrations of a drug in solution. For example, a 1:100 concentration of a drug means that there is 1 part of the drug in 100 parts of the solution (1 g per 100 mL). It is also common to reverse the order of the values written in a ratio.

250 mg:1 tablet   or   1 tablet:250 mg
1 g:100 mL   or   100 mL:1 g
500 mg:20 mL   or   20 mL:500 mg

The ratio may be manipulated by multiplying or dividing both parts of the ratio by ... ...e factor. This ... ...ation is used when ... ...g the volume of a medication

15

TABLES encapsulate pertinent information related to the chapter topics and serve as a study aid for students.

determining the relationship of parts to each other.

TABLE 2.3 Steps for Solving for *x* in the Ratio-Proportion Method **15**

Step 1. Create the proportion by placing the ratios in fraction form so that the *x* is in the upper-left corner.

Step 2. Check that the unit of measurement in the numerators is the same and the unit of measurement in the denominators is the same.

Step 3. Solve for *x* by multiplying both sides of the proportion by the denominator of the ratio containing the unknown, and cancel.

Step 4. Check your answer by seeing if the product of the means equals the product of the extremes.

16

HANDOUT REFERENCES *New!* are scattered throughout each chapter and signal students to obtain handouts from their instructors to complete certain exercises.

Chapter Practice Test

 STUDY PARTNER Additional Practice Questions

To put your pharmacy calculation skills to the test, read the following questions and then record your answers on a separate sheet of paper.

Determine the volume to prepare for each ordered injectable solution using the labels provided. (Round to the hundredths place.)

16 *Note: Questions 1–4 have accompanying handouts that must be obtained from your instructor.*

1. How many milliliters of solution are needed to provide 2 g of cefazolin? On the handout that you obtained from your instructor, indicate the correct volume on the measuring device.

3. How many milliliters of solution are needed to provide 25 mg of diphenhydramine HCl? On the handout that you obtained from your instructor, indicate the correct volume on the measuring device.

17

CHAPTER SUMMARY *New!* provides an overview of the key points of the chapter.

Chapter Summary **17**

- Ratios are used to describe the amount of medication per dose or unit.
- Ratios may also be written as fractions.
- Ratios may be written in reverse order (1:100 or 100:1) or may be written flipped upside down (1/100 or 100/1).
- Ratios may be multiplied when a larger dose is desired or divided when a smaller dose is desired.
- Percent is the number of parts per 100 parts.
- Ratios, percents, fractions, and decimals may all be used to express the same value.

- Proportions are an expression of equivalency between two ratios (or fractions).
- A proportion with one missing value may be solved if three of the four values are known.
- When using the ratio-proportion method to solve for a missing value, the numerators must have the same unit of measure, and the denominators must have the same unit of measure.
- The ratio-proportion method may be used to convert between units of measure by

18

ASSESSING COMPREHENSION provides 10 multiple-choice questions that cover important concepts from the chapter. *New!*

Chapter Review

18 Assessing Comprehension

To check your comprehension of this chapter's key concepts, read the following multiple-choice questions and then record your answers on a separate sheet of paper. Write your answers as modeled in these examples: 1d; 2c; 3b; etc.

1. For a pharmacy technician, the most useful ratio form for setting up a pharmacy calculation is a
   a. ratio (a:b).
   b. fraction (a/b).
   c. decimal with a trailing zero.
   d. percentage.

2. When 2 doses or units of medication are given, you manipulate the ratio strength by
   a. multiplying the numerator by 2.
   b. dividing the numerator by 2.
   c. multiplying both the numerator and denominator by 2.
   d. dividing both the numerator and denominator by 2.

6. When converting a percentage to a numerical value or a decimal, you should
   a. drop the percent symbol.
   b. drop the percent symbol and move the decimal point two places to the right.
   c. drop the percent symbol and move the decimal point two places to the left.
   d. subtract 100 from the number and insert a zero if needed.

7. The ratio-proportion method is used in pharmacy calculations when
   a. all four values are known.
   b. three of four values are known.
   c. the units of measure are all the same.
   d. the unknown value is in a unit not written on the drug label.

19

FINDING SOLUTIONS
presents real-world
scenarios to help
pharmacy technician
students gain practice
in handling challenging
workplace situations.

New!

10. The percentage of error is
   a. calculated by dividing the actual
     amount by the desired amount.
   b. calculated by multiplying the quantity
     desired by 5%.
   c. always expressed as a positive value.
   d. determined by comparing a weighed
     amount of drug to a standard brass
     weight.

19 Finding Solutions

To gain practice in handling challenging situations in the workplace, consider the following real-world scenarios and then use the guiding questions to help you formulate your responses.

Note: To indicate your answer for Scenario A, Question 1, ask your instructor for the handout depicting measuring devices.

Scenario A: A patient with poison ivy has been taking over-the-counter (OTC) Benadryl for itching. The doctor has told her to take 50 mg every six hours. The medication is available in a 12.5 mg/5 mL

4. What is the infant's weight in kilograms?

Scenario C: You have been asked to reorder and restock a special order lip balm that your pharmacy carries. A carton of 24 tubes costs the

20

**SAMPLING THE
CERTIFICATION
EXAM** provides
students with
five practice prob-
lems that model the
test format of the
Certification Exam.

New!

20 Sampling the Certification Exam

To provide you with practice for the Certification Exam, read the following questions that have been patterned after the test format and then record your answers on a separate sheet of paper. Write your answers as modeled in these examples: 1d; 2c; 3b; etc.

1. A medication label reads 300 mg/5 mL.
   How many milligrams of medication are
   in 15 mL?
   a. 150 mg
   b. 450 mg
   c. 500 mg
   d. 900 mg

2. How many grams of medication are in
   200 g of a 1% ointment?
   a. 0.2 g
   b. 1 g
   c. 1.2 g
   d. 2 g

3. A solution that is 1:20 is also the
   concentration:

   c. 5%
   d. 20%

4. A medication is available in a 250 mg/5 mL
   concentration. How many milliliters
   contain 750 mg?
   a. 1.5 mL
   b. 7.5 mL
   c. 10 mL
   d. 15 mL

5. A patient needs to pay 20% of the cost of
   his medications. If his medications are
   $12.79 and $81.24, how much will he pay?
   a. $18.81
   b. $37.62
   c. $47.02

21

CHAPTER PRACTICE TEST
allows students to demon-
strate their understanding
of the math concepts and
calculations skills presented
in the chapter by solving
real-world pharmacy prob-
lems.

21 Chapter Practice Test

STUDY PARTNER   **Additional Practice Questions**

To put your pharmacy calculation skills to the test, read the following questions and then record your answers on a separate sheet of paper.

State the ratio for the following doses.

1. 10 mg tablet of glipizide

2. 5 mL dose of azithromycin
   containing 250 mg

3. 5 mL dose of diphenhydramine
   containing 12.5 mg

4. 2 mL ampule containing 500 mg

5. A 1:10 solution contains _____
   g of active ingredient and _____ mL
   of product, and 1000 mL of that solution
   contains _____ g.

Choose the appropriate solution from the
available stock.

11. A 1:5 solution has been ordered.
   You have a 5% solution, a 10% solution,
   and a 20% solution in stock. Which
   solution will you choose?

12. A 1:250 solution has been ordered.
   You have a 0.4% solution, a 0.05%
   solution, and a 4% solution in stock.
   Which solution will you choose?

Convert the following using the ratio
1 g:1000 mg.

13. 120 mg = _____ g

14. 1800 m _____ g

Resources for the Student

To support their study of the textbook, students have access to additional print and electronic resources that enhance the development of pharmacy technician skills and address different learning styles.

Key to Body System Icons

Throughout each chapter, body system icons have been placed next to generic and brand name medications. These icons help students to make connections between the drugs and the body systems they are prescribed to treat. Although many of the medications discussed in the text are used on multiple systems, the body system icons chosen fit the context of the problems and examples presented.

The key below provides a snapshot of the body system icons and their meanings. Students should be aware that two icons—those for the Reproductive System and the Sensory System—are used to refer to more than one component of each system, depending on the particular drug and its use. That is, the Reproductive System icon will refer to either the male or female symbol and the Sensory System icon will refer to either the eye, ear, or nose. In each case, the relevant component remains sharp and vivid whereas the irrelevant components are faded out.

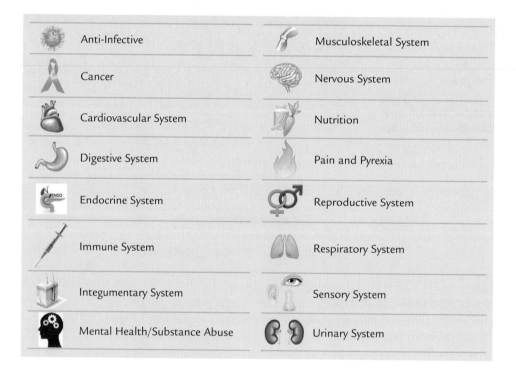

Anti-Infective	Musculoskeletal System
Cancer	Nervous System
Cardiovascular System	Nutrition
Digestive System	Pain and Pyrexia
Endocrine System	Reproductive System
Immune System	Respiratory System
Integumentary System	Sensory System
Mental Health/Substance Abuse	Urinary System

Appendices

Four appendices provide important resources for pharmacy technician students:

- **Appendix A:**
  Problem Set Answers
- **Appendix B:**
  Additional Practice with Fractions and Percents
- **Appendix C:**
  Common Pharmacy Abbreviations and Acronyms
- **Appendix D:**
  Measures and Conversions

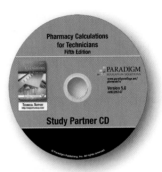

Study Partner CD

The Study Partner CD included with each textbook offers the following tools to support student learning:

- **Chapter Terms and Flash Cards**—to help students learn key terminology
- **Matching Activities**—to provide students with a fun, interactive way to learn chapter content
- **Quizzes**—to test students' understanding of important chapter concepts, provided in both practice and reported modes
- **Link to Internet Resource Center**—to allow students access to additional course-related resources

Student Internet Resource Center

The Internet Resource Center for this title at www.paradigmcollege.net/pharmcalc5e provides additional reference information and resources for students.

 One of these resources is the *Canadian Pharmacy Technician Supplement*. This supplement presents general information about the Canadian healthcare system, including drug regulation, the top 100 dispensed drugs in Canada, and the role of the pharmacy technician in the practice setting. For students who may have the option to work in Canada, this supplement provides valuable insights into the differences between the U.S. and Canadian healthcare systems. To indicate content areas that are different in Canadian pharmacy practice, we have placed the Canadian flag icon in the page margin near Supplement-relevant content.

eBook

For students who prefer studying with an eBook, this text is available in an electronic form. The Web-based, password-protected eBook features dynamic navigation tools, including bookmarking, a linked table of contents, and the ability to jump to a specific page. The eBook format also supports helpful study tools, such as highlighting and note taking.

Resources for the Instructor

Pharmacy Calculations for Technicians, Fifth Edition is supported by several tools to help instructors plan their courses and assess student learning.

Instructor's Guide with Instructor Resources CD

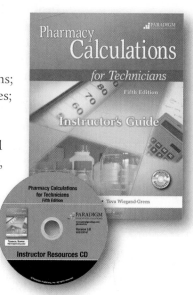

In addition to course planning tools and syllabus models, the *Instructor's Guide* provides chapter lessons; handouts that accompany specific textbook exercises; and answer keys for all end-of-chapter exercises, Chapter Practice Tests, and Appendix B problems. The *Instructor's Guide* also offers a pretest, additional practice tests that parallel the Chapter Practice Test, and a multiple-choice final exam. Included in the package is the Instructor Resources CD, which offers PowerPoint® presentations as well as the **Exam**View® Assessment Suite. **Exam**View® is a full-featured, computerized test generator that provides both print and online tests and the option for instructors to create customized tests using the chapter item banks.

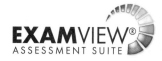

Instructor Internet Resource Center

Many of the features that appear in the *Instructor's Guide* also are available on the password-protected instructor section of the Internet Resource Center for this title at www.paradigmcollege.net/pharmcalc5e. An additional posted resource to be aware of is the *Canadian Pharmacy Technician Supplement*. This supplement presents general information about the Canadian healthcare system, including drug regulation, the top 100 dispensed drugs in Canada, and the role of the pharmacy technician in the practice setting. For students who may have the option to work in Canada, this supplement provides valuable insights into the differences between the U.S. and Canadian healthcare systems. To indicate content areas that are different in Canadian pharmacy practice, we have placed the Canadian flag icon in the page margin near Supplement-relevant content.

Distance Learning Cartridges

Distance learning cartridges are available for this program.

Textbooks in the Pharmacy Technician Series

In addition to *Pharmacy Calculations for Technicians, Fifth Edition*, Paradigm Publishing, Inc. offers other titles designed specifically for the pharmacy technician curriculum:

- *Pharmacology for Technicians, Fifth Edition*

- *Pharmacology for Technicians Workbook, Fifth Edition*

- *Pharmacy Labs for Technicians, Second Edition*

- *Pharmacy Practice for Technicians, Fifth Edition*

- *Certification Exam Review for Pharmacy Technicians, Third Edition*

- *Sterile Compounding and Aseptic Technique*

- *Pharmacology Essentials for Technicians*

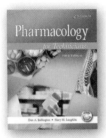 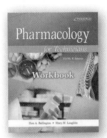 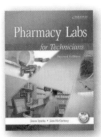 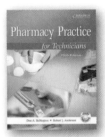

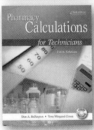 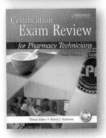 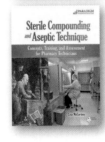 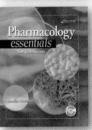

About the Authors

Don A. Ballington, MS, served as program coordinator of the pharmacy technician training program at Midlands Technical College in Columbia, South Carolina, for 27 years. He has also served as president of the Pharmacy Technician Educators Council and in 2005 received the council's Educator of the Year award. Mr. Ballington has conducted site visits for pharmacy technician accreditation and helped develop the American Society of Health-System Pharmacists' model curriculum. He has also been a consulting editor for the *Journal of Pharmacy Technology*. Over the course of his career at Midlands Technical College, he developed a set of high-quality training materials for pharmacy technicians. These materials became the foundation for Paradigm's Pharmacy Technician series.

Tova Wiegand-Green, MS, is the dean of the School of Health Sciences at Ivy Tech Community College Northeast in Fort Wayne, Indiana. She began her college education at Coastal Carolina Community College in North Carolina studying pre-pharmacy. A native Hoosier, she transferred back home to Purdue University and graduated in 1992. After working in the pharmacy industry for five years, Ms. Wiegand-Green transitioned to teaching at the community college level. Serving first as the coordinator of the Pharmacy Technician program and later as the chair for the Medical Assisting program, she developed and used many applied math activities to effectively transition students in both vocational and community college programs to new occupations that required applied math and offered richer career development options. These students continue to be an inspiration to Ms. Wiegand-Green as she promotes all types of hands-on learning, applied mathematics, and place-based learning.

In addition, Ms. Wiegand-Green has been involved in distance-learning technologies since 1999 and was the first faculty member to teach on-campus students as well as distance learners using a two-way video/face-to-face/Internet hybrid combination all in one course. She views distance learning as an exciting, always-evolving field and values it as a supplement to face-to-face and hybrid classes while strongly advocating 24/7 learning opportunities for all students.

In 2010, Ms. Wiegand-Green graduated from Ball State University with a Master of Arts in Environmental and Natural Resource Management. She has recently spent time researching and conducting place-based learning residential camps for children in Lagrange County, Indiana.

Author's Acknowledgments

I would like to thank my family! Like so many authors, writing is done in the home, amid the schoolwork, family activities, soccer, cooking, laundry, and all the hectic business that is our life. I am so thankful for the teachers that have encouraged me along the way to becoming a writer and helping me to learn to love math. I grew up hating math; in fact, I missed all of the afternoon recess sessions in the fourth grade because I couldn't remember my times tables! But my instructors along the way have helped me to appreciate the exactness of math and to embrace it as a means to explore and understand science. I would like to offer a special thank-you to two of those instructors—Professor Ben Chen and Professor Mary Losey. I would also like to thank the reviewers, contributing authors, and faculty members who have helped shape the text and improve it. Lastly, thanks go to Nancy Papsin for her helpful suggestions and questions about even the minutest things! Her attention to detail is wonderful! Thank you, Nancy!

Tova Wiegand-Green

Acknowledgments

The quality of this body of work is a testament to the feedback we have received from the many contributors and reviewers who participated in *Pharmacy Calculations for Technicians, Fifth Edition.*

Robert W. Aanonsen, CPhT
Platt College
Tulsa, Oklahoma

Harold S. Bender, PharmD, RPh
National College of Business
  and Technology
Spring Hill, Tennessee

Diana Vasquez Broome, BS, CPhT, PhTR
Lone Star College
Tomball, Texas

Christina Cox, BS, CPhT
Heald College
Honolulu, Hawaii

Erika D'Arezzo, BS, CPhT
Sanford-Brown
Cranston, Rhode Island

Elizabeth Garcia, AA, CPhT
San Joaquin Valley College
Visalia, California

Aldo Gatti, BSc Pharm, RPh
Centennial College
Toronto, Ontario, Canada

Joseph P. Gee, PharmD
Cosumnes River College
Sacramento, California

Mary Good, AA, CPhT
National College
Harrisonburg, Virginia

Jeff Gricar, MEd, CPhT, PhTR
HCC Coleman College
Houston, Texas

Lisa Homburg, RPh
College of the Mainland
Texas City, Texas

Susan Howell, BS, CPhT
Ivy Tech Community College
Muncie, Indiana

Kent LaFary, CPhT

Belva J. Matherly, BA, BA, CPhT
National College
Salem, Virginia

Marcy May, MEd, CPhT, PhTR
Austin Community College
Austin, Texas

Lisa McCartney, BAAS, CPhT, PhTR
Austin Community College
Austin, Texas

Shawn McPartland, MD, JD
Harrison College
Indianapolis, Indiana

Lynda Melendez, AS, CPhT, PhTR
Texas State Technical College
Waco, Texas

Mary Stende Miller, BS, RPh
Minnesota State Community &
  Technical College
Wadena, Minnesota

Michael T. Mockler, MBA, RPh
Heald College
Portland, Oregon

Jody Myhre-Oechsle, MS, CPhT
Chippewa Valley Technical College
Eau Claire, Wisconsin

Elina Pierce, MS, CPhT
Southeast Community College
Beatrice, Nebraska

Vickey L. Rose, CPhT

Becky Schonscheck, BS
Maricopa, Arizona

Julia B. Sherwood, AA, CPhT
Spartanburg Community College
Spartanburg, South Carolina

Shahriar Siddiq, MBBS (MD), DNM
Algonquin Careers Academy
Ottawa, Ontario, Canada

Jacqueline T. Smith, RN, CPhT
National College
Princeton, West Virginia

Jason P. Sparks, MEd, CPhT, PhTR
Consultant and Instructional Designer
Austin, Texas

Maureen Simmons Sparks, CPhT
Clover Park Technical College
Lakewood, Washington

Bobbi Steelman, MEd, CPhT
Daymar College
Bowling Green, Kentucky

Cynthia J. Steffen, MS, RPh
Milwaukee Area Technical College
Milwaukee, Wisconsin

Dawn M. Tesner, DHEd, MSHA, CPhT
Mid Michigan Community College
Mt. Pleasant, Michigan

Sandi Tschritter, MEd, CPhT
Spokane Community College
Spokane, Washington

Terry Walker, RN (retired)
Selkirk College
Castlegar, British Columbia, Canada

Jeremy Watson, BS, CPhT, RT
National College
Knoxville, Tennessee

Elaine Young, MEd, CPhT
Angelina College
Lufkin, Texas

The author and editors would like to say a special thank-you to **Lisa McCartney** for her writing contributions to Chapters 7, 8, and 9. Her extensive knowledge and experience as both a practitioner and an instructor in the pharmacy technician field—particularly, in the area of sterile compounding and aseptic technique—have shaped the content of these chapters.

We also offer a special thank-you to **Marcy May**, **Bobbi Steelman**, **Shawn McPartland**, and **Jason Sparks** for their expert chapter reviews and to **Dr. Shahriar Siddiq** for his creation of the online *Canadian Pharmacy Technician Supplement* that addresses topics specific to Canadian pharmacy technicians. Finally, we would like to thank **Diana Vasquez Broome** for her writing of the ExamView test banks and **Andrea Redman** for her creation of the PowerPoint presentations.

The authors and editorial staff invite your feedback on the text and its supplements. Please reach us by clicking the "Contact us" button at www.emcp.com.

Understanding Subdivisions of Numbers, Number Systems, Estimating, and Accuracy

1

Learning Objectives

- Understand fractions and be able to compare them, express them as decimals, and find common denominators.

- Manipulate fractions by adding, subtracting, multiplying, and dividing them.

- Interpret Roman and Arabic numbers and convert values between the two systems.

- Read scientific notation and convert large and small numbers to scientific notation.

- Determine the value of a decimal and accurately round off decimal values.

- Estimate drug doses to check the accuracy of final calculations.

- Perform calculations while retaining accuracy and the correct number of significant figures.

- Understand conversions between standard time and 24-hour time.

For a key to the body system icons that appear in each chapter of this textbook, refer to the Preface.

STUDY PARTNER

Preview chapter terms and definitions.

1.1 Fractions

When something is divided into parts, each part is considered a **fraction** of the whole. For example, a pie might be divided into eight slices, each of which is a fraction, or ⅛, of the whole pie. The pie is still whole but has been divided into eight slices. Each slice is a selection—an eighth—of the whole pie, or 1 (the number of slices in the selection) over 8 (the number of slices in the whole pie). In the fraction ⅜, the selection is for 3 of the 8 slices (see Figure 1.1).

Just as a pie can be divided into parts, so can a tablet, a common procedure for both pharmacist and patient. Figure 1.2 on the following page shows how cutting a tablet into smaller parts relates to fractions.

FIGURE 1.1
Fractions of the Whole Pie

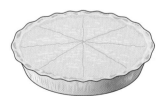

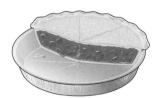

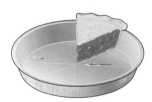

8 slices = 1 whole pie = $\frac{8}{8}$ of the whole pie   3 slices = $\frac{3}{8}$ of the whole pie   1 slice = $\frac{1}{8}$ of the whole pie

FIGURE 1.2   **Fractions of a Tablet**

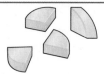

1 tablet = 1000 mg $\frac{1}{2}$ tablet = 500 mg $\frac{1}{4}$ tablet = 250 mg

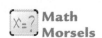 **Math Morsels**

The numerator and denominator can be remembered by recalling that the **d**enominator is **d**own below the line in the fraction.

Fractions are either common (½, ⅔, etc.) or decimal (0.5, 0.66, etc.). A common fraction is composed of a **numerator** (top number) and a **denominator** (bottom number). The numerator represents the portion (1 piece in the case of the pie), and the denominator represents the whole (8 pieces of the pie).

$$\text{numerator} \longrightarrow \frac{1}{8} \\ \text{denominator} \longrightarrow$$

A fraction with the same numerator and denominator has a value equivalent to 1.

$$\frac{8}{8} = \frac{5}{5} = \frac{3}{3} = \frac{10}{10} = \frac{15}{15} = 1$$

A fraction with a value less than 1 (numerator smaller than denominator) is called a **proper fraction**.

$$\frac{1}{4} \quad \frac{2}{3} \quad \frac{7}{8} \quad \frac{9}{10}$$

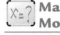 **For Good Measure**

Proper fractions always have a value less than 1, or less than the "whole" of what is being talked about.

A fraction with a value greater than 1 (numerator greater than denominator) is called an **improper fraction**.

$$\frac{6}{5} \quad \frac{7}{5} \quad \frac{9}{6} \quad \frac{15}{8}$$

A **mixed number** consists of a whole number and a fraction and can be converted to an improper fraction by multiplying the whole number by the denominator and adding the numerator.

$$5\frac{1}{2} = \frac{(5 \times 2) + 1}{2} = \frac{11}{2}$$

A fraction in which both the numerator and the denominator are fractions is called a **complex fraction**.

$$\frac{\frac{1}{4}}{\frac{1}{8}}$$

Math Morsels

The symbol > means "is greater than," and the symbol < means "is less than."

Comparing Fraction Size

When fractions that have the same numerator are compared, the fraction with the smaller denominator will have the larger value.

$$\frac{1}{10} > \frac{1}{25}$$

If two fractions have the same denominator, the fraction with the larger numerator will have the larger value.

$$\frac{3}{6} > \frac{2}{6}$$

When medications are dosed using fractions, it is important to recognize which strengths are largest and smallest.

Example 1.1.1

Which of the following nitroglycerin tablets is the smallest dose?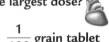

$$\frac{3}{10} \text{ mg tablet} \qquad \frac{4}{10} \text{ mg tablet} \qquad \frac{6}{10} \text{ mg tablet}$$

The $^{3}/_{10}$ mg tablet is the smallest dose because when fractions have the same denominator, the fraction with the smallest numerator will have the smallest value.

Example 1.1.2

Which of the following nitroglycerin tablets is the largest dose?

$$\frac{1}{200} \text{ grain tablet} \qquad \frac{1}{150} \text{ grain tablet} \qquad \frac{1}{100} \text{ grain tablet}$$

The $^{1}/_{100}$ grain tablet is the largest dose because when fractions have the same numerator, the fraction with the smallest denominator will have the largest value.

Safety in Numbers

Medication labels for nitroglycerin tablets—a medication prescribed for chest pain—may contain either decimals or fractions. Therefore, be sure to check the label carefully before proceeding.

Expressing Fractions as Decimals

As the section on decimals later in the chapter will explain, in decimal fractions, the denominator is not written but is represented by the location of the number in relation to the decimal point. For now, it is sufficient to know that any fraction may be expressed in decimal form by dividing the numerator by the denominator.

$$\frac{1}{2} = 1 \div 2 = 0.5$$

$$\frac{7}{10} = 7 \div 10 = 0.7$$

Adding and Subtracting Fractions

When adding or subtracting fractions with unlike denominators, it is necessary to create a **common denominator**, a number into which each of the unlike denominators can be divided evenly. Think of it as making both fractions into the same kind of "pie." Creating a common denominator requires transforming each fraction by multiplying it by a form of 1 that represents one entire "pie."

Multiplying a number by 1 does not change the value of the number ($5 \times 1 = 5$). Therefore, if you multiply a fraction by a fraction that equals 1 (such as $5/5$), you do not change the value of the fraction. It is this mathematical rule that allows for the conversions in the following examples.

Example 1.1.3

Find the sum of $\frac{1}{2} + \frac{3}{5}$.

The lowest number that can be divided evenly by both 2 and 5 is 10. A quick way to determine a possible common denominator is to multiply the two denominators together ($5 \times 2 = 10$). Thus, tenths will be the common denominator for the two fractions, and each fraction must be converted to tenths.

To convert $1/2$ to tenths, multiply $1/2$ by $5/5$ (one "pie" of fifths), which equals $5/10$.

$$\frac{1}{2} = \frac{1}{2} \times \frac{5}{5} = \frac{5}{10}$$

To convert $3/5$ to tenths, multiply $3/5$ by $2/2$ (one "pie" of halves), which equals $6/10$.

$$\frac{3}{5} = \frac{3}{5} \times \frac{2}{2} = \frac{6}{10}$$

Then add $5/10 + 6/10$, which equals $11/10$ or 1 and $1/10$.

$$\frac{5}{10} + \frac{6}{10} = \frac{11}{10} = 1\frac{1}{10}$$

Example 1.1.4

Find the sum of $\frac{1}{4} + \frac{3}{7}$.

The common denominator is 28, since $4 \times 7 = 28$.

$$\frac{1}{4} = \frac{1}{4} \times \frac{7}{7} = \frac{7}{28} \qquad \frac{3}{7} = \frac{3}{7} \times \frac{4}{4} = \frac{12}{28}$$

$$\frac{7}{28} + \frac{12}{28} = \frac{19}{28}$$

$$\frac{1}{4} + \frac{3}{7} = \frac{19}{28}$$

Sometimes, especially when there are three or more fractions, multiplying the denominators is not the best method to use to find a common denominator. In that case, follow the basic steps given in Table 1.1.

TABLE 1.1 Steps for Finding a Common Denominator

Step 1. Examine each denominator in the given fractions for its divisors, or factors.

$$\frac{1}{15} = \frac{1}{3 \times 5} \qquad \frac{5}{6} = \frac{5}{2 \times 3} \qquad \frac{11}{36} = \frac{11}{2 \times 2 \times 3 \times 3}$$

Step 2. See what factors any of the denominators have in common.

$$\frac{1}{15} = \frac{1}{3 \times 5} \text{ has a 3 in its denominator}$$

$$\frac{5}{6} = \frac{5}{2 \times 3} \text{ and } \frac{11}{36} = \frac{11}{2 \times 2 \times 3 \times 3} \text{ both have 2 and 3 in their denominators.}$$

Step 3. Form a common denominator by multiplying all the factors that occur in all of the denominators. If a factor occurs more than once, use it the largest number of times it occurs in any denominator.

$$\begin{aligned} \text{Common denominator} &= 5 \times 2 \times 2 \times 3 \times 3 \\ &= 5 \times 4 \times 9 \\ &= 180 \end{aligned}$$

Note: The product of all of the original denominators is $15 \times 6 \times 36 = 3240$.

After two fractions have been converted to a common denominator and added together, it may be necessary to reduce the fraction. This requires canceling. To understand why this works, remember that multiplying a fraction by 1 will not change its value.

$$\frac{a}{b} \times 1 = \frac{a}{b}$$

Rewrite 1 as $\frac{c}{c}$.

$$\frac{a}{b} = \frac{a}{b} \times 1 = \frac{a}{b} \times \frac{c}{c} = \frac{ac}{bc}$$

$$\frac{a\cancel{c}}{b\cancel{c}} = \frac{a}{b}$$

Once the largest number possible has been canceled out of the numerator and denominator, the fraction is said to be in its lowest terms.

Example 1.1.5

Simplify the fraction $\dfrac{3}{27}$.

$$\frac{3 \div 3}{27 \div 3} = \frac{1}{9}$$

When subtracting fractions that have the same denominator, subtract the numerators and place the number over the common denominator. It may be necessary to reduce the answer fraction to its lowest terms.

Example 1.1.6

Perform the following subtraction.

$$\frac{5}{6} - \frac{3}{6}$$

Since these fractions already have the common denominator 6, subtract the numerators.

$$\frac{5}{6} - \frac{3}{6} = \frac{2}{6}$$

$$\text{Reduce: } \frac{2}{6} = \frac{1}{3}$$

Example 1.1.7

Simplify the following subtraction.

$$3\frac{3}{4} - \frac{1}{2}$$

Math Morsels

A mixed fraction has a whole number in front of the fraction.

Change the mixed fraction to an improper fraction.

$$3\frac{3}{4} = \frac{15}{4}$$

Replace the mixed fraction with the improper fraction in the subtraction, and confirm that the denominators are the same. Because the second denominator is 2, it must be changed to a fraction with a denominator of 4. To do this, you multiply the numerator and denominator by 2.

$$\frac{1}{2} \times \frac{2}{2} = \frac{2}{4}$$

Then,

$$3\frac{3}{4} - \frac{2}{4} = \frac{15}{4} - \frac{2}{4} \quad \text{(Both denominators are 4.)}$$

Solve the problem by subtracting the numerators.

$$\frac{15}{4} - \frac{2}{4} = \frac{13}{4}$$

Change the improper fraction to a mixed fraction.

$$\frac{13}{4} = 3\frac{1}{4}$$

Safety in Numbers

When working with fractions, always include the units (if known) after the number—for example, a ½ mg tablet.

When subtracting fractions that have different denominators, find the lowest common denominator, convert to equivalent fractions, subtract the numerators, and place the number over the denominator. It may be necessary to reduce the answer fraction to its lowest terms.

Example 1.1.8

Perform the following calculation.

$$\frac{3}{4} - \frac{2}{3}$$

The lowest common denominator is 12, so to convert to equivalent fractions, ³⁄₄ must be multiplied by ³⁄₃ and ²⁄₃ by ⁴⁄₄.

$$\frac{3}{4} = \frac{9}{12}$$

$$\frac{2}{3} = \frac{8}{12}$$

Replace the original fractions and subtract the numerators.

$$\frac{9}{12} - \frac{8}{12} = \frac{1}{12}$$

Example 1.1.9

Subtract the two given fractions.

$$2\frac{1}{2} - \frac{6}{3}$$

Change the mixed number to a fraction.

$$2\frac{1}{2} = \frac{(2 \times 2) + 1}{2} = \frac{5}{2}$$

Replace the mixed fraction with the improper fraction.

$$2\frac{1}{2} - \frac{6}{3} = \frac{5}{2} - \frac{6}{3}$$

The lowest common denominator is 6; convert to equivalent fractions.

$$\frac{5}{2} \times \frac{3}{3} = \frac{15}{6}$$

$$\frac{6}{3} \times \frac{2}{2} = \frac{12}{6}$$

Rewrite the original problem and subtract the numerators.

$$\frac{15}{6} - \frac{12}{6} = \frac{3}{6}$$

Simplify the answer.

$$\frac{3}{6} = \frac{1}{2}$$

So $2\frac{1}{2} - \frac{6}{3} = \frac{1}{2}$.

Multiplying and Dividing Fractions

The basic step in multiplying fractions is to multiply numerators by numerators and denominators by denominators. Another way to state this rule is the following: Multiply all numbers above the line; then multiply all numbers below the line. Finally, cancel if possible and reduce to lowest terms.

$$\frac{1}{8} \times \frac{1}{2} = \frac{1 \times 1}{8 \times 2} = \frac{1}{16}$$

$$\frac{1}{8} \times \frac{1}{2} \times \frac{2}{3} = \frac{1 \times 1 \times 2}{8 \times 2 \times 3} = \frac{2}{48} = \frac{1}{24}$$

$$5 \times \frac{3}{4} = \frac{5}{1} \times \frac{3}{4} = \frac{15}{4} = 3\frac{3}{4}$$

When partial doses such as ½ tablet or ¾ teaspoonful are prescribed, it may become necessary to multiply fractions as part of the calculations needed to determine the amount of medication to dispense. The following examples will demonstrate these calculations.

For Good Measure

A whole number can be written as an improper fraction in order to multiply the fractions.

Example 1.1.10

A patient needs to take ½ of a furosemide 40 mg tablet each day for 30 days. How many tablets will the patient need to last 30 days?

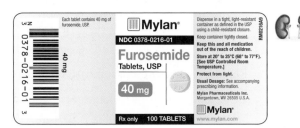

This problem may be solved by multiplying the number of days by the amount of medication taken per day.

$$\frac{30 \text{ days}}{1} \times \frac{1 \text{ tablet}}{2} = \frac{30 \times 1}{1 \times 2} = \frac{30}{2} = 15 \text{ tablets will last 30 days}$$

Example 1.1.11

How many milligrams are in ½ of a furosemide tablet shown in the following label?

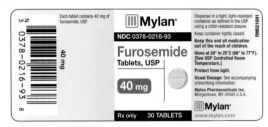

$$\frac{40 \text{ mg}}{1 \text{ tablet}} \times \frac{1 \text{ tablet}}{2} = \frac{40 \times 1}{1 \times 2} = \frac{40}{2} = 20 \text{ mg}$$

Alternatively, you can divide the strength of the tablet by 2, because ²/₁ is the reciprocal of ½.

$$40 \text{ mg} \div 2 = 20 \text{ mg}$$

Tables 1.2 and 1.3 list guidelines for multiplying and dividing fractions. To divide by a fraction, turn it upside down, multiply by the result (called the reciprocal of the original fraction), and then reduce if necessary.

TABLE 1.2   Guidelines for Multiplying Fractions

1. Multiplying the numerator by a number increases the value of a fraction.

$$\frac{1}{4} \times \frac{2}{1} = \frac{1 \times 2}{4 \times 1} = \frac{2}{4} = \frac{1}{2}$$

2. Multiplying the denominator by a number decreases the value of a fraction.

$$\frac{1}{4} \times \frac{1}{2} = \frac{1 \times 1}{4 \times 2} = \frac{1}{8}$$

3. The value of a fraction is not altered by multiplying or dividing both the numerator and the denominator by the same number.

$$\frac{1}{4} \times \frac{4}{4} = \frac{1 \times 4}{4 \times 4} = \frac{4}{16} = \frac{1}{4}$$

TABLE 1.3   Guidelines for Dividing Fractions

1. Dividing the denominator by a number is the same as multiplying the numerator by that number.

$$\frac{3}{\frac{20}{5}} = \frac{3}{4} \qquad \frac{3 \times 5}{20} = \frac{15}{20} = \frac{3}{4}$$

2. Dividing the numerator by a number is the same as multiplying the denominator by that number.

$$\frac{\frac{6}{3}}{4} = \frac{2}{4} = \frac{1}{2} \qquad \frac{6}{3 \times 4} = \frac{6}{12} = \frac{1}{2}$$

Circle the fraction with the highest value.

1. $\dfrac{1}{2}$ $\dfrac{1}{3}$ $\dfrac{1}{4}$

2. $\dfrac{3}{10}$ $\dfrac{3}{12}$ $\dfrac{3}{8}$

Circle the fraction with the lowest value.

3. $\dfrac{3}{1}$ $\dfrac{4}{1}$ $\dfrac{2}{1}$

4. $\dfrac{2}{6}$ $\dfrac{3}{6}$ $\dfrac{4}{6}$

5. $\dfrac{1}{10}$ $\dfrac{1}{8}$ $\dfrac{1}{6}$

Complete the following operations.

6. $\dfrac{5}{6} + \dfrac{7}{10} + \dfrac{2}{5} =$

7. $\dfrac{21}{32} + \dfrac{1}{12} + \dfrac{31}{48} =$

Reduce the following fractions to their lowest form.

8. $\dfrac{25}{100}$

9. $\dfrac{67}{10}$

10. $\dfrac{11}{5}$

11. $\dfrac{27}{30}$

12. $\dfrac{12}{30}$

13. $\dfrac{\frac{1}{2}}{6}$

Express the following fractions in decimal form.

14. $\dfrac{1}{5}$

15. $\dfrac{1}{20}$

16. $4\dfrac{2}{4}$

17. $\dfrac{30}{100}$

18. $\dfrac{1}{200}$

19. $\dfrac{1}{500}$

20. $1\dfrac{8}{10}$

21. $\dfrac{1}{25}$

22. $\dfrac{1}{125}$

Applications

23. A patient has taken ¼ tablet, ½ tablet, 1½ tablets, and ¾ tablet. In total, how many tablets has the patient taken?

24. Which dose contains the largest amount of medication: one tablet containing $^1/_{150}$ grain or two tablets containing $^1/_{100}$ grain in each tablet?

25. You are to measure ¼ grain of medication each into unit dose oral containers. Your bulk container holds 375 grains. How many containers will be prepared?

Table sugar is needed for making simple syrup. One formula calls for ½ lb to make enough syrup; a second formula requires ⅘ lb; a third formula needs ¼ lb; and the last formula requires 2½ lb. You need to make one batch of all four formulas.

26. How many bags should you buy if the sugar is packaged in 2 lb bags?

27. How many bags must be purchased if the sugar is packaged in 5 lb bags?

Self-check your work in Appendix A.

1.2 Number Systems

Two types of numbers are used in pharmaceutical calculations: Roman and Arabic. The Arabic system is more commonly used in health care, although the Roman system is used on a limited basis.

Roman Numerals

Safety in Numbers

Roman numerals are often used on prescriptions because they are harder to alter than Arabic numbers.

The Roman numbering system (numerals) can be traced back to ancient Rome. This system uses letters to represent quantities or amounts, whereas the Arabic system uses numbers, fractions (such as ³⁄₈), and decimals. **Roman numerals** are expressed as either lowercase letters (particularly in calculations) or as capital letters. The most frequently used numerals are the uppercase *I*, *V*, and *X*, which represent 1, 5, and 10, respectively. In writing prescriptions, however, the lowercase letter *i* is often used to represent the number one, *ii* to represent two, and so on. To prevent errors in interpretation, a line is drawn above the symbol, with the dot above the line (for example: *ī*, *īī*, *īīī*). The symbol for ½, if placed after a Roman numeral, is *ss* (for example: 5½ is *vss*). Roman numerals are used to record amount or quantity but have little use in calculations.

Table 1.4 lists the common units and their values in the Roman system. The following example shows a prescription that uses Roman numerals to indicate both the amount to take at each dose and the quantity to dispense.

TABLE 1.4 Comparison of Roman and Arabic Numerals

Roman		Arabic	Roman		Arabic
ss	=	½	L or l	=	50
I or i or ī	=	1	C or c	=	100
V or v	=	5	D or d	=	500
X or x	=	10	M or m	=	1000

Example 1.2.1

The following prescription is received in the pharmacy. According to this prescription, how many tablets are in a daily dose and how many tablets are to be dispensed?

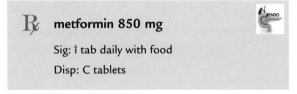

℞   metformin 850 mg

Sig: ī tab daily with food

Disp: C tablets

Determine the dose.

$$\bar{i} \text{ tablet per day} = 1 \text{ tablet}$$

Determine the quantity to dispense.

$$C \text{ tablets} = 100 \text{ tablets}$$

Roman numerals may be grouped together to express different quantities. To interpret these numbers, addition and subtraction must be used, as specified in the guidelines shown in Table 1.5. Example 1.2.2 will demonstrate reading grouped Roman numerals.

TABLE 1.5   Guidelines for Interpreting Roman Numerals

1. When a numeral is repeated or a smaller numeral follows a larger one, the values are added together.

ii or II = 1 + 1 = 2	VII = 5 + 2 = 7
LVII = 50 + 5 + 1 + 1 = 57	XXI = 10 + 10 + 1 = 21
CXIII = 100 + 10 + 1 + 1 + 1 = 113	LXV = 50 + 10 + 5 = 65

2. When a smaller numeral comes before a larger numeral, subtract the smaller value.

IV = 5 − 1 = 4	IX = 10 − 1 = 9
CD = 500 − 100 = 400	

3. Numerals are never repeated more than three times in sequence.

III = 3   IV = 4   XXX = 30   XL = 40

4. When a smaller numeral comes between two larger numerals, subtract the smaller numeral from the numeral that follows.

XIX = 10 + (10 − 1) = 19   XIV = 10 + (5 − 1) = 14

Example 1.2.2

Name Exchange

Diphenhydramine is generic for Benadryl. It is an over-the-counter (OTC) medication but will still need a prescription written in some cases.

The following prescription is received in the pharmacy. How many milligrams are in a dose and how many tablets are to be dispensed?

> ℞   **diphenhydramine XXV mg**
>
> Sig: ii tab each night
>
> Disp: XXXII tablets

To calculate the number of milligrams in a dose, start by calculating the amount of milligrams in a tablet. Add the Roman numerals on the prescription.

$$\frac{XXV \text{ mg}}{1 \text{ tablet}} = 10 + 10 + 5 = \frac{25 \text{ mg}}{1 \text{ tablet}}$$

Then, determine the number of tablets taken each night.

$$\text{ii tab} = 1 + 1 = 2 \text{ tablets}$$

Determine the daily dose by multiplying the amount of milligrams in each tablet by the number of tablets taken each night.

$$\frac{25 \text{ mg}}{1 \text{ tablet}} \times 2 \text{ tablets} = 50 \text{ mg}$$

Calculate the number to dispense by adding the Roman numerals on the prescription.

$$\text{XXXII tablets} = 10 + 10 + 10 + 1 + 1 = 32 \text{ tablets}$$

The Arabic Number System

The Arabic number system is also called the decimal system. Ten figures are used: 0, 1, 2, 3, 4, 5, 6, 7, 8, 9. The decimal point serves as the anchor. Each place to the left of the decimal point signals a tenfold increase, and each place to the right signals a tenfold decrease. Figure 1.3 illustrates the relative value of each unit. Memorize the **place values**, which describe each numeral's relationship to the decimal point, for future reference.

FIGURE 1.3   Decimal Units and Values

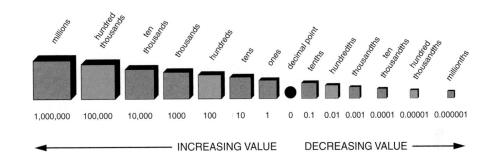

In expressions using **Arabic numbers**, the whole numbers are to the left of the decimal point, whereas the fractions are on the right. The positions for the numbers to the right of the decimal point are called decimal places. Table 1.6 on the following page provides guidelines for interpreting Arabic numbers.

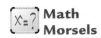 **Math Morsels**

An exponent is a number that is written in the space just above the number and to the right. It may have a negative or a positive value.

Scientific Notation

Scientific notation is a method used to write numbers that have a very large or very small numerical value. Because of space issues as well as readability, it is not practical to write out numbers that have a large number of zeros, such as 5,200,000,000,000, or very small numbers, such as 0.00000025. Numbers such as these are written as a group of significant figures multiplied by 10 with an exponent. The number in the exponent indicates how many places the decimal has been moved, and the value of the exponent (positive or negative) indicates the direction the decimal was moved. A positive exponent indicates a number greater than 1, and a negative exponent indicates a number less than 1. Table 1.7 shows examples of values written in Arabic numbers and in scientific notation.

TABLE 1.6 Guidelines for Interpreting Arabic Numbers

1. The value of a decimal equal to 1 or more depends on the size of the whole numbers. The higher the value of the whole numbers, the higher the overall value.

   8.2 > 6.2
   20.1 > 14.6
   3.08 > 2.39

2. If the decimal fraction does not have a whole number preceding the decimal point, a zero is used in front of the decimal point. This is called a *leading zero*. The fraction with the highest tenth will have the highest value.

   0.4 > 0.3
   2.41 > 2.39

3. When the tenths are identical, a number with a decimal fraction that is higher in hundredths will have a higher value.

   0.17 > 0.15
   0.35 > 0.30
   10.66 > 10.64

4. Look at the tenths first. If these are identical, the hundredths will determine the value unless they are also identical. Then the value will be determined by the thousandths.

   0.125 > 0.124

5. The total value of a number is therefore the sum of the different parts, depending on their position.

   467.43 represents   400.00 = four hundreds
                          +60.00 = six tens
                          + 7.00 = seven ones
                          + 0.40 = four tenths
                          + 0.03 = three hundredths

TABLE 1.7 Scientific Notation Equivalences

Arabic Number	Scientific Notation	Decimal Place Movement
6500	6.5×10^3	3 places to the left
120,000	1.2×10^5	5 places to the left
921,000,000	9.21×10^8	8 places to the left
4,800,000,000,000	4.8×10^{12}	12 places to the left
0.109	1.09×10^{-1}	1 place to the right
0.000587	5.87×10^{-4}	4 places to the right
0.00000026	2.6×10^{-7}	7 places to the right
0.000000000049	4.9×10^{-11}	11 places to the right

1.2 Problem Set

Give the equivalent Arabic number for each of the following Roman numerals.

1. X

2. V

3. DCXXIV

4. MML

5. XLVIII

Give the equivalent Roman numeral for each of the following Arabic numbers.

6. 17

7. 67

8. 1995

In each group of numbers, circle the highest value.

9. 3.1   1.7   4.1

10. 0.5   0.56   0.6

In each group of numbers, circle the lowest value.

11. 2.02   2.12   2.1

12. 0.16   0.167   0.017

Using the following number, list the value of each numeral in the named places.

92,375.046

13. tenths place

14. thousandths place

15. hundreds place

State the place value of the underlined digit.

16. 18,240.6

17. 7.2391

18. 621.508

19. 0.98

20. 40.023

Write the following numbers without using scientific notation.

21. 6.8×10^4

22. 1.87×10^6

23. 1.03×10^7

24. 8.4×10^{-4}

25. 7.68×10^{-3}

26. 6.239×10^{-5}

Write the following numbers using scientific notation.

27. 0.00000000329

28. 390,000,000,000

29. 0.0038

30. 52,000,000,000,000,000

31. 3,779,000

32. 0.000000000202

Applications

33. A patient is to take "VIIss tablets three times daily." How many tablets must be dispensed to last seven days?

34. Using the prescription below, answer the following questions.

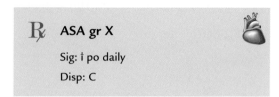

℞ ASA gr X

Sig: ĭ po daily

Disp: C

a. What is the strength of the tablet?

b. What is the daily dose?

c. What is the quantity to be dispensed?

35. Using the prescription below, answer the following questions.

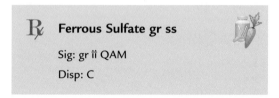

℞ Ferrous Sulfate gr ss

Sig: gr ĭĭ QAM

Disp: C

Note: QAM (or qam or q am) means "every morning."

a. What is the dosage strength of the drug XYZ?

b. How many grains are ordered each day?

c. How many tablets will be needed for 7 days?

d. How long will C tablets last the patient?

36. Using the prescription below, answer the following questions.

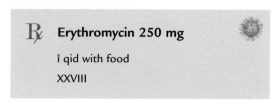

℞ Erythromycin 250 mg

ĭ qid with food

XXVIII

Note: qid (or QID) means "four times a day."

a. How many tablets will be dispensed?

b. How many days will the prescription last?

37. Using the prescription below, answer the following questions.

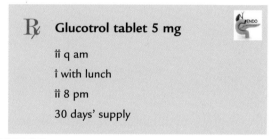

℞ Glucotrol tablet 5 mg

ĭĭ q am

ĭ with lunch

ĭĭ 8 pm

30 days' supply

a. How many tablets are taken each day?

b. How many tablets will be dispensed?

c. How long would C tablets last?

Self-check your work in Appendix A.

1.3 Decimals

A fraction in which the denominator is 10 or some multiple of 10 is a decimal fraction or, more simply, a **decimal**. In decimal fractions, the denominator is not written but is represented by the location of the number in relation to the decimal point. (Refer to the previous section titled "The Arabic Number System" and to Figure 1.3.) The decimal point represents the center. Numbers written to the right of the decimal point are decimal fractions with a denominator of 10 or a multiple of 10 and so have a value of less than 1. Numbers written to the left of the decimal point have a value of 1 or greater (whole numbers).

An understanding of decimals is *crucial* to pharmacy calculations because most medication orders are written in metric, which uses decimals. Remember, numbers to the left of the decimal point are whole numbers; numbers to the right of the decimal point are decimal fractions (parts of a whole).

Safety in Numbers

For a decimal value less than 1, use a leading zero to prevent errors.

Reading and Writing Decimals

A decimal is read by first reading the whole number, if there is one, to the left of the decimal point, then the decimal point (say "and" or "point"), and then the decimal fraction, to the right of the decimal point.

A decimal is written as a whole number or a zero, then the decimal point (indicating the value of the number to the right of the decimal), and then the fractional portion. The values to the right of the decimal point are multiples of one-tenth: tenths, hundredths, thousandths, ten thousandths, and so on. Figure 1.4 illustrates this relationship in terms of medication.

To further emphasize the value of the calculation when there is no whole number, a zero should be placed to the left of the decimal point. This zero is called a **leading zero**. Using a leading zero will help prevent errors by ensuring a correct reading of the value.

For Good Measure

The size of tablets does not always represent the amount of drug in a tablet. Many tablets contain large amounts of fillers to make the tablets a size that is easy for patients to handle.

FIGURE 1.4   Decimal Places

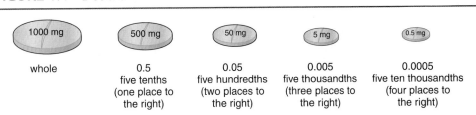

| whole | 0.5 five tenths (one place to the right) | 0.05 five hundredths (two places to the right) | 0.005 five thousandths (three places to the right) | 0.0005 five ten thousandths (four places to the right) |

Adding and Subtracting Decimals

When adding or subtracting decimals, place the numbers in columns so that the decimal points are aligned directly under each other. Add or subtract from the far-right column to the far-left column.

$$
\begin{array}{r} 20.4 \\ +21.8 \\ \hline 42.2 \end{array}
\qquad
\begin{array}{r} 11.2 \\ 13.6 \\ +16.0 \\ \hline 40.8 \end{array}
\qquad
\begin{array}{r} 15.36 \\ -3.80 \\ \hline 11.56 \end{array}
$$

Multiplying and Dividing Decimals

Multiply the two decimals as whole numbers. Add the total number of decimal places that are in the two numbers being multiplied (count from right to left), count that number of places from right to left in the answer, and insert a decimal point.

$$
\begin{array}{r} 1.23 \\ \times 2.3 \\ \hline 369 \\ +2460 \\ \hline 2.829 \end{array}
$$

(A zero is added to align the columns. Note that no value is added to the number.)

To divide decimal numbers, change both the divisor (the number doing the dividing; the denominator) and the dividend (the number being divided; the numerator) to whole numbers by moving their decimal points the same number of places to the right. If the divisor and the dividend have a different number of digits after the decimal point, choose the one that has more digits and move its decimal point a sufficient number of places to make it a whole number. Then move the decimal point in the other number the same number of places, adding a zero at the end if necessary. In the first example below, the divisor has more digits after the decimal point, so move its decimal point three places to the right to make it a whole number. Then move the decimal point in the dividend the same number of places, adding a zero at the end. In the second example below, the dividend has more digits after the decimal point, so move its decimal point three places to the right to make it a whole number. Then move the decimal point in the divisor three places to the right also.

$$1.45 \div 3.625 = 0.4 \qquad 1.617 \div 2.31 = 0.7$$

$$\frac{1.45}{3.625} = \frac{1450}{3625} = 0.4 \qquad \frac{1.617}{2.31} = \frac{1617}{2310} = 0.7$$

Rounding Decimals

Rounding numbers is essential for daily use of mathematical operations. The purpose of rounding is to keep the number you are working with to a manageable size. It is important to recognize, however, that rounding will affect the **accuracy** to which a medication can be measured. In some cases, it may be appropriate to calculate a dose to the nearest whole milliliter and, in other cases, to round to the nearest tenth or hundredth of a milliliter. Depending on the drug and strength prescribed, it may not be possible to accurately measure a very small quantity such as a hundredth of a milliliter.

When numbers with decimals are used to calculate a volumetric dose, a number with multiple digits beyond the decimal often results. It is not practical to retain all of these numbers, as a dose cannot be accurately measured beyond the hundredths or thousandths place for most medications. Most commonly, the dose is rounded to the nearest tenth. It is common practice to round the weight of a dose at the hundredths or thousandths place, or as accurate as the particular measuring device (or medication) will permit.

To round off an answer to the nearest tenth, carry the division out two places, to the hundredths place. If the number in the hundredths place is 5 or greater, add 1 to the tenths place number. If the number in the hundredths place is less than 5, round the number down by omitting the digit in the hundredths place.

$$5.65 \text{ becomes } 5.7 \qquad\qquad 4.24 \text{ becomes } 4.2$$

The same procedure may be used when rounding to the nearest hundredths place or thousandths place.

$$3.8421 = 3.84 \qquad \text{(hundredths place)}$$
$$41.2674 = 41.27 \qquad \text{(hundredths place)}$$
$$0.3928 = 0.393 \qquad \text{(thousandths place)}$$
$$4.1111 = 4.111 \qquad \text{(thousandths place)}$$

As mentioned earlier, when rounding numbers used in pharmacy calculations, it is common to round off to the nearest tenth. However, there are times when a dose is very small and rounding to the nearest hundredth or thousandth may be more appropriate.

The exact dose calculated is 0.08752 g
Rounded to nearest tenth: 0.1 g
Rounded to nearest hundredth: 0.09 g
Rounded to nearest thousandth: 0.088 g

When a number that has been rounded to the tenths place is multiplied or divided by a number that was rounded to the hundredths or thousandths place, the answer must be rounded back to the tenths place. The reason is that the answer can only be accurate to the place to which the highest rounding was made in the original numbers.

Example 1.3.1

Round off the answer of the following equation to the appropriate decimal. Note that 7.1 is a rounded figure.

$$3.46 \times 7.1 = 24.566$$

The answer must be rounded to the tenths place.

Answer = 24.6

Safety in Numbers

Do not use a trailing zero unless it indicates accuracy of a number (i.e., is significant).

Example 1.3.2

Round off the answer of the following equation to the appropriate decimal. Note that 1.349 is a rounded figure.

$$0.3563 \times 1.349 = 0.4806487$$

The answer must be rounded to the thousandths place.

Answer = 0.481

In most cases, a zero occurring at the end of a string of digits is not written. This zero is called a **trailing zero**. The exception to this rule occurs when rounding results in a zero as the last place value. When the last digit resulting from rounding is a zero, this zero should be written because it is considered significant to that particular problem or dosage. In such cases, the amount can be measured out to an exact zero as the place value.

Example 1.3.3

Round 9.98 to the nearest tenths place.

Answer = 10.0

Example 1.3.4

Round 0.599 to the nearest hundredths place.

Answer = 0.60

1.3 Problem Set

Write the following decimals.

1. seven hundred eighty-four and thirty-six hundredths

2. nine tenths

Add the following decimals.

3. 0.34 + 1.54 =

4. 1.39 + 1.339 =

Subtract the following decimals.

5. 15.36 − 0.987 =

6. 3.09875 − 0.00045 =

7. 12.901 − 0.903 =

Multiply the following decimals and round to the hundredths place.

8. 21.62 × 21.62 =

9. 0.9 × 500 =

Divide the following decimals and round to the thousandths place.

10. 12 ÷ 6.5 =

11. 0.8 ÷ 0.6 =

Round the following to the nearest hundredths place.

12. 3.872

13. 0.138

14. 0.076

Round the following to the nearest thousandths place.

15. 0.1961

16. 0.0488

Multiply the following and round to the appropriate place.

17. 6.7 × 5.21 =

18. 0.45 × 3.1 =

Applications

19. Using the prescription below, answer the following questions.
    Note: QID means "four times a day."

 Alprazolam 0.25 mg

Sig: 3 tabs po QID

Disp: 100 tablets

a. How many milligrams is the patient taking with each dose?

b. How many milligrams is the patient taking each day?

c. How many tablets will the patient need for 14 days?

d. Is the prescription written for enough tablets to last the patient until the next office visit in two weeks?

e. The pharmacy plans to charge $7.59 plus the cost of the medication. The available products include:

alprazolam 0.25 mg #100/$14.95
alprazolam 0.5 mg #100/$17.46
alprazolam 1 mg #100/$23.87

Select the appropriate product and calculate the price for the patient.
Based on the prescription provided, the pharmacy can only dispense 100 tablets.

20. The physician changes the prescription at the patient's next visit. The prescription is shown below.

 R̸ Alprazolam 0.25 mg

    Sig: 4 tabs po QID

    Disp: 175 tablets

The available products include:

alprazolam 0.25 mg #100/$14.95
alprazolam 0.5 mg #100/$17.46
alprazolam 1 mg #100/$23.87

a. How many milligrams at each dose is this?

b. How much would #125 alprazolam 0.5 mg tablets cost the pharmacy?

c. How much would #50 alprazolam 1 mg tablets cost the pharmacy?

d. How many days would #50 alprazolam 1 mg tablets taken QID last?

21. Sterile water comes in bottles of 1 L. You will need to pour out 120 mL bottles for each patient.

a. How many 120 mL bottles will you get from a 1 L bottle? (1 L = 1000 mL)

b. How much will be left over?

22. How many total milliliters will need to be dispensed for the following prescription? *Note:* bid means "twice a day."

 R̸ Augmentin 125 mg/5 mL susp

    8.5 mL bid days 1–2

    5.75 mL bid days 3–7

23. Round the following to the nearest whole dollar.

a. $46.92

b. 12 @ $1.26

c. $7.37 divided by 2

24. Calculate the following dollar amounts and round to the nearest cent.

a. $5.84 × 12 =

b. $0.415 × 269 =

25. Calculate the following test scores to the nearest tenth of a percent.

a. 34 of 38 questions correct

b. 51 of 60 questions correct

c. 83 of 90 questions correct

Self-check your work in Appendix A.

1.4 Estimates

Estimating an answer before calculating the solution is a simple way of checking to see whether the answer you arrive at is reasonable. Estimating can be used in both simple mathematical equations and more complicated algebraic equations.

There are no set mathematical rules for estimating. Most commonly, estimating is performed by rounding to the nearest whole unit that makes sense for the numbers involved. This may be the ones place, tens place, hundreds place, or even larger. A common estimate that is used daily is rounding to the nearest whole dollar while shopping.

Estimating Sums

A **sum** is the result of adding two or more numbers together. When estimating sums, it is common to round the numbers to be added to the nearest ten or hundred or thousand first and then add these rounded numbers. When this is done, the values in the ones place and lower are often ignored. The following calculations compare an actual mathematical computation with a corresponding estimate.

$$\text{Actual} \qquad 73.8 + 42.03 + 18.3 + 87.32 = 221.45$$
$$\text{Estimate} \qquad 70 \ \ + 40 \ \ \ + 20 \ \ + 90 \ \ \ \ = 220$$

$$\text{Actual} \qquad 623 + 1493 + 1631 + 794 + 86 \ \ \ = 4627$$
$$\text{Estimate} \qquad 600 + 1500 + 1600 + 800 + 100 = 4600$$

$$\text{Actual} \qquad 6425 + 2652 + 2328 + 4490 = 15{,}895$$
$$\text{Estimate} \qquad 6000 + 3000 + 2000 + 4000 = 15{,}000$$

Safety in Numbers

Estimated values can be used to double-check doses but cannot be relied on for accuracy.

Another common method of estimating sums is to stack the numbers by aligning them on their decimal points; add the numbers in the far left column using their place value (6428 would be 6000 because the 6 is in the thousands place, for example); and then add one-half of the place value of the far-left column for each number with a value in the second-from-the-left column. If the second-from-the left column is the hundreds column, each number that had a numeral in the column would represent 500 (one-half of the next left column of 1000). This is loosely based on the assumption that, on average, each of the entries with a numeral in the column will contribute about half of the next place value.

Estimating is a process that becomes easier and more accurate with practice. A small list of numbers will often generate a fairly accurate estimate, whereas longer lists of numbers may require more practice and may be less accurate. For a long list of numbers, it is helpful to estimate the sums on paper using the method shown in Table 1.8. The following examples demonstrate this stepped method for estimating. The sum determined by estimating cannot be relied on as accurate when dispensing prescriptions.

TABLE 1.8   Steps for Estimating Sums

Step 1. Stack the numbers whose sum is to be estimated so that their decimal points are aligned.

Step 2. Add the numbers in the far-left column using their column place value. For example, if the first number is 735, use 700 as that number's value.

Step 3. Multiply one-half of the place value of the far-left column by the total number of numbers that have place values in the second-from-the-left column.

Step 4. Add the totals determined in Steps 2 and 3 to estimate the sum.

Example 1.4.1

Estimate the sum of 73.80, 42.05, 18.30, and 87.32.

Step 1. Stack these four numbers so that their decimal points are aligned.

$$73.80$$
$$42.05$$
$$18.30$$
$$87.32$$

Step 2. Add the numbers in the far-left column using their place value, in this case, the tens column.

$$70 + 40 + 10 + 80 = 200$$

Step 3. Multiply one-half of the place value of the far-left column by the total number of numbers that have place values in the second-from-the-left column in the original problem.

$$(10 \text{ far-left column value} \div 2) \times 4 \text{ numbers} = 20$$

Step 4. Add the totals determined in Steps 2 and 3 to determine the estimate.

$$200 + 20 = 220$$

Compare the estimate with the actual sum of the original numbers, which is 221.47.

Example 1.4.2

Estimate the sum of 623, 1493, 1631, 794, and 86.

Step 1. Stack these five numbers so that their decimal points are aligned.

$$\begin{array}{r} 623 \\ 1493 \\ 1631 \\ 794 \\ 86 \end{array}$$

Step 2. Add the numbers in the far-left column using their place value, in this case, the thousands column.

$$1000 + 1000 = 2000$$

Step 3. Multiply one-half of the place value of the far-left column by the total number of numbers that have place values in the second-from-the-left column in the original problem.

$$(1000 \text{ far-left column value} \div 2) \times 4 \text{ numbers} = 2000$$

Note: Because 86 does not have a hundreds place value, the number 4, not 5, is used in this step.

Step 4. Add the totals determined in Steps 2 and 3 to determine the estimate.

$$2000 + 2000 = 4000$$

Compare the estimate with the actual sum of the original numbers, which is 4627.

Example 1.4.3

Estimate the sum of 6425, 2652, 2328, and 4490.

Step 1. 6425
            2652
            2328
            4490

Step 2. 6000 + 2000 + 2000 + 4000 = 14,000

Step 3. (1000 far-left column value ÷ 2) × 4 numbers = 2000

Step 4. 14,000 + 2000 = 16,000

Compare the estimate with the actual sum of the original numbers, which is 15,895.

Estimating Products and Quotients

A **product** is the result of multiplying two numbers together. A **quotient** is the result of dividing one number by another number. When estimating products or quotients, it is common to round each of the original numbers, divided by the place value of its leftmost column, to the nearest whole number. The rounded numbers can be quickly multiplied or divided, and the appropriate number of zeros can be added to the answer.

Example 1.4.4

Estimate the product of 325 × 618.

Round the two numbers and multiply the leftmost digits.

$$3 \times 6 = 18$$

Add four zeros to this answer to account for the four places of "25" and "18" in the original problem.

$$180,000$$

Compare the estimate to the actual product, which is 200,850.

Example 1.4.5

Estimate the product of 843 × 41.

Round the two numbers and multiply them.

$$8 \times 4 = 32$$

Add three zeros for the "43" and "1."

$$32,000$$

Compare the estimate to the actual product, which is 34,563.

Example 1.4.6

Estimate the product of 843 × 56.

Round the two numbers, and multiply them. Note that 56 is rounded up to 6, not down to 5.

$$8 \times 6 = 48$$

Add three zeros for the "43" and "6."

$$48,000$$

Compare the estimate to the actual product, which is 47,208.

Example 1.4.7

Estimate the quotient of 5355 ÷ 4.79.

Round the two numbers and divide them.

$$5 \div 5 = 1$$

Add three zeros for the "355." Do not add zeros for the numbers to the right of the decimal place in 4.79.

$$1000$$

Compare the estimate to the actual quotient, which is 1117.95.

Example 1.4.8

Estimate the product of 14.3 × 0.19.

Round the two numbers.

14.3 is rounded to 14
0.19 is rounded to 0.2

To avoid the decimal in the estimate operation, simplify 0.2 to 2. The decimal point will be inserted after you have multiplied the two rounded numbers.

$$14 \times 2 = 28$$

You ignored one decimal place to perform the estimating process quickly, so now you must account for the decimal. To do this, move the decimal point the same number of places that you ignored—in this case, one place. Thus, 28 becomes 2.8.

Compare the estimate to the actual product, which is 2.717.

In other cases, it may make sense to round to a near factor of 10 or 100 or even larger.

Actual	$18.79 × 6 = $112.74
Estimate	$20.00 × 6 = $120.00
Actual	$424.00 × 2 = $848.00
Estimate	$420.00 × 2 = $840.00
Actual	4326 ÷ 3.78 = 1144.44
Estimate	4000 ÷ 4 = 1000
Actual	820 ÷ 42 = 19.52
Estimate	800 ÷ 40 = 20

Example 1.4.9

A patient needs to take 3.75 mL daily for 30 days. Estimate the total number of milliliters needed. The pharmacy technician can select between a 120 mL bottle and 180 mL bottle for dispensing this liquid medication. Which bottle should the technician use?

Estimate	4 mL × 30 days = 120 mL for 30 days
Actual	3.75 mL × 30 days = 112.5 mL for 30 days

Because the 120 mL bottle has more than enough room, the 180 mL bottle is not necessary, and the 120 mL bottle will be used to dispense the medication.

Safety in Numbers

As stated before, an estimated value can be used to double-check a dose but cannot be relied on for accuracy.

Estimating a Drug Dose

Estimating a drug dose before calculating the actual dose is helpful because the estimate can be used to double-check the accuracy of the calculated actual dose. If the amounts do not match, then the answer should be checked carefully. When estimating a drug dose, the first step is to determine whether the dose is going to be more or less than the unit dose or available drug strength. Continue estimating the dose by rounding the given dose to simplify the problem and dividing this rounded dose by the available drug strength.

Example 1.4.10

An order for 12.5 mg of a drug needs to be filled using a 5 mg tablet. Estimate the number of tablets needed for this dose.

The medication on hand has 5 mg of drug for each tablet. Since the order is for 12.5 mg of drug, the dose to be measured out will be larger than 1 tablet.

Simplify the estimation by rounding 12.5 mg down to 10 mg. This will make it easier to use the available dose to determine the value of the requested dose.

$$10 \text{ mg (estimated requested amount)} \times \frac{1 \text{ tablet}}{5 \text{ mg}} \text{ (available amount)} = 2 \text{ tablets}$$

Therefore, the estimate indicates that the dose will be at least 2 tablets.

The actual calculated dose of 2.5 tablets can then be checked by comparing it with the estimate. If an actual dose of 0.25 tablet or 25 tablets was calculated instead, then a quick comparison with the estimated dose of 2 tablets would immediately indicate that the actual dose was calculated incorrectly.

In addition to drug doses, the volume to be dispensed and the size of the container needed can be useful estimates when preparing a drug for dispensing.

Example 1.4.11

The pharmacy receives an order for a 10-day supply of a liquid antibiotic to be taken in a dose of 8.5 mL of medication three times a day. The pharmacy has 100 mL, 200 mL, and 300 mL bottles of this antibiotic in stock. Which size bottle of antibiotic should be dispensed?

Begin by simplifying the problem, rounding the dose of 8.5 mL/dose to 10 mL/dose. It is important to round up to make sure the patient has enough drug.

Using this rounded value, calculate the amount of drug needed per day by multiplying the estimated dose by the number of doses each day.

$$\frac{10 \text{ mL}}{1 \text{ dose}} \times \frac{3 \text{ doses}}{1 \text{ day}} = \frac{30 \text{ mL}}{1 \text{ day}}$$

In other words, the patient will need about 30 mL of drug a day.

Since the patient needs to take this drug for 10 days, multiply the amount of drug per day by the number of days of therapy.

$$\frac{30 \text{ mL}}{\text{day}} \times 10 \text{ days} = 300 \text{ mL}$$

Therefore, the patient will need about 300 mL of the medication. The actual amount needed is 255 mL, but the 300 mL bottle is the correct choice to fill this prescription.

1.4 Problem Set

Using the stack-up process described in Table 1.7, estimate the sum to the nearest tens place and then calculate the actual value.

1. 231 + 718 + 357 + 609 =

2. 176 + 34 + 49 + 16 =

3. 12.38 + 6.26 + 18.95 + 16.52 =

4. 93.7 + 16 + 48.7 + 12.02 =

5. 0.95 + 6.96 + 0.49 + 12.42 =

Use rounding to estimate the dollar amounts to the nearest whole dollar, and then calculate the actual value.

6. $12.53 − $6.15 =

7. $6.28 + $1.99 + $3.98 =

8. $40 − $34.81 =

9. $100 − $18.29 =

10. $100 − $17.52 − $31.90 =

Estimate the products by rounding the two numbers and then multiplying them. Also calculate the actual value.

11. 6.8 × 7656 =

12. 4.02 × 350.07 =

13. 598.4 × 0.015 =

14. 4569 × 0.0972 =

15. 6183 × 18 =

16. 1253 × 9.1 =

Estimate the quotients by rounding the two numbers and then dividing them. Also calculate the actual value.

17. 185 ÷ 18 =

18. 18,015 ÷ 56 =

19. 584.0 ÷ 8 =

20. 844.23 ÷ 4.4 =

21. 123 ÷ 14 =

Applications

Round and estimate to find the following.

22. An employee of the pharmacy is being sent to the grocery store to buy the following items. Estimate how much petty cash he will need.

Food dye	$1.89
Sugar, 2@	$4.25
Baking soda	$0.79
Cherry flavoring	$2.39
1 gallon bleach	$1.97
Distilled water, 4@	$0.89

23. Estimate how much sterile water for injection (SWFI) you will need for the following reconstitutions: 3.2 mL, 7.6 mL, 1.6 mL, and 4.1 mL. Choose the appropriate vial from the available vials (15 mL SWFI, 30 mL SWFI, and 50 mL SWFI).

24. A patient is receiving the following fluids: IV fluids, 1723 mL; juice, 150 mL; coffee, 126 mL. Estimate the patient's intake to the nearest 10 mL.

25. The following is a patient's parenteral fluid intake for the first 24 hours of admittance: 780 mL normal saline (NS), 3 × 50 mL piggybacks, 250 mL NS, 3 × 1000 mL NS. Estimate the total to the nearest 100 mL amount.

Self-check your work in Appendix A.

1.5 Significant Figures and Measurement Accuracy

Rounding and estimating have been discussed as a practical way of using numbers to calculate and measure a dose. In the process, you should not lose sight of the mathematical principle that each numerical value has a certain number of **significant figures**. These significant figures consist of those that are known to be accurate plus the digit in the lowest place value, which is approximate.

The **lowest known place value** is the last digit on the right of a written numeral. This lowest known value is approximate because of many sources of error including the limitation of the instrument used to measure, operator error, temperature variation, and the need to round at a certain point to make the number practical for calculations.

Significant figures are digits that have a practical meaning or value. A leading zero that marks the place of the decimal is not significant because it only marks the place value of the numbers that follow the decimal. Counting of significant figures begins at the first nonzero digit. Table 1.9 provides a short list of "rules" to follow when counting significant figures. Table 1.10 shows several numbers and indicates how many significant figures they have.

In certain cases, when the accuracy of the measurement is known, the trailing zero to the right of the apparent last significant figure may also be considered significant. For example, if the device used to measure a substance is accurate to the nearest tenth,

Safety in Numbers

Do not use a trailing zero unless it indicates accuracy of a number (i.e., is significant).

TABLE 1.9   Rules for Counting Significant Figures

Rule 1.   Begin counting at the first nonzero digit.

Rule 2.   Continue counting to the right until you reach the place value that is last (or rounded).

Rule 3.   Zeros that are located between digits are significant and should be counted.

Rule 4.   Do not count zeros that are placed to the left of the first digit. They only mark the place of the decimal.

Rule 5.   One or more final zeros may or may not be significant depending on the accuracy to which the number is held.

TABLE 1.10   Counting Significant Figures

Number	Number of Significant Figures	Rule Applied
1.8	2	1, 2
18.3	3	1, 2
183	3	1, 2
1.832	4	1, 2
1832	4	1, 2
0.183	3	1, 2, 4
0.108	3	1, 2, 3, 4
0.0108	3	1, 2, 3, 4
0.01	1	1, 2, 4
0.8	1	1, 2, 4
8	1	1, 2

the tenths place may be considered significant even if the last digit is a zero. The zero may be retained to indicate the accuracy of the number. For example,

1.0 has two significant figures.

Larger numbers have significant figures based on their accuracy to the nearest factor of 10. If a very large amount of a substance is measured, at some point the person doing the measuring must "estimate" the closest amount represented by the device being used. As a result, the last digit recorded cannot be considered to be accurate and is thus not significant. For example, if 2788 is considered accurate from 2780 to 2790, it has only three significant figures. Similarly, if 8,341,274 is considered accurate from 8,341,270 to 8,341,280, it has only six significant figures.

When the degree of accuracy is known to a certain place value, the significant figures are counted only to that place value. Knowing the level of accuracy is important when considering the weighing capacity and sensitivity of a scale or balance in the pharmacy.

Example 1.5.1

An item is weighed on a balance with a degree of accuracy to the nearest tenth when measuring milligrams. The balance indicates that an item weighs 1.459 mg. How many significant figures does this weight have? What would the rounded value be?

Because the accuracy of the scale can only be relied on to the tenths place, the number of significant figures is two. The "59" is not considered significant because of the sensitivity of the scale being used.

The weight would be rounded to 1.5 mg.

More significant digits indicate a greater accuracy of known values. A number that is accurate to within two figures has a practical 5% error from the actual measurement. Table 1.11 demonstrates these accuracy translations.

In studying mathematics, numbers may be considered accurate for an infinite number of figures. In the study of pharmacy, however, for practical purposes, a range of two to five figures is common. Additionally, it is important to recognize that a quantity measured to a certain degree of accuracy has a number of significant figures that are more relevant than a number that that quantity may be multiplied or divided by. The resulting product when multiplying two numbers is typically considered accurate only to the number of significant figures of the number with the lesser significant figures. In pharmacy, we recognize the measured dose as the more important of the two factors. For example, if 6.25 mg is measured exactly and then multiplied by 2 for a twice a day

TABLE 1.11 Accuracy Ranges

Accuracy Level	Example
Two-figure accuracy is within 5%	100 mg is in the range of 95 mg to 105 mg
Three-figure accuracy is within 0.5%	100 mg is in the range of 99.5 mg to 100.5 mg
Four-figure accuracy is within 0.05%	100 mg is in the range of 99.95 mg to 100.05 mg
Five-figure accuracy is within 0.005%	100 mg is in the range of 99.995 mg to 100.005 mg

administration, the resulting daily dose is exactly 12.5 mg. In pharmacy applications, it is typical to use the number with the most accurately measured significant figures as the guide for determining the final number of relevant significant figures as most instances involve a dose multiplied or divided by a dosage frequency. Therefore, dosages should be determined as accurately as possible based on the available measurement.

Numbers greater than 100 have significant figures based on the relative accuracy of the measurement. If a number over 100 is accurate to the nearest 10, the first two digits are considered significant, and the last zero is considered an estimate and thus not significant. This is also true for numbers that are accurate to the nearest 100 or 1000. For example, if the following numbers are accurate to the nearest 10, they will have the indicated number of significant figures.

200 has two significant figures
1800 has three significant figures
30,000 has four significant figures

Similarly, if the following numbers are accurate to the nearest 100, they will have the indicated number of significant figures.

200 has one significant figure
1800 has two significant figures
30,000 has three significant figures

Just as with rounding, when performing calculations with numbers that have a different number of significant figures or have been rounded to different place values, the answer must be rounded to the place value of the least number of decimals.

Example 1.5.2

Determine the product of 6.5 mg × 4.18 using the appropriate number of accurate and significant figures.

Note the number of significant figures and the level of accuracy for each number: 6.5 has two significant figures and is accurate to the tenths place, whereas 4.18 has three significant figures and is accurate to the hundredths place.
Now, determine the product of the two numbers.

$$6.5 \times 4.18 = 27.17$$

Because 6.5 is accurate only to the tenths place, the answer is only accurate to the tenths place. Therefore, 27.17 needs to be rounded to the tenths place. The answer, 27.2, has three significant figures.

Example 1.5.3

Determine the product of 12.59 × 1572 using the appropriate number of accurate and significant figures.

Note the number of significant figures and the accuracy of the numbers. Both factors have four significant figures. The number 12.59 is accurate to the hundredths place, but 1572 is accurate only to the ones place.

Now, determine the product of the two numbers.

$$12.59 \times 1572 = 19{,}791.48$$

The accuracy of the product is considered only to the ones place. Therefore, the answer must be rounded to that place, and the acceptable answer is 19,791.

1.5 Problem Set

Identify the number of significant figures in the following amounts. Assume that all final zeros are not significant.

1. 15.4324 grains

2. 1500 mL

3. 0.21 mg

4. $1.07

5. 100,000 mcg

6. 507.2 mg

7. 1.0 kg

8. 0.001 mg

9. 21,204.075 mcg

10. 100 mL

Round the following numbers to three significant figures.

11. 42.75

12. 100.19

13. 0.04268

14. 18.426

15. 0.003918

Round the following numbers to two decimal places and state how many significant figures each has.

16. 0.3479

17. 0.056921

18. 1.9947

19. 0.00986

20. 1.0277

Calculate the following and retain the correct number of decimal places in the calculation.

21. $0.67 \times 95.2 =$

22. $1.26 \times 24 =$

23. $325 \times 0.5 =$

Applications

24. You are to prepare capsules that contain 0.125 g of a drug. You have four partial containers of medication, which weigh 3.2 g, 1.784 g, 2.46 g, and 5.87 g. Assume you have weighed each of the four containers with the same scale, and the accuracy is known to the hundredth gram.

    a. Which amount will need to be rounded?

    b. Which amount is not as accurate as it should be?

    c. What is the amount of the medication that will be left over after making the 0.125 g capsules?

25. A unit dose of an oral medication requires 21.65 mg. You are to prepare 45 doses.

    a. How many milligrams will you need?

    b. How many significant figures does this amount have?

Self-check your work in Appendix A.

1.6 Time of Day

Telling time is a skill that you learn as a child. For many individuals, this skill was taught using a clock with movable hands: one hand indicating the hours and one hand indicating the minutes. In addition to these traditional clocks, digital clocks that display the hours and minutes as numbers separated by a colon are also used to tell time. Digital clocks are commonly seen on computer software programs. Both types of clocks typically indicate what is known as **standard time**—a system of time that relates to the natural day and is based on a 12-hour format. Standard time, also known as *civilian time*, uses the designations of "a.m." and "p.m."

However, the pharmacy profession uses a different method to indicate time: military time. **Military time** is based on a 24-hour format and, as its name indicates, is used among military personnel to avoid confusion between "a.m." and "p.m." In fact, most countries—with the exception of the United States and Canada—have adopted the military time system as their official time standard. The military time system is now commonly referred to as the *24-hour system*.

In the healthcare setting, the 24-hour system is used for accuracy. This system prevents ambiguity and provides a simple means of documenting the exact time in a 24-hour day. The 24-hour system may be used to document what time a medication is to be administered, what time an event (such as an adverse reaction) occurs, or what time an intravenous (IV) medication runs out. Exact minutes are also used, so if a medication is to be given at 6:30 a.m., it would be recorded as 06:30 to indicate the exact time.

The 24-hour system uses the numbers 0–24 to represent the 24-hour day. To provide consistency and prevent confusion, the 24-hour system uses two digits for the hour (followed by a colon) and then two digits for the minutes. If seconds are indicated, a colon will follow and also use two digits. Times between 1:00 a.m. and 10:00 a.m. will often be preceded by a leading zero so that the hour has two digits. Table 1.12 provides a comparison of standard time and 24-hour time.

The start of each day is designated as 00:00, and midnight is designated as 24:00. These two designations are actually the same time, so some computer systems will accept times up to 24:00 and then require the first minute after midnight to be entered as 00:01, thereby skipping the 00:00 time display.

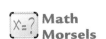 **Math Morsels**

Computer systems do not always permit the use of a colon when entering time. Consequently, you may see a time entry as a four-digit entry—for example, 0430 rather than 04:30. Be aware that both time entries indicate 4:30 a.m.

TABLE 1.12 Standard Time and 24-Hour Time (Military Time) Equivalents

Standard Time	24-Hour Time	Standard Time	24-Hour Time
1:00 a.m.	01:00 hours	1:00 p.m.	13:00 hours
2:00 a.m.	02:00 hours	2:00 p.m.	14:00 hours
3:00 a.m.	03:00 hours	3:00 p.m.	15:00 hours
4:00 a.m.	04:00 hours	4:00 p.m.	16:00 hours
5:00 a.m.	05:00 hours	5:00 p.m.	17:00 hours
6:00 a.m.	06:00 hours	6:00 p.m.	18:00 hours
7:00 a.m.	07:00 hours	7:00 p.m.	19:00 hours
8:00 a.m.	08:00 hours	8:00 p.m.	20:00 hours
9:00 a.m.	09:00 hours	9:00 p.m.	21:00 hours
10:00 a.m.	10:00 hours	10:00 p.m.	22:00 hours
11:00 a.m.	11:00 hours	11:00 p.m.	23:00 hours
12:00 p.m.	12:00 hours	12:00 a.m.	24:00 hours

It is important for pharmacy personnel to become familiar with the time equivalents and be able to accurately convert times without looking at a chart. The times that occur in the morning hours are simple and straightforward because they are similar to the display on a typical digital clock. The times that occur in the afternoon and evening (1:00 p.m. to 12:00 a.m.) have numbers that many individuals are not accustomed to seeing when telling time: 13:00 to 24:00. For these 24-hour times, remember this simple rule: These designations can quickly be converted back to standard time by subtracting 12. So, for example, if you subtract 12 from 19:00 hours, you get 7:00—the standard time designation.

 Math Morsels

Depending on which type of time conversion you are doing, you will either add or subtract 12 hours.

Example 1.6.1

Convert the following times from standard time to 24-hour time using the conversion chart:

3:45 a.m.	becomes 03:45
9:20 a.m.	becomes 09:20
6:13 p.m.	becomes 18:13
11:56 p.m.	becomes 23:56

Example 1.6.2

Convert the following times from 24-hour time to standard time using the conversion chart:

01:28	becomes 1:28 a.m.
04:56	becomes 4:56 a.m.
15:30	becomes 3:30 p.m.
22:15	becomes 10:15 p.m.

Example 1.6.3

According to her electronic health record, a patient has received medication at the following times: 0700, 1300, and 1900. Convert these 24-hour times to standard times.

0700	becomes 7:00 a.m.
1300	becomes 1:00 p.m.
1900	becomes 7:00 p.m.

1.6 Problem Set

Convert the followng standard times to 24-hour times:

1. 7:30 a.m.

2. 4:28 p.m.

3. 12:45 a.m.

4. 9:20 p.m.

5. 2:24 a.m.

6. 10:58 p.m.

7. 11:50 p.m.

8. 1:20 a.m.

9. 12:03 a.m.

10. 12:20 p.m.

Convert the following 24-hour times to standard times:

11. 17:30

12. 23:49

13. 15:22

14. 00:34

15. 12:04

16. 0355

17. 2245

18. 1719

19. 1300

20. 0145

Applications

21. Sun Ng, a patient who arrived in the emergency room around midnight, stated that he took his pain medication three times during the day: at 8:15 in the morning, at 1:15 with his lunch, and at 7:00 in the evening. Using the 24-hour system, what times should be reflected in the patient's health record?

22. A prescription states that Lucy Andrews, a pediatric patient in the intensive care unit, is to take medication three times a day, every eight hours, beginning at 5:00 a.m. Using the 24-hour system, what time should the medication therapy begin?

23. Dr. Dominic Estores has written a prescription for a patient to take a preoperative medication at 22:00 on the evening before his scheduled surgery. Using the standard time system, what time should you tell the patient to take his medication?

24. The IV medications prepared each afternoon for overnight administration have to be delivered to the floors between 1800 and 1900. According to the clock in the pharmacy, when should you deliver the medications?

25. Mrs. Singh has just been brought to the hospital via ambulance. During admittance, she said that before calling for an ambulance she had taken two sublingual nitroglycerin tablets for chest pain: one at 3:00 p.m. and one at 3:05 p.m. Because her pain didn't go away, she reported that she took a third nitroglycerin tablet five minutes later. Using 24-hour time, at what times did she take the medication?

Self-check your work in Appendix A.

Chapter Summary

- Fractions are part of a whole.
- The upper number in a fraction is the numerator.
- The lower number in a fraction is the denominator.
- When adding or subtracting fractions, you need to have a common denominator first.
- When multiplying fractions, you multiply the numerators together and the denominators together.
- When dividing fractions, you multiply the first fraction by the reciprocal of the second fraction.
- Common denominators can be found by factoring the denominators and comparing them.
- Roman numerals are used on prescriptions, and they may be written as either uppercase or lowercase letters.
- Roman numerals are never repeated more than three times in sequence.
- Roman numerals that have a smaller value in front of a larger value should be subtracted before determining the final value.
- Arabic numbers use a decimal as a place value holder.
- Scientific notation is a way to write very large or very small numbers.
- Decimals may use a leading zero in front of the decimal point to avoid calculation errors.
- A trailing zero should only be used when indicating accuracy or significant figures.
- Estimation is helpful in double-checking results but should never be considered accurate.
- Significant figures can be used to determine accuracy.
- Time can be recorded using a standard time system or a 24-hour system.
- The 24-hour system uses the numbers 0–24 to designate the 24 hours of a day.
- Hours before 10:00 a.m. have a leading zero in the 24-hour system.
- Hours and minutes may be separated by a colon.

Key Terms

accuracy the correctness of a number in its representation of a given value

Arabic numbers a numbering system that uses numeric symbols to indicate numbers, fractions, and decimals; uses the numerals 0, 1, 2, 3, 4, 5, 6, 7, 8, 9

common denominator a number into which each of the unlike denominators of two or more fractions can be divided evenly

complex fraction a fraction in which both the numerator and the denominator are fractions

decimal a fraction value in which the denominator is 10 or some power of 10

denominator the number in the bottom part of a fraction

fraction a portion of a whole that is represented as a ratio

improper fraction a fraction with a value greater than 1 (the value of the numerator is larger than the value of the denominator)

leading zero a zero that is placed to the left of the decimal point, in the ones place, in a number that is less than 1 and is being represented by a decimal value

lowest known place value the last digit on the right of a written numeral

military time a system of time based on a 24-hour format

mixed number a whole number and a fraction

numerator the number in the top part of a fraction

place value the location of a numeral in a string of numbers that describes the numeral's relationship to the decimal point

product the result of multiplying one number by another

proper fraction a fraction with a value of less than 1 (the value of the numerator is smaller than the value of the denominator)

quotient the result of dividing one number by another

Roman numerals a numbering system that uses alphabetic symbols to indicate a quantity; uses the letters I, V, and X to represent 1, 5, and 10, respectively

scientific notation a method used to write numbers that have a very large or very

small numerical value; uses "× 10" with an exponent

significant figures the figures in a numeral that are known values and have not been rounded or estimated in the process of mathematical calculation, plus the digit in the lowest place value, which is approximate

standard time a system of time that relates to the natural day and is based on a 12-hour format

sum the result of adding two or more numbers together

trailing zero a zero that appears at the end of a decimal string and is not needed except when considered significant

Chapter Review

Assessing Comprehension

To check your comprehension of this chapter's key concepts, read the following multiple-choice questions and then record your answers on a separate sheet of paper. Write your answers as modeled in these examples: 1d; 2c; 3b; etc.

1. Which of the following is the number located on the top part of a fraction?
   a. denominator
   b. numerator
   c. common denominator
   d. whole number

2. When finding a common denominator, you should
   a. find the sum of the numerators.
   b. multiply by the reciprocal of the second fraction.
   c. subtract the numerators.
   d. factor the denominators.

3. When multiplying fractions, you should
   a. always change mixed fractions into whole fractions first.
   b. multiply the denominators by the least common denominator.
   c. multiply the first fraction by the reciprocal of the second fraction.
   d. reduce all fractions so that a 1 is in the numerator.

4. Roman numerals require
   a. adding all numerals together, regardless of their order.
   b. adding uppercase numerals together and subtracting lowercase numerals.
   c. adding numerals together unless a smaller numeral precedes a larger numeral.
   d. subtracting the series of three from the numeral immediately following.

5. The decimal point
   a. holds the place between the ones and tenth places.
   b. indicates where a zero should be placed.
   c. holds the place where a number should be rounded up or down.
   d. holds the place between the ones and tens places.

6. Scientific notation is used to write
   a. Roman numerals that need to be converted.
   b. Arabic numbers that are very large or very small.
   c. notes to the pharmacist about an estimated dose.
   d. drug doses when they are very small.

7. Leading zeros are used to
   a. indicate that a number has been rounded down.
   b. indicate that a number has been rounded up.
   c. keep the column aligned when multiplying without a calculator.
   d. prevent errors with numbers that are less than 1.

8. Estimates are useful for
   a. charging the patient for a liquid medication.
   b. checking that your calculated amount is in the correct range.

   c. finding the exact dose for a patient.
   d. aligning decimal points when adding numbers without a calculator.

9. Significant figures are used for
   a. determining accuracy.
   b. estimating a drug dose.
   c. eliminating zeros to the left of a decimal.
   d. calibrating the sensitivity of a pharmacy scale.

10. Converting standard time to 24-hour time requires
   a. the hour to be converted to a two-digit number between 00 and 24.
   b. the minutes to be rounded up to the nearest quarter hour.
   c. the number 12 to be added to each hour after 6 a.m.
   d. the number 12 to be subtracted from each hour after noon.

Finding Solutions

To gain practice in handling challenging situations in the workplace, consider the following real-world scenarios and then use the guiding questions to help you formulate your responses.

Note: To indicate your answer for Scenario D, Question 9, ask your instructor for the handout depicting a dosing spoon.

Scenario A: A patient has brought in the following prescription:

R℘ **Lasix 40 mg**

Sig: Take ī tablet by mouth each M, W, F and īī tablets on other days.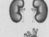

Dispense: 30-day supply

Refills: 2

1. How many tablets does the patient take on MWF?

2. Estimate how many tablets a patient will need to last 30 days.

3. Calculate exactly how many tablets the patient will need in a 30-day period if the patient begins taking the medication on a Sunday.

Scenario B: The maximum dose for an OTC medication is 4000 mg per day. A patient tells you that she has taken 4 whole tablets and ½ tablet today but wants to know if she can take more. The package indicates that there are 500 mg in each tablet.

4. How many milligrams of medication did the patient receive from the ingestion of the whole tablets?

5. How many milligrams did she receive from the ingestion of the ½ tablet?

6. How many total milligrams of medication did the patient take?

7. How many more tablets can she take before she exceeds the maximum dose?

Scenario C: Dr. Ingrid Johansson has written a prescription for a patient to take an antibiotic three hours before a cardiac procedure. The operating room schedule indicates the procedure is slated for 1430.

8. What standard time will you tell the patient to take his medication?

Scenario D: A mother has come to the pharmacy and is confused about the markings on her daughter's dosage spoon. The prescription drug label states that she is to give ¾ of a teaspoon to her daughter.

9. On the handout that you obtained from your instructor, indicate the amount of medication that the mother should administer to her child.

Sampling the Certification Exam

To provide you with practice for the Certification Exam, read the following questions that have been patterned after the test format and then record your answers on a separate sheet of paper. Write your answers as modeled in these examples: 1d; 2c; 3b; *etc.*

1. How many tablets should be dispensed for a furosemide 40 mg prescription with a quantity of XXI?
   a. 12
   b. 21
   c. 35
   d. 51

2. Which of the following has an underlined digit in the tenths place?
   a. 41<u>2</u>.678
   b. 41<u>2</u>.678
   c. 412.<u>6</u>78
   d. 412.6<u>7</u>8

3. Which of the following decimal values represents the fraction ⅕?
   a. 0.05
   b. 0.15
   c. 0.2
   d. 1.5

4. Sterile water is purchased in containers of 1000 mL. How many 125 mL containers could be poured out of the large container?
   a. 5
   b. 8
   c. 10
   d. 12

5. If a 100-count bottle of alprazolam 1 mg costs the pharmacy $23.87, how much would 75 tablets cost the pharmacy?
   a. $12.56
   b. $17.90
   c. $21.45
   d. $27.91

To put your pharmacy calculation skills to the test, read the following questions and then record your answers on a separate sheet of paper.

Circle the fraction with the highest value.

1. $\dfrac{4}{8}$ $\dfrac{3}{8}$ $\dfrac{2}{8}$

2. $\dfrac{1}{100}$ $\dfrac{1}{400}$ $\dfrac{1}{500}$

Express the following fractions in decimal form. Round to the nearest thousandths place or zero.

3. $\dfrac{1}{5}$

4. $\dfrac{7}{8}$

Give the equivalent Arabic number for each of the following Roman numerals.

5. XXXIX

6. CCXVI

Give the equivalent Roman numeral for each of the following Arabic numbers.

7. 1200

8. 473

Write the following numbers without using scientific notation.

9. 9.1×10^8

10. 7.2×10^2

11. 2.538×10^{-5}

12. 2.01×10^{-4}

Write the following numbers using scientific notation.

13. 375,940,000,000

14. 0.000000109

15. 1,800,000

16. 920

In each group of numbers, circle the highest value.

17. 0.31   0.61   0.91

18. 0.33   0.3   0.31

State the place value of the underlined digit.

19. 1.3̲6

20. 56.7̲8̲

21. 0.231̲

22. 1̲4.02

Write the following decimals.

23. one thousand ninety and six tenths

24. twelve and nine thousand six hundred and forty-seven millionths

Add the following decimals.

25. $12.2 + 19.7 + 16.57 =$

26. $3.89 + 0.257 + 9.023 =$

Multiply the following decimals.

27. $6.08 \times 3.24 =$

28. $10.728 \times 4.23 =$

Calculate the following, retaining the correct number of decimal places.

29. $15.432 \times 3 =$

30. $208 \times 62.1 =$

Round the following to the nearest tenths place.

31. 6.52

32. 83.97

Round the following to the nearest thousandths place.

33. 643.7308

34. 4.2619

Multiply the following and round to the appropriate place.

35. $8.23 \times 0.23 =$

36. $0.8015 \times 0.9921 =$

Calculate the following test scores to the nearest tenth of a percent.

37. 34 of 38 questions correct

38. 51 of 60 questions correct

Convert the following standard times to 24-hour times:

39. 10:30 a.m.

40. 7:50 p.m.

41. 12:25 a.m.

42. A prescription is to be filled for a patient who needs to take 11 mL of medication two times daily. She needs a 7-day supply. You have amber ovals (bottles) in three sizes: 120 mL, 240 mL, and 360 mL. Estimate the total volume needed and choose the appropriate container size.

43. The following list indicates the value of various drugs that were destroyed: $41.71, $11.50, $8.93, $10.50, $3.29, $14.34, $68.20. Estimate the total dollar amount to the nearest tens place ($10), to be documented for the loss.

44. Dr. Daniel Reyes has written a prescription for a patient to take a preoperative suppository at 1800 on the evening before his scheduled surgery. Using the standard time system, what time should you tell the patient to take his medication?

45. The outpatient pharmacy receives daily deliveries for hospital medications that are "stat" orders. They are delivered each day between 7:00 a.m. and 8:30 a.m. How would you express this time range in 24-hour time?

Using Ratios, Percents, and Proportions

2

Learning Objectives

- Describe the use of ratios and proportions in the pharmacy.
- Solve pharmacy calculations by using ratios and proportions.

- Calculate percentage of error in measurements.

For a key to the body system icons that appear in each chapter of this textbook, refer to the Preface.

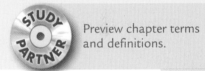

Preview chapter terms and definitions.

2.1 Numerical Ratios

A **ratio** is a numerical representation of the relationship between two parts of a whole or of the relationship of one part to the whole. Ratios are written with a colon (:) between the numbers, which may be read as *per*, *of*, *to*, or *in*. The ratio 1:2 could mean that the second part has twice the value (e.g., size, number, weight, volume) of the first part, or it could mean that one part is something within a total of two parts. Ratios may also be written as fractions, and it is the ratio in fraction form that is most useful to the pharmacy technician.

Math Morsels

The ratio written in the form of a fraction is most useful in pharmacy calculations.

1:2	is read as	1 part to 2 parts	and may also be written as $\frac{1}{2}$
3:4	is read as	3 parts to 4 parts	and may also be written as $\frac{3}{4}$
1:20	is read as	1 part to 20 parts	and may also be written as $\frac{1}{20}$
1:10	is read as	1 part to 10 parts	and may also be written as $\frac{1}{10}$

In the above ratios, any unit of description may be substituted for the word *part* or *parts*. For example, you say there are 250 mg per tablet. Other common unit labels include capsule, bottle, gram, milligram, microgram, and liter.

A ratio can be any numerical relation you wish it to be. With medications, you commonly use a ratio to express the weight or strength of a drug per dose or

FIGURE 2.1   Ratios on an Ampule Label

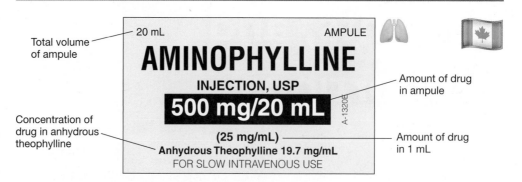

Total volume
of ampule

20 mL   AMPULE

AMINOPHYLLINE
INJECTION, USP
500 mg/20 mL

A-1320E

Amount of drug
in ampule

Concentration of
drug in anhydrous
theophylline

(25 mg/mL)
Anhydrous Theophylline 19.7 mg/mL
FOR SLOW INTRAVENOUS USE

Amount of drug
in 1 mL

volumetric measurement. Ratios are commonly used to express concentrations of a drug in solution. For example, a 1:100 concentration of a drug means that there is 1 part of the drug in 100 parts of the solution (1 g per 100 mL). It is also common to reverse the order of the values written in a ratio.

250 mg:1 tablet	or	1 tablet:250 mg
1 g:100 mL	or	100 mL:1 g
500 mg:20 mL	or	20 mL:500 mg

The ratio may be manipulated by multiplying or dividing both parts of the ratio by the same factor. This application is used when calculating the volume of a medication to be given or, in some cases, the amount of drug per volume of drug given. See the drug label above when reviewing the following examples.

Some drug labels, especially those of injectable drugs, have more than one ratio listed. For example, the aminophylline label shown in Figure 2.1 includes three ratios, each descriptive of the drug's concentration. The first ratio, 500 mg/20 mL, represents the total amount of drug in the ampule. The second ratio, 25 mg/mL, represents the amount of drug in 1 mL. The third ratio, 19.7 mg/mL, describes the concentration of drug in its anhydrous-theophylline state. The pharmacist may use this concentration to further analyze the dosage. The ratio indicating the total amount of drug in the ampule is of the most importance to the pharmacy technician. Typically, this ratio is the most prominent one on the label, as is the case for this label.

Medication labels indicate the ratio of the active ingredient and, as mentioned earlier, the ratio may be manipulated by multiplying or dividing both parts of the ratio by the same factor. If the dose needs to be increased, you multiply the ratio by a factor. If the dose needs to be decreased, you divide the ratio by a factor.

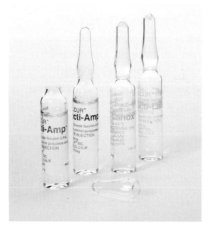

Ampules are small, single-dose containers of medication that are opened at the time of use.

Example 2.1.1

How much aminophylline was ordered if two ampules were administered and each ampule contained 500 mg/20 mL?

For two ampules, you multiply both parts of the ratio by 2.

$$\frac{500 \text{ mg} \times 2}{20 \text{ mL} \times 2} = \frac{1000 \text{ mg}}{40 \text{ mL}}$$

So, 1000 mg were given.

Example 2.1.2

How much aminophylline was ordered if half an ampule was administered and each ampule contained 500 mg/20 mL?

For half of an ampule, you divide both parts of the ratio by 2.

$$\frac{500 \text{ mg} \div 2}{20 \text{ mL} \div 2} = \frac{250 \text{ mg}}{10 \text{ mL}}$$

So, 250 mg were given.

Example 2.1.3

The physician has ordered that a patient take ½ of a levothyroxine tablet that is 137 mcg. How many micrograms is this?

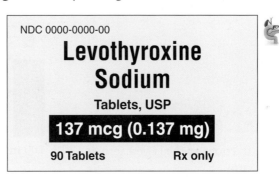

NDC 0000-0000-00

Levothyroxine Sodium

Tablets, USP

137 mcg (0.137 mg)

90 Tablets   **Rx only**

$$\frac{1 \text{ tablet}}{2} = \tfrac{1}{2} \text{ tablet}$$

$$\frac{137 \text{ mcg}}{2} = 68.5 \text{ mcg}$$

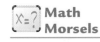

Math Morsels

When the dose is written as a typical ratio (1:1000), the amount of drug is very small.

Some medications are ordered in concentrations that are expressed in a ratio. Typically, these medications are available in a very small percentage (less than 1%). The dose form (such as a cream, solution, or liquid mixture) will influence the ratio. The following examples use a 1:10,000 ratio.

1 g active ingredient:10,000 g product for a solid such as a cream
1 g active ingredient:10,000 mL solution for a solution
1 mL active ingredient:10,000 mL mixture for a liquid

A 1:100 solution has 1 g active ingredient in 100 mL. How much active ingredient is present in 300 mL of this solution?

Set up a ratio and solve for x. In this problem, x equals the active ingredient.

$$\frac{x \text{ g}}{300 \text{ mL}} = \frac{1 \text{ g}}{100 \text{ mL}}$$

$$\frac{(\cancel{300 \text{ mL}}) \, x \text{ g}}{\cancel{300 \text{ mL}}} = \frac{(\cancel{300 \text{ mL}}) \, 1 \text{ g}}{100 \cancel{\text{ mL}}}$$

$$x \text{ g} = 3 \text{ g}$$

Therefore, there are 3 g of active ingredient in 300 mL of this solution.

2.1 Problem Set

Express the following ratios as fractions and reduce to the lowest terms.

1. 3:7

2. 8:6

3. 3:4

4. 4:6

5. 1:7

Reduce the following fractions to the lowest terms and express each as a ratio.

6. $\dfrac{2}{3}$

7. $\dfrac{6}{8}$

8. $\dfrac{5}{10}$

9. $\dfrac{1}{9}$

10. $\dfrac{1}{10,000}$

Applications

State the ratio for the following doses.

11. 30 mg capsule Cymbalta

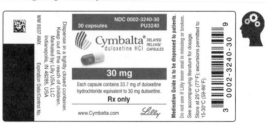

12. 100 mg capsule Dilantin

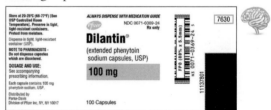

13. 5 mL dose of oral suspension containing 250 mg amoxicillin

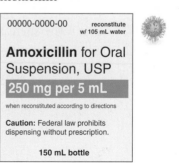

Use the ratios calculated in the preceding problems to calculate how much drug is in the following doses. Write your answer as a ratio and then write a sentence explaining how you calculated each answer.

14. 3 capsules of Cymbalta

15. 2 capsules of Dilantin

16. 15 mL of amoxicillin suspension, 250 mg in 5 mL

Fill in the blanks.

17. A 10:1000 solution contains _____ g of active ingredient in _____ mL of product, and 100 mL of that solution contains _____ g.

18. A 1:100 solution contains _____ g of active ingredient in _____ mL of product, and 500 mL of that solution contains _____ g.

19. A 1:250 solution contains _____ g of active ingredient in _____ mL of product, and 1000 mL of that solution contains _____ g.

20. A 1:1000 solution contains _____ g of active ingredient in _____ mL of product, and 50 mL of that solution contains _____ g. As indicated on the label below, this can be reduced to 1 mg/1 mL.

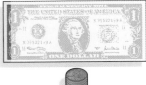

NDC 0517-1071-25
EPINEPHRINE
INJECTION, USP
1:1000 (1 mg/mL)

1 mL AMPULE
FOR SC AND IM USE. FOR IV
AND IC USE AFTER DILUTION.
Rx Only
CONTAINS NO SULFITES.
PRESERVATIVE FREE.
Store below 23°C (73°F). Do not freeze.
AMERICAN REGENT, INC.
SHIRLEY, NY 11967   Rev. 5/05

Self-check your work in Appendix A.

2.2 Percents

Put Down Roots

The word *percent* comes from the Latin term *per centum*, meaning "by the hundred." Therefore, *percent* literally means "per 100."

Percent expresses the number of parts compared with a total of 100 parts. The word *percent* means "per 100" or "hundredths" and is the same as a fraction in which the denominator is 100. Percent is represented by the symbol %. Percents can be visualized by comparing a stack of 100 pennies (equivalent to $1) next to smaller stacks of pennies (see Figure 2.2). A stack of 5 pennies equals 5 cents and represents 5% of a dollar. Similarly, a stack of 40 pennies equals 40 cents and represents 40% of a dollar.

A percent can be written as a ratio, a fraction, or a decimal. For example, 30% means there are 30 parts in a total of 100 parts.

$$30:100, \quad \frac{30}{100}, \quad \text{or } 0.30$$

FIGURE 2.2   **Comparison of Percents**

100% of a dollar   40% of a dollar   5% of a dollar

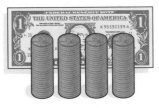 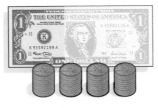

100 pennies   40 pennies   5 pennies

If a test has 100 questions and you receive a score of 89%, you got 89 of the 100 questions correct.

$$89{:}100, \quad \frac{89}{100}, \text{ or } 0.89$$

Percent strengths are often used to describe intravenous (IV) solutions and topically applied drugs. The higher the percentage of dissolved substances (in a solute or a topical drug), the greater the strength. Both of the following examples may be expressed as 1:100, $\frac{1}{100}$, or 0.01.

A 1% solution contains 1 g of drug per 100 mL of fluid.

A 1% hydrocortisone cream contains 1 g of hydrocortisone per 100 g of cream.

By multiplying the first number in the ratio (the solute) while keeping the second number unchanged, you can increase the strength. Conversely, by dividing the first number in the ratio while keeping the second number unchanged, you can decrease the strength.

Example 2.2.1

A 5% solution contains 5 g of solute per 100 mL of solution. If the patient is to receive a 10% solution, how many grams of solute will the solution have to contain?

$$\frac{5 \text{ g} \times 2}{100 \text{ mL}} = \frac{10 \text{ g}}{100 \text{ mL}} = 10\% \text{ solution}$$

Thus, a 10% solution contains 10 g of solute per 100 mL of solution.

Example 2.2.2

A 2% solution contains 2 g of solute per 100 mL of solution. If the patient is to receive a 1% solution, how many grams of solute will the solution have to contain?

$$\frac{2 \text{ g} \div 2}{100 \text{ mL}} = \frac{1 \text{ g}}{100 \text{ mL}} = 1\% \text{ solution}$$

Thus, a 1% solution contains 1 g of solute per 100 mL of solution.

Example 2.2.3

Convert the percent Xylocaine to a ratio and then convert the grams to milligrams.

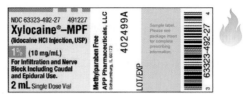

A 1% solution of Xylocaine contains 1 g of Xylocaine in 100 mL solution. This could also be written as 1000 mg solute per 100 mL solution (1 g is equivalent to 1000 mg). Equivalent to this ratio is the strength indicated on the label above (10 mg/mL). The label uses both percentage and milligrams per milliliter expressions to describe the concentration of the drug.

$$1\% = \frac{1 \text{ g}}{100 \text{ mL}} = \frac{1000 \text{ mg}}{100 \text{ mL}} = \frac{10 \text{ mg}}{1 \text{ mL}}$$

When working in the pharmacy, the technician will need to know how to convert between ratios, percents, and decimals. The values in each row of Table 2.1 are equivalent. They are simply expressed in different ways.

TABLE 2.1   Equivalent Values

Percent	Fraction	Decimal	Ratio
45%	$\frac{45}{100}$	0.45	45:100
0.5%	$\frac{0.5}{100}$	0.005	0.5:100

Converting a Ratio to a Percent

To express a ratio as a percent, designate the first number of the ratio as the numerator and the second number as the denominator. Multiply the fraction by 100 and add a percent sign after the number.

$$5:1 = \frac{5}{1} \times 100 = \frac{500}{1} = 500\%$$

$$1:5 = \frac{1}{5} \times 100 = \frac{100}{5} = 20\%$$

$$1:2 = \frac{1}{2} \times 100 = \frac{100}{2} = 50\%$$

Example 2.2.4

A 1:1000 solution has been ordered. You have a 1% solution, a 0.5% solution, and a 0.1% solution in stock. Will one of these work to fill the order?

$$1{:}1000 = \frac{1}{1000} \times 100 = \frac{100}{1000} = 0.1\%$$

The 0.1% solution is the same concentration as the ordered 1:1000 solution.

Converting a Percent to a Ratio

To convert a percent to a ratio, first change it to a fraction by dividing it by 100 and then reduce the fraction to its lowest terms. Express this as a ratio by making the numerator the first number of the ratio and the denominator the second number.

$$2\% = 2 \div 100 = \frac{2}{100} = \frac{1}{50} = 1{:}50$$

$$10\% = 10 \div 100 = \frac{10}{100} = \frac{1}{10} = 1{:}10$$

$$75\% = 75 \div 100 = \frac{75}{100} = \frac{3}{4} = 3{:}4$$

$$\frac{1}{2}\% = \frac{1}{2} \div 100 = \frac{\frac{1}{2}}{100} = \frac{1}{2} \times \frac{1}{100} = \frac{1}{200} = 1{:}200$$

Example 2.2.5

A 0.02% solution has been ordered. You have a 1:1000 solution, a 1:5000 solution, and a 1:10,000 solution in stock. Will one of these work to fill the order?

$$0.02\% = \frac{0.02}{100} = 0.02{:}100$$

Simplify the ratio by dividing both sides of the ratio by 0.02.

$$0.02 \div 0.02 = 1$$
$$100 \div 0.02 = 5000$$

The percent 0.02% is represented by the ratio 1:5000. The supply of 1:5000 solution may be used to fill this order.

A solution commonly used for cleaning in healthcare facilities is a 1:10 solution of bleach and water. This solution is available commercially or may be made fresh daily using regular bleach. Figure 2.3 shows the recipe for making a 1:10 bleach solution. In the recipe, one part bleach is mixed with nine parts of water. The amounts can be adjusted, but the ratio should not change. Because it chemically degrades, a bleach solution prepared according to this recipe is good for only one day.

FIGURE 2.3   10% Bleach Solution

> **1:10 Bleach Solution**
>
> **Materials:** *Storage container, measuring cup or graduated cylinder, bleach, water, label*
>
> **Instructions:** *Measure one quantity of bleach (such as 1 cup) and place it into the storage container. Measure the same quantity of water nine times (9 cups) and place it into the storage container. Mix well, label, and date the container.*

Example 2.2.6

You have been asked to prepare a 480 mL (1 pint) of 1:10 bleach solution. How much bleach and water will you need to measure out?

Determine the size of a "part" by dividing 10 parts into the total volume.

$$\text{total volume} \div \text{number of parts} = \text{volume per one part}$$

$$480 \text{ mL} \div 10 \text{ parts} = \frac{48 \text{ mL}}{1 \text{ part}}$$

You know from the recipe for a 10% bleach solution that the bleach volume is equal to one part, or 48 mL. Determine the amount of water needed by subtracting the known amount of bleach from the total volume.

$$\text{total volume} - \text{bleach volume} = \text{water volume}$$
$$480 \text{ mL} - 48 \text{ mL} = 432 \text{ mL}$$

The following ratio and fractions show the relationship of the 1:10 solution.

$$1:10 = \frac{1 \text{ part bleach}}{10 \text{ parts water and bleach solution}} = \frac{48 \text{ mL bleach}}{480 \text{ mL water and bleach solution}}$$

---

x=? Math Morsels

When converting a percent to a decimal, always remember to insert zeros—including a leading zero—if necessary.

Converting a Percent to a Decimal

To convert a percent to a decimal, drop the percent symbol and divide the number by 100. Dividing a number by 100 is equivalent to moving the decimal point two places to the left and inserting zeros if necessary.

$$4\% = 4 \div 100 = 0.04$$
$$15\% = 15 \div 100 = 0.15$$
$$200\% = 200 \div 100 = 2.0$$

Math Morsels

Converting a decimal to a percent means the decimal point will need to move two places to the right.

Converting a Decimal to a Percent

To change a decimal to a percent, multiply by 100 or move the decimal point two places to the right and add a percent symbol.

$$0.25 = 0.25 \times 100 = 25\%$$
$$1.35 = 1.35 \times 100 = 135\%$$
$$0.015 = 0.015 \times 100 = 1.5\%$$

2.2 Problem Set

Express the following fractions as percents.

1. $\dfrac{6}{7}$

2. $\dfrac{5}{12}$

3. $\dfrac{1}{4}$

4. $\dfrac{2}{3}$

5. $\dfrac{0.5}{10}$

Express the following ratios as percents.

6. 2:3

7. 1.5:4.65

8. 1:250

9. 1:10,000

10. 1:6

Convert the following percents to fractions; then reduce to lowest terms.

11. 50%   12. 2%

Convert the following percents to decimals.

13. 6%   15. 126%

14. 12.5%

Calculate the following, rounding off to the nearest hundredth when necessary.

16. 5% of 20   19. 110% of 70

17. 20% of 60   20. 0.2% of 50

18. 19% of 63

Fill in the missing values.

	Percent	Fraction	Ratio	Decimal
21.	33%	$\dfrac{1}{3}$	_____	_____
22.	2.5%	_____	1:40	_____
23.	_____	$\dfrac{1}{2}$	_____	0.5
24.	_____	_____	1:100	0.01
25.	90%	_____	_____	0.90
26.	67%	_____	_____	0.67
27.	_____	$\dfrac{1}{500}$	1:500	_____
28.	0.45%	_____	_____	0.0045
29.	5%	_____	1:20	_____
30.	20%	$\dfrac{1}{5}$	_____	_____

Applications

Choose the appropriate solution from the available stock.

31. A 1:10,000 solution has been ordered. You have a 0.05% solution, a 0.01% solution, and a 1% solution in stock. Which will you choose?

32. A 1:20 solution has been ordered. You have a 5% solution, a 10% solution, and a 20% solution in stock. Which will you choose?

33. A 1:25 solution has been ordered. You have a 0.4% solution, a 0.05% solution, and a 4% solution in stock. Which will you choose?

34. A 1:800 solution has been ordered. You have a 0.01% solution, a 0.125% solution, and a 1.25% solution in stock. Which will you choose?

35. A 1:10 solution has been ordered. You have a 0.09% solution, a 0.01% solution, and a 10% solution in stock. Which will you choose?

Self-check your work in Appendix A.

2.3 Proportions

A **proportion** is an expression of equality between two ratios. A proportion can be visualized by thinking of two triangles that resemble one another in shape but are different sizes. The triangles in Figure 2.4 have equal proportions.

A proportion is notated by an equal sign or a double colon (::) between the ratios. It can also be noted by using fractions.

$$3:4 = 15:20 \qquad \text{or} \qquad 3:4 :: 15:20 \qquad \text{or} \qquad \frac{3}{4} = \frac{15}{20}$$

In a proportion, the first and fourth, or outside, numbers are called the *extremes*. The second and third, or inside, numbers are called the *means*.

$$3:4 \quad = \quad 15:20$$

    means
    extremes

The product of the means must always equal the product of the extremes in a proportion. You can check for the correctness of the proportion by using this formula.

Given a proportion

$$a{:}b = c{:}d$$

the product of means = the product of extremes

or

$$b \times c = a \times d$$

FIGURE 2.4 **Triangles with Equal Proportions**

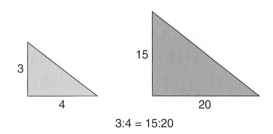

3:4 = 15:20

Example 2.3.1

Confirm that the proportion 3:4 equals the proportion 15:20.

$$3{:}4 = 15{:}20$$
$$4 \times 15 = 3 \times 20$$
$$60 = 60$$

 Put Down Roots

The word *ratio* comes from the Latin term *ratio* meaning "to reason or calculate." The word *proportion* also has its roots in Latin, with the phrase *pro portione* meaning "for or according to the relation of parts." Thus, a ratio-proportion calculation is based on determining the relationship of parts to each other.

The **ratio-proportion method** is one of the most frequently used methods for calculating drug doses in the pharmacy. You can use this method any time one ratio is complete and the other one has a missing component. In other words, if you know three of the four values in a proportion, you can solve for the missing value. When setting up ratios in the proportion, it is important that the numbers remain in the correct ratio and that the numbers have the correct units of measurement in both the numerator and the denominator. Table 2.2 lists the rules for using the ratio-proportion method. Table 2.3 lists the steps for solving for an unknown quantity, typically designated by the letter *x*.

TABLE 2.2   Rules for Using the Ratio-Proportion Method

Rule 1. Three of the four amounts must be known.

Rule 2. The numerators must have the same unit of measurement.

Rule 3. The denominators must have the same unit of measurement.

TABLE 2.3   Steps for Solving for *x* in the Ratio-Proportion Method

Step 1. Create the proportion by placing the ratios in fraction form so that the *x* is in the upper-left corner.

Step 2. Check that the unit of measurement in the numerators is the same and the unit of measurement in the denominators is the same.

Step 3. Solve for *x* by multiplying both sides of the proportion by the denominator of the ratio containing the unknown, and cancel.

Step 4. Check your answer by seeing if the product of the means equals the product of the extremes.

Example 2.3.2

A drug is available as 250 mg/5 mL. How many milliliters represent a dose of 375 mg?

In this case, set the ordered dose ratio equal to the pharmacy stocked drug ratio. In setting up a proportion, the ratios on the two sides of the equal sign may be flipped over as long as *both* ratios are reversed.

$$\text{prescription order ratio} = \text{pharmacy shelf ratio}$$

$$\frac{x\ \text{mL}}{375\ \text{mg}} = \frac{5\ \text{mL}}{250\ \text{mg}}$$

Be sure to check that the unit of measurement in the numerators is the same (both are milliliters) and that the unit of measurement in the denominators is the same (both are milligrams). Multiply both sides by 375 mg to cancel the milligram unit and isolate the unknown.

$$\frac{(\cancel{375\ mg})\ x\ mL}{\cancel{375\ mg}} = \frac{(\cancel{375\ mg})\ 5\ mL}{250\ \cancel{mg}}$$

$$x\ mL = \frac{1875\ mL}{250}$$

Simplify the fraction by dividing 1875 by 250.

$$x\ mL = 7.5\ mL$$

Check that the product of the means equals the product of the extremes.

$$7.5\ mL{:}375\ mg = 5\ mL{:}250\ mg$$
$$375 \times 5 = 7.5 \times 250$$
$$1875 = 1875$$

Example 2.3.3

The label shown below is the stock your pharmacy has available for gentamicin. How many milliliters will need to be prepared if the patient is prescribed 50 mg?

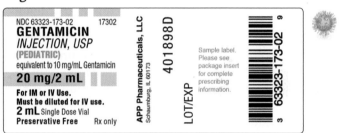

$$\frac{x\ mL}{50\ mg} = \frac{2\ mL}{20\ mg}$$

$$\frac{(\cancel{50\ mg})\ x\ mL}{\cancel{50\ mg}} = \frac{(\cancel{50\ mg})\ 2\ mL}{20\ \cancel{mg}}$$

$$x\ mL = \frac{100\ mL}{20}$$

$$x\ mL = 5\ mL$$

Check that the product of the means equals the product of the extremes.

$$5\ mL{:}50\ mg = 2\ mL{:}20\ mg$$
$$50 \times 2 = 5 \times 20$$
$$100 = 100$$

Example 2.3.4

The label shown below is the stock available at your pharmacy. How many milligrams of diazepam will need to be dispensed to the patient if the prescription is for 4 mL?

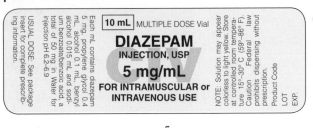

$$\frac{x \text{ mg}}{4 \text{ mL}} = \frac{5 \text{ mg}}{1 \text{ mL}}$$

$$\frac{(4 \text{ mL}) \, x \text{ mg}}{4 \text{ mL}} = \frac{(4 \text{ mL}) \, 5 \text{ mg}}{1 \text{ mL}}$$

$$x \text{ mg} = 20 \text{ mg}$$

Check that the product of the means equals the product of the extremes.

$$20 \text{ mg}{:}4 \text{ mL} = 5 \text{ mg}{:}1 \text{ mL}$$
$$4 \times 5 = 20 \times 1$$
$$20 = 20$$

In addition to being useful for calculating drug doses in the pharmacy, the ratio-proportion method can be used for converting between units of measure. To solve a conversion problem, put the unknown and the specific value that is to be converted on the left side of the proportion. On the right side of the proportion, put the conversion factor. The **conversion factor** is an equivalency equal to 1. For example, since 1 g = 1000 mg, an example of a conversion factor is 1 g/1000 mg or 1000 mg/1 g. Additional conversion factors are presented in Appendix D.

Example 2.3.5

How many milligrams are equivalent to 3 g?

Begin the solution by setting up a ratio and solving for x, using the conversion factor 1000 mg = 1 g.

$$x \text{ mg}{:}3 \text{ g} = 1000 \text{ mg}{:}1 \text{ g}$$

$$\frac{x \text{ mg}}{3 \text{ g}} = \frac{1000 \text{ mg}}{1 \text{ g}}$$

The unit of measurement in the numerators is the same (both are milligrams), and the unit of measurement in the denominators is the same (both are grams). Multiply both sides by 3 g to cancel the grams and isolate the unknown.

For Good Measure

When setting up a proportion to solve a conversion, the units in the numerators must match, and the units in the denominators must match.

$$\frac{(3\cancel{g})\, x\, \text{mg}}{3\cancel{g}} = \frac{(3\cancel{g})\, 1000\, \text{mg}}{1\cancel{g}}$$

$$x\, \text{mg} = \frac{3000\, \text{mg}}{1} = 3000\, \text{mg}$$

$$x\, \text{mg} = 3000\, \text{mg}$$

Check that the product of the means equals the product of the extremes.

$$3000\, \text{mg:3 g} = 1000\, \text{mg:1 g}$$
$$3 \times 1000 = 3000 \times 1$$
$$3000 = 3000$$

Example 2.3.6

Change 44 lb to kilograms. Your conversion chart in Appendix D states that 1 kg = 2.2 lb.

$$\frac{x\, \text{kg}}{44\, \text{lb}} = \frac{1\, \text{kg}}{2.2\, \text{lb}}$$

$$\frac{(44\,\cancel{\text{lb}})\, x\, \text{kg}}{44\,\cancel{\text{lb}}} = \frac{(44\,\cancel{\text{lb}})\, 1\, \text{kg}}{2.2\,\cancel{\text{lb}}}$$

$$x\, \text{kg} = \frac{44\, \text{kg}}{2.2}$$

$$x\, \text{kg} = 20\, \text{kg}$$

Make sure the product of the means equals the product of the extremes.

$$20\, \text{kg:44 lb} = 1\, \text{kg:2.2 lb}$$
$$44 = 44$$

The ratio-proportion method can also be used to solve many types of percentage problems. When setting up the ratios, remember that a percentage may be written in fraction form, with the percent value over 100. For example, 95% is equivalent to $^{95}/_{100}$.

Example 2.3.7

A patient needs to take 75% of a recommended dose before it may be discontinued. The recommended dose is 650 mg. How much must the patient take before it is discontinued?

Write the percentage (75%) as a fraction ($^{75}/_{100}$) and solve for x.

$$\frac{x \text{ mg}}{650 \text{ mg}} = \frac{75 \text{ mg}}{100 \text{ mg}}$$

$$\frac{(650 \text{ mg}) \, x \text{ mg}}{650 \text{ mg}} = \frac{(650 \text{ mg}) \, 75 \text{ mg}}{100 \text{ mg}}$$

$$x \text{ mg} = 487.5 \text{ mg}$$

Example 2.3.8

A patient has taken 85% of a recommended dose. If the amount taken is 320 mg, what was the recommended dose?

Another way of phrasing this question is "320 mg is 85% of what?"

$$\frac{x \text{ mg}}{320 \text{ mg}} = \frac{100 \text{ mg}}{85 \text{ mg}}$$

$$\frac{(320 \text{ mg}) \, x \text{ mg}}{320 \text{ mg}} = \frac{(320 \text{ mg}) \, 100 \text{ mg}}{85 \text{ mg}}$$

$$x \text{ mg} = 376.47 \text{ mg}$$

2.3 Problem Set

Solve for x for each of the following ratios. Round your answers to the nearest hundredth when necessary.

1. $\dfrac{x}{10} = \dfrac{20}{40}$

2. $\dfrac{x}{0.6} = \dfrac{0.8}{6.12}$

3. $\dfrac{x}{9} = \dfrac{5}{10}$

4. $\dfrac{x}{1} = \dfrac{0.5}{5}$

5. $\dfrac{x}{50} = \dfrac{0.4}{125}$

6. $\dfrac{13}{15} = \dfrac{5}{x}$

7. $\dfrac{x}{68} = \dfrac{72}{90}$

8. $\dfrac{14}{3} = \dfrac{x}{52}$

9. $\dfrac{x}{27} = \dfrac{49}{51}$

10. $\dfrac{13}{x} = \dfrac{52}{64}$

11. $\dfrac{14}{23} = \dfrac{27}{x}$

12. $\dfrac{31}{13} = \dfrac{51}{x}$

13. $\dfrac{47}{9} = \dfrac{x}{15}$

14. $\dfrac{9}{26} = \dfrac{x}{31}$

15. $\dfrac{37}{x} = \dfrac{11}{23}$

Set up proportions and solve for x to answer the following questions. Round your answers to the hundredths place.

16. 72 is what percent of 254?

17. 90% of what number is 44?

18. 44% of what number is 100?

19. 28% of what number is 34?

20. 24.5 is what percent of 45?

Change the following weights using the conversion factor 1 g = 1000 mg.

21. 100 mg = _____ g

22. 247 mg = _____ g

23. 1420 mg = _____ g

24. 495 mg = _____ g

25. 3781 mg = _____ g

26. 0.349 g = _____ mg

27. 1.5 g = _____ mg

28. 0.083 g = _____ mg

29. 0.01 g = _____ mg

30. 2.1 g = _____ mg

Change the following weights using the conversion factor 1 kg = 2.2 lb. Round your answer to the tenths place.

31. 6.3 lb = _____ kg

32. 15 lb = _____ kg

33. 97 lb = _____ kg

34. 115 lb = _____ kg

35. 186 lb = _____ kg

36. 7.5 kg = _____ lb

37. 3.6 kg = _____ lb

38. 79.2 kg = _____ lb

39. 90 kg = _____ lb

40. 0.5 kg = _____ lb

Applications

Set up a proportion using x as the unknown and solve the following. Explain in your own words how you set up your proportion.

41. A drug is available as 50 mg/mL. The order calls for 100 mg. How many milliliters will you prepare?

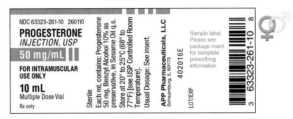

42. Capicillin is available as a 125 mg tablet. How many tablets are needed to give a dose of 375 mg?

43. Soakamycin is available as a concentration of 20 mg/mL. How many milliliters are needed to prepare a foot soak that contains 300 mg?

44. You are going to buy some folders to file your orders. After checking around, you find that the most cost-effective price is $7.40 per box of 100 folders. You have $15 to spend. How many folders can you buy? (The boxes may not be broken.)

47. A dose of 60 mg famotidine is ordered. The drug is available as a 40 mg/4 mL solution. How many milliliters are needed to provide the ordered dose?

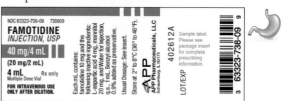

45. The patient is to get an intramuscular injection of 10,000 units of Musclesporin. You have a bottle containing 250,000 units per 15 mL. How many milliliters must be prepared to administer this dose?

48. A dose of 300 mg is ordered. The drug is available as a 500 mg/10 mL solution. How many milliliters are needed to provide the ordered dose?

49. A dose of 30 mg lamivudine oral solution is ordered. The drug is available in a 5 mg/mL oral solution. How many milliliters are needed to provide the ordered dose?

46. A dose of 60 mg gentamicin is ordered. The drug is available as a 20 mg/2 mL solution. How many milliliters are needed to provide the ordered dose?

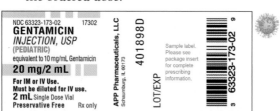

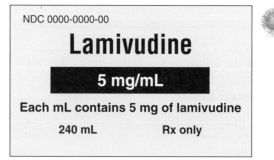

50. A dose of 30 mg is ordered. The drug is available as a 20 mg/mL solution. How many milliliters are needed to provide the ordered dose?

51. The order calls for 5 mL. How many milligrams is this?

52. The order calls for 80 mg. How many milliliters is this?

53. The order calls for 50 mg. How many milliliters is this?

Use the following drug label to determine the dose needed for questions 51–55.

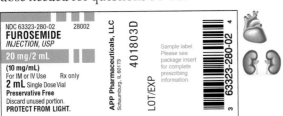

54. The order calls for 12.5 mg. How many milliliters is this?

55. The order calls for 3.5 mL. How many milligrams is this?

Self-check your work in Appendix A.

2.4 Percentage of Error

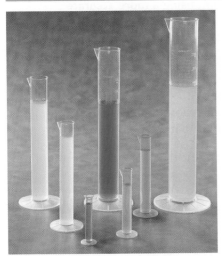

Graduated cylinders are used to accurately measure liquids in the pharmacy.

Percentages are used in a variety of ways when preparing medication doses. In the compounding pharmacy, percentages are used to determine the possible percentage of error and the least weighable quantity of a substance for safe preparation. Percentages are also used when doing the business of the pharmacy, such as calculating the percentage of sales, percentage of discount, and percentage of markup. These applications will be covered in Chapter 9, "Using Business Math in the Pharmacy."

When measuring a liquid or weighing a solid ingredient in the pharmacy, a certain amount of error is expected. Not all graduated cylinders used in the pharmacy are equally accurate, although they are usually much more accurate than the measuring devices found in patients' homes. Graduated cylinders used in pharmacies may be conical or cylindrical, with the cylindrical shape being more accurate. Similarly, pharmacy balances, though generally very accurate when compared with

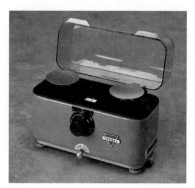

A Class III prescription balance can accurately weigh small quantities.

other small scales, may exhibit slight variations. A Class III prescription balance is a type of balance commonly used to weigh very small quantities in the pharmacy. Regardless of the measuring tool being used, it is important to know the margin of error that a particular balance or graduated cylinder has.

When weighing any substance, the balance will appear to have weighed correctly. A very small sample, however, may have an unacceptable margin of error. Pharmacy balances are generally marked with their degree of accuracy. This degree of accurateness has been determined by comparing quantities weighed on the balance with the weights obtained from another balance whose accuracy is known. This determination of accuracy is performed in the factory and typically is not done in the pharmacy.

If a substance was weighed or measured incorrectly, and you have something that will allow you to more accurately measure the amount in question, then you can determine the **percentage of error** by using the following formula:

$$\frac{\text{amount of error}}{\text{quantity desired}} \times 100 = \text{percentage of error}$$

In this equation, the amount of error is the difference between the actual amount and the quantity desired, or

$$\text{actual amount} - \text{quantity desired} = \text{amount of error}$$

The percentage of error is considered to be a range both above and below the target measurement. It is inconsequential whether the result is over or under the target (i.e., whether it is positive or negative). Percentage of error is always expressed as a positive value.

Example 2.4.1

You are to dispense 120 mL of a liquid. The original measurement is 120 mL. When you double-check the amount, using a more accurate graduated cylinder, the actual amount is 126 mL. What is the percentage of error of the first measurement?

Calculate the difference in the two measurements to determine the amount of error.

$$\text{actual amount} - \text{quantity desired} = \text{amount of error}$$
$$126 \text{ mL} - 120 \text{ mL} = 6 \text{ mL}$$

Use the percentage of error equation to determine the percentage of error of the measurement.

$$\frac{\text{amount of error}}{\text{quantity desired}} \times 100 = \frac{6 \text{ mL}}{120 \text{ mL}} \times 100 = 5\%$$

The percentage of error is 5%.

Example 2.4.2

You are to dispense 30 g of a powder. The original measurement is 30 g. When you double-check the amount, using a more accurate balance, the actual amount is 31.8 g. What is the percentage of error of the first measurement?

Calculate the difference in the two amounts to determine the amount of error.

$$31.8\ g - 30\ g = 1.8\ g$$

Use the percentage of error equation to determine the percentage of error of the measurement.

$$\frac{\text{amount of error}}{\text{quantity desired}} \times 100 = \frac{1.8\ g}{30\ g} \times 100 = 6\%$$

The percentage of error is 6%.

Example 2.4.3

You are to dispense 453 mg of a powder. The original measurement is 453 mg. When you double-check the amount, using a more accurate balance, the actual amount is 438 mg. What is the percentage of error of the first measurement?

Calculate the difference in the two measurements to determine the amount of error.

$$453\ mg - 438\ mg = 15\ mg$$

Use the percentage of error equation to determine the percentage of error of the measurement.

$$\frac{\text{amount of error}}{\text{quantity desired}} \times 100 = \frac{15\ mg}{453\ mg} \times 100 = 3.3\%$$

The percentage of error is 3.3%.

Example 2.4.4

You are to weigh 60 g of a cream base for a topical compound. Your error range is 3%. What will be the least amount and the largest amount acceptable?

Multiply the percentage (in decimal form) by the target weight.

$$60\ g \times 0.03 = 1.8\ g$$

Determine the range.

$$60 \text{ g} - 1.8 \text{ g} = 58.2 \text{ g} \qquad 60 \text{ g} + 1.8 \text{ g} = 61.8 \text{ g}$$

Therefore, the acceptable range is 58.2 g to 61.8 g.

Example 2.4.5

You are preparing an order by measuring 800 mL from a 1 L normal saline IV bag. When you check the volume of the fluid in a graduated cylinder, the amount measured is actually 820 mL. You have an acceptable range of 2%. What is the percentage of error in this measurement? Did you meet your target?

Determine the difference in the two measurements to determine the amount of error.

$$820 \text{ mL} - 800 \text{ mL} = 20 \text{ mL}$$

Use the percentage of error equation to determine the percentage of error of the measurement.

$$\frac{\text{amount of error}}{\text{quantity desired}} \times 100 = \frac{20 \text{ mL}}{800 \text{ mL}} \times 100 = 2.5\%$$

Because 2.5% is larger than the acceptable percentage of error, the target range was not met.

2.4 Problem Set

Calculate the percentage of error for the following measurements; then round to the nearest hundredths place. Assume that the measured amount is equal to the quantity desired.

1. The measured weight was 185 mg, but the actual weight is 189 mg.

2. The measured weight was 500 mg, but the actual weight is 476 mg.

3. The measured weight was 1200 mg, but the actual weight is 1507 mg.

4. The measured weight was 15 mg, but the actual weight is 12.5 mg.

5. The measured weight was 400 mcg, but the actual weight is 415 mcg.

6. The measured volume was 5 mL, but the actual volume is 6.3 mL.

7. The measured volume was 15 mL, but the actual volume is 13 mL.

8. The measured volume was 15 mL, but the actual volume is 20 mL.

9. The measured volume was 1.5 L, but the actual volume is 1.45 L.

10. The measured volume was 700 mL, but the actual volume is 726 mL.

Determine the percentage of error for the following measurements, and identify those within a percentage of error of 3%.

11. The measured volume was 3 mL, but the actual volume is 2.6 mL.

12. The measured volume was 12.5 mL, but the actual volume is 12.1 mL.

13. The measured volume was 1.8 mL, but the actual volume is 1.5 mL.

14. The measured volume was 3.2 mL, but the actual volume is 3.29 mL.

Determine the percentage of error for the following measurements, and identify those within a percentage of error of 6%.

15. The measured weight was 150 mg, but the actual weight is 149 mg.

16. The measured weight was 200 mg, but the actual weight is 192 mg.

17. The measured weight was 30 mg, but the actual weight is 31.5 mg.

18. The measured weight was 454 mg, but the actual weight is 450 mg.

State the acceptable range of error for each of the following. Round to the nearest hundredths place.

19. The desired volume is 200 mL, and the percentage of error is 0.5%.

20. The desired volume is 10.3 mL, and the percentage of error is 0.75%.

21. The desired volume is 830 mL, and the percentage of error is 2%.

22. The desired weight is 18 g, and the percentage of error is 0.15%.

23. The desired weight is 750 mg, and the percentage of error is 0.4%.

Applications

24. If a generic drug manufacturer meets a bioavailability comparison to within 20% and a drug normally has a bioavailability of 100 mg, what is the range of accuracy?

25. A new brand of vitamins claims to have bioavailability within 12% of a national brand of vitamin C. The national brand has 500 mg of vitamin C per tablet. What is the range of vitamin C contained in the tablet?

Self-check your work in Appendix A.

Chapter Summary

- Ratios are used to describe the amount of medication per dose or unit.
- Ratios may also be written as fractions.
- Ratios may be written in reverse order (1:100 or 100:1) or may be written flipped upside down (1/100 or 100/1).
- Ratios may be multiplied when a larger dose is desired or divided when a smaller dose is desired.
- Percent is the number of parts per 100 parts.
- Ratios, percents, fractions, and decimals may all be used to express the same value.
- When converting a percent to a numerical value, divide by 100, or move the decimal point two places to the left.
- When converting a numerical value to a percent, multiply by 100, or move the decimal point two places to the right.

- Proportions are an expression of equivalency between two ratios (or fractions).
- A proportion with one missing value may be solved if three of the four values are known.
- When using the ratio-proportion method to solve for a missing value, the numerators must have the same unit of measure, and the denominators must have the same unit of measure.
- The ratio-proportion method may be used to convert between units of measure by setting the ratio desired to be converted equal to a unit of "1."
- Percentage of error is calculated by dividing the amount of error by the quantity desired, and multiplying by 100.
- Error range is the amount above or below the target.

Formulas for Success

Pages 51–52	Decimals to Percent	Page 54	Rx Order Ratio = Pharmacy Shelf Ratio
Page 53	Means and Extremes in a Proportion	Page 62	Percentage of Error

Key Terms

conversion factor an equivalency equal to 1 that can be used when converting units of measure using the ratio-proportion method

percent the number of parts per 100; can be written as a fraction, a decimal, or a ratio

percentage of error the percentage by which a measurement is inaccurate

proportion an expression of equality between two ratios

ratio a numerical representation of the relationship between two parts of the whole or between one part and the whole

ratio-proportion method a conversion method based on comparing a complete ratio to a ratio with a missing component

Chapter Review

Assessing Comprehension

To check your comprehension of this chapter's key concepts, read the following multiple-choice questions and then record your answers on a separate sheet of paper. Write your answers as modeled in these examples: 1d; 2c; 3b; *etc.*

1. For a pharmacy technician, the most useful ratio form for setting up a pharmacy calculation is a
   a. ratio (a:b).
   b. fraction (a/b).
   c. decimal with a trailing zero.
   d. percentage.

2. When 2 doses or units of medication are given, you manipulate the ratio strength by
   a. multiplying the numerator by 2.
   b. dividing the numerator by 2.
   c. multiplying both the numerator and denominator by 2.
   d. dividing both the numerator and denominator by 2.

3. By multiplying the first number in a ratio while keeping the second number unchanged, you can
   a. increase the strength of the medication.
   b. decrease the strength of the medication.
   c. convert the ratio to a percentage.
   d. rewrite the ratio strength as a decimal.

4. Percentage of medication means
   a. the amount of medication per 100 doses.
   b. the amount of medication per 100 parts (grams or milliliters).
   c. the amount of medication purchased for $100.
   d. the ratio strength of 100 mg medication.

5. Which of the following has the highest concentration of medication?
   a. 0.05%
   b. 0.5%
   c. 5%
   d. 50%

6. When converting a percentage to a numerical value or a decimal, you should
   a. drop the percent symbol.
   b. drop the percent symbol and move the decimal point two places to the right.
   c. drop the percent symbol and move the decimal point two places to the left.
   d. subtract 100 from the number and insert a zero if needed.

7. The ratio-proportion method is used in pharmacy calculations when
   a. all four values are known.
   b. three of four values are known.
   c. the units of measure are all the same.
   d. the unknown value is in a unit not written on the drug label.

8. You can check the accuracy of your ratio-proportion calculations by
   a. verifying that the product of the means equals the product of the extremes.
   b. subtracting the product of the means from the product of the extremes.
   c. inverting one ratio in the proportion and recalculating.
   d. converting all of the units to one common measure.

9. Percentage of error is calculated to
   a. determine the amount of error that may occur in the measurement or weighing process in the pharmacy.
   b. verify the accuracy of the prescription balance.
   c. verify the accuracy of the dose calculated by the physician.
   d. determine the amount that the patient will be charged for a prescription that is compounded in the pharmacy.

10. The percentage of error is
   a. calculated by dividing the actual amount by the desired amount.
   b. calculated by multiplying the quantity desired by 5%.
   c. always expressed as a positive value.
   d. determined by comparing a weighed amount of drug to a standard brass weight.

Finding Solutions

To gain practice in handling challenging situations in the workplace, consider the following real-world scenarios and then use the guiding questions to help you formulate your responses.

Note: *To indicate your answer for Scenario A, Question 1, ask your instructor for the handout depicting measuring devices.*

Scenario A: A patient with poison ivy has been taking over-the-counter (OTC) Benadryl for itching. The doctor has told her to take 50 mg every six hours. The medication is available in a 12.5 mg/5 mL solution.

1. On the handout that you obtained from your instructor, indicate how many milliliters the patient will need for each dose.

2. If the patient uses three doses per day, how many milliliters will she need to last three days?

3. How many 4 fluid ounce bottles (120 mL) will the patient need to purchase?

Scenario B: A patient has brought her newborn infant into the pharmacy. She said the baby weighs 9½ pounds.

4. What is the infant's weight in kilograms?

Scenario C: You have been asked to reorder and restock a special order lip balm that your pharmacy carries. A carton of 24 tubes costs the pharmacy $21.50. You know that you may not spend more than $100 and that you may not purchase a partial carton.

5. How many cartons can you buy?

6. What will the cost be for this quantity of cartons?

7. How many tubes of lip balm will this provide?

8. How much money will be left over after the cost of the lip balm?

9. The company charges an additional 4% of the cost of the product for shipping. How much is this?

Sampling the Certification Exam

To provide you with practice for the Certification Exam, read the following questions that have been patterned after the test format and then record your answers on a separate sheet of paper. Write your answers as modeled in these examples: 1d; 2c; 3b; etc.

1. A medication label reads 300 mg/5 mL. How many milligrams of medication are in 15 mL?
   a. 150 mg
   b. 450 mg
   c. 500 mg
   d. 900 mg

2. How many grams of medication are in 200 g of a 1% ointment?
   a. 0.2 g
   b. 1 g
   c. 1.2 g
   d. 2 g

3. A solution that is 1:20 is also the concentration:
   a. 1.2%
   b. 2%
   c. 5%
   d. 20%

4. A medication is available in a 250 mg/5 mL concentration. How many milliliters contain 750 mg?
   a. 1.5 mL
   b. 7.5 mL
   c. 10 mL
   d. 15 mL

5. A patient needs to pay 20% of the cost of his medications. If his medications are $12.79 and $81.24, how much will he pay?
   a. $18.81
   b. $37.62
   c. $47.02
   d. $94.03

Chapter Practice Test

Additional Practice Questions

To put your pharmacy calculation skills to the test, read the following questions and then record your answers on a separate sheet of paper.

State the ratio for the following doses.

1. 10 mg tablet of glipizide

2. 5 mL dose of azithromycin containing 250 mg

3. 5 mL dose of diphenhydramine containing 12.5 mg

4. 2 mL ampule containing 500 mg

5. A 1:10 solution contains _____ g of active ingredient and _____ mL of product, and 1000 mL of that solution contains _____ g.

6. A 1:100 solution contains _____ g of active ingredient and _____ mL of product, and 250 mL of that solution contains _____ g.

Convert the following percents to fractions; then reduce to lowest terms.

7. 12.5%

8. 66.67%

Convert the following percents to decimals.

9. 0.5%

10. 93%

Choose the appropriate solution from the available stock.

11. A 1:5 solution has been ordered. You have a 5% solution, a 10% solution, and a 20% solution in stock. Which solution will you choose?

12. A 1:250 solution has been ordered. You have a 0.4% solution, a 0.05% solution, and a 4% solution in stock. Which solution will you choose?

Convert the following using the ratio 1 g:1000 mg.

13. 120 mg = _____ g

14. 1800 mg = _____ g

Use the ratio-proportion method to determine the unknown quantity.

15. A dose of 50 mg is ordered. The drug is available as a 1 mg tablet. How many whole tablets are needed to provide the ordered dose?

16. A dose of 30 mg is ordered. The drug is available as a 20 mg/mL solution. How many milliliters are needed to provide the ordered dose?

Determine the percentage of error for the following measurements. Round to the hundredths place when needed. Assume the measured amount is equal to the quantity desired.

17. The measured weight was 325 mg, but the actual weight is 343 mg.

18. The measured weight was 850 mg, but the actual weight is 790 mg.

19. The measured volume was 480 mL, but the actual volume is 473 mL.

20. The measured volume was 30 mL, but the actual volume is 32 mL.

21. The measured volume was 125 mL, but the actual volume is 119 mL.

    a. What is the actual percentage of error?

    b. Is the percentage of error within the 3% range?

22. The measured volume was 50 mL, but the actual volume is 57 mL.

    a. What is the actual percentage of error?

    b. Is the percentage of error within the 3% range?

State the acceptable range of error for the following situations. Round to the nearest hundredths place.

23. The desired volume is 467 mL, and the percentage of error is 1%.

24. The desired weight is 30 g, and the percentage of error is 0.25%.

Developing Literacy Skills

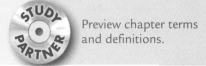

3

Learning Objectives

- Identify the elements of a complete prescription order.
- Apply calculation operations in handling prescription orders.
- Recognize the elements of a medication label.
- Apply calculation operations to information on medication labels.

Preview chapter terms and definitions.

3.1 Elements of a Prescription Order

Put Down Roots

The word *prescription* is derived from the Latin word *praescriptio* meaning "order, direction, a writing before." Therefore, a prescription is an order for a medication that is written before the medication is given or dispensed to the patient.

A **prescription** is an order for a medication or mixture of medications written (or otherwise recorded and/or transmitted) by a practitioner to be filled by a pharmacist. Prescriptions may be received in the pharmacy by several means: a handwritten order, a digital or computerized order, or a phone order. The pharmacy technician will need to interpret the prescription to determine which calculations will be necessary to fill this order correctly and appropriately. Although the legal requirements for information necessary on a prescription are regulated by state law and vary from one state to another, the following elements will appear on every prescription: patient information, prescriber information, and drug designation. Figure 3.1 illustrates the parts of a prescription written for a community pharmacy, and Figure 3.2 illustrates the parts of a medication order written for a hospital pharmacy. (These figures are shown on the following pages.)

Patient Information

Every prescription order must have enough information to uniquely identify the patient. In addition to the patient's full name (first and last), most states also require outpatient prescriptions to include the patient's address (street, city, state). It is also good practice to include the patient's age or date of birth on every prescription, and some states and most insurers require this information.

Prescriptions for inpatients, often referred to as "orders," usually substitute the patient's hospital identification number and room number for the address and are typically written on a form prestamped with the patient's admission date, the admitting physician's name, and the patient's date of birth in addition to the patient's

FIGURE 3.1   Elements of a Prescription for a Community Pharmacy

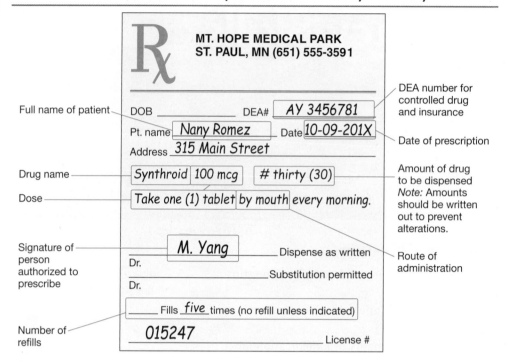

Full name of patient

Drug name

Dose

Signature of person authorized to prescribe

Number of refills

DEA number for controlled drug and insurance

Date of prescription

Amount of drug to be dispensed
Note: Amounts should be written out to prevent alterations.

Route of administration

MT. HOPE MEDICAL PARK
ST. PAUL, MN (651) 555-3591

DOB _____ DEA# *AY 3456781*
Pt. name *Nany Romez*   Date *10-09-201X*
Address *315 Main Street*

Synthroid *100 mcg*   *# thirty (30)*
Take one (1) tablet *by mouth* *every morning.*

M. Yang   Dispense as written
Dr. _____
_____   Substitution permitted
Dr. _____

_____ Fills *five* times (no refill unless indicated)
015247
_____ License #

name and hospital number. Hospital medication order forms frequently require a notation of the patient's allergy information as well.

Many pharmacies require that the patient's height and weight be available, either on the prescription itself or in the patient's file. (Hospital order forms, as well as outpatient prescription forms, frequently have blanks where the height and weight are to be written.) If height and weight are included, it is important to know the units in which they were determined. Patient weights may be measured in either kilograms (kg) or pounds (# or lb); heights are generally measured in centimeters (cm) or inches (sometimes abbreviated as ″ or in.). These measurements are quite different from one another: A 100 kg patient is more than twice the size of a 100 lb patient; a 76 cm patient is most likely a child under three years of age, whereas a 76″ patient is a very tall adult! (Conversions of height and weight units are covered in Chapters 4 and 5.)

Safety in Numbers

The appropriate unit should always be indicated with each number.

Prescriber Information

In most states, outpatient prescription orders must include the name, authority (medical doctor, doctor of osteopathy, etc.), and address of the prescribing practitioner. Frequently, the prescriber's telephone number is noted. Prescriptions for controlled substances must also bear a registration code known as a **DEA number**. DEA numbers are issued by the Drug Enforcement Administration (DEA), an agency of the federal government, and signify the authority of the holder to prescribe or handle controlled substances. They are *always* formatted to begin with two letters, which are followed by seven digits. The last of the seven digits is a "checksum" digit, calculated by following the steps in Table 3.1.

The first two letters of the DEA number provide information about the prescriber. The first letter usually (but not always) designates the level of authority of the holder. For example, A, B, and F are used for primary-level practitioners such as physicians and dentists, and M is used to indicate mid-level practitioners such as nurse midwives and

FIGURE 3.2   Elements of a Hospital Medication Order

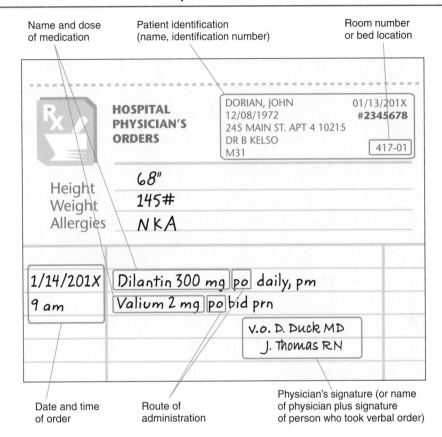

Name and dose of medication — Patient identification (name, identification number) — Room number or bed location — Date and time of order — Route of administration — Physician's signature (or name of physician plus signature of person who took verbal order)

Safety in Numbers

The checksum digit calculation is a necessary but not sufficient condition for the validity of a DEA number.

advanced practice nurses. The second letter in the DEA number is the first letter of the prescriber's last name. So, the first two letters of the DEA number for Dr. Mary Smith might be AS or BS, whereas the first two letters for nurse practitioner David Jones might be MJ.

DEA numbers are carefully regulated, and a DEA number that does not have a correct checksum digit (as determined by the steps in Table 3.1) is considered to be invalid. The checksum digit gives pharmacists and pharmacy technicians one way to check whether a DEA number was falsified. Note that passing the checksum test does not necessarily mean that a DEA number is valid. Many unethical or criminally minded people know the formula and are able to compose DEA numbers that *look* valid but were not issued by the government authority. If a pharmacy technician discovers an invalid DEA number or suspects a problem with the authenticity of a prescription, he or she should notify a pharmacist immediately.

The following examples demonstrate how the steps in Table 3.1 can be used to check for false DEA numbers.

TABLE 3.1   DEA Checksum Formula

Step 1. Add the first, third, and fifth digits of the DEA number.

Step 2. Add the second, fourth, and sixth digits of the DEA number.

Step 3. Double the sum obtained in Step 2 (i.e., multiply it by 2).

Step 4. Add the results of Steps 1 and 3. The last digit of this sum should match the checksum digit, the last digit of the DEA number.

Example 3.1.1

A patient brings a prescription for methylphenidate tablets to the pharmacy, signed by Dr. Johnson and bearing a DEA number of BJ 2345678. Is this DEA number valid?

Begin by reviewing the letters of the DEA number. The first letter is consistent with the prescriber's level of authority (A or B for a primary practitioner), and the second letter matches the last name of the physician (J).

Now, check the validity of the checksum digit.

Step 1. Add the first, third, and fifth digits of the DEA number.

$$2 + 4 + 6 = 12$$

Step 2. Add the second, fourth, and sixth digits of the DEA number.

$$3 + 5 + 7 = 15$$

Step 3. Multiply the sum obtained in Step 2 by 2.

$$15 \times 2 = 30$$

Step 4. Add the results of Steps 1 and 3. The last digit of this sum should match the checksum digit, the last digit of the DEA number.

$$12 + 30 = 42$$

Because the checksum digit is 8, not 2, this DEA number is invalid.

Example 3.1.2

A patient brings a prescription for oxycodone to the pharmacy, signed by nurse-midwife Ann Johnson and bearing a DEA number of MJ 3456781. (In the state where the prescription is received, advanced practice nurses are authorized to prescribe narcotic analgesics.) Is this DEA number valid?

Begin by reviewing the letters of the DEA number. The first letter is consistent with the prescriber's level of authority (M for a nurse practitioner), and the second letter matches the last name of the prescriber (J).

Now, check the validity of the checksum digit.

Step 1. Add the first, third, and fifth digits of the DEA number.

$$3 + 5 + 7 = 15$$

Step 2. Add the second, fourth, and sixth digits of the DEA number.

$$4 + 6 + 8 = 18$$

Step 3. Multiply the sum obtained in Step 2 by 2.

$$18 \times 2 = 36$$

Step 4. Add the results of Steps 1 and 3. The last digit of this sum should match the checksum digit, the last digit of the DEA number.

$$15 + 36 = 51$$

Because the checksum digit is 1, this DEA number meets the criteria for a valid registration.

Inpatient prescriptions are most often written or transcribed on the premises where the patient is located and where the medication will be administered; such prescriptions may be ordered only by practitioners with privileges within that institution. Physician addresses and DEA numbers are generally not required on the actual medication orders because the institutional pharmacy that will fill the orders usually has this information on file for each authorized practitioner.

Put Down Roots

The word *nomenclature*—a term used in pharmacy to indicate naming guidelines for medications—has its beginnings in the Roman Empire. The word means the "calling or assigning of names" and comes from the Latin roots *nomen* meaning "name" and *calare* meaning "to call out."

Drug Designation

A prescription order must always designate the medication that is intended for the patient. Medications may have three names: a chemical name, a generic name, and a brand name. These naming guidelines are referred to as *nomenclature*. Sometimes, the drug will be identified by its **generic name**, the name by which it was approved by the Food and Drug Administration (FDA) as a unique chemical product safe and effective for use in its approved indication. The generic name of a drug is the same, regardless of the company that manufactures it or the dosage form or packaging in which it is supplied. At other times, a physician will specify a brand name drug. The **brand name** is a registered trademark of the manufacturer and may indicate the dose form or packaging of the drug as well. State law and (in the case of inpatients) institutional policy govern the extent to which generic products can be substituted for brand name drugs. In some instances, the pharmacy can automatically substitute an equivalent product with the same generic name (but a different brand name) for cost savings or convenience. In other situations, the pharmacy must supply the exact brand prescribed, unless the pharmacist has discussed a substitution with the prescriber.

Figure 3.3 identifies the standard parts of a drug label for Cleocin Phosphate. As shown in this example, the label of a brand name drug will indicate both the trade and generic names. Medications with a given name (brand or generic) are frequently

Name Exchange

Cleocin Phosphate is a brand name for the generic drug clindamycin.

FIGURE 3.3 Parts of a Drug Label

Although medication labels from different manufacturers vary slightly in format, the labels' components remain the same. Pharmacy technicians must be able to identify and interpret all parts of a drug label.

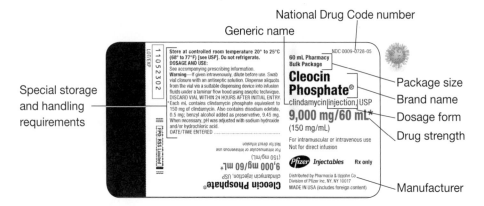

FIGURE 3.4   Comparison of Dosage Forms

(a) 20 mg tablet
(b) 40 mg tablet
(c) 40 mg/4 mL solution

Name Exchange

Furosemide is the generic name for the brand name drug Lasix.

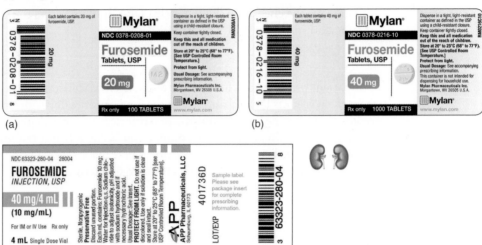

(a)

(b)

(c)

available in a variety of strengths, doses, or dosage forms, and information about the particular strength, dose, and dosage form is also clearly stated on the drug label. Digoxin, for instance, is available as a generic product and as several branded preparations. It is available as a tablet in two different strengths (0.125 mg and 0.25 mg), a capsule in three strengths (0.05 mg, 0.1 mg, and 0.2 mg), an elixir of 0.05 mg/mL, and injections of 0.1 mg/mL and 0.25 mg/mL. Many other drugs present a similar array of choices (brand names, dosage forms, strengths, or concentrations), and the proper product to select must be made clear in the prescription order. Figure 3.4 shows labels for the same drug in different dosage forms. Note how the labels use color to help distinguish the unique information.

It is important to correctly match a prescription order with the appropriate medication available in the pharmacy. The following example demonstrates this procedure.

Example 3.1.3

The pharmacy receives an order for epinephrine 1 mg/mL. Epinephrine 1:10,000, 1:2000, and 1:1000 injections are available in stock. Which one matches the order?

As discussed in Chapter 2, the available drug concentrations are 1:10,000, or 1 g/10,000 mL; 1:2000, or 1 g/2000 mL; and 1:1000, or 1 g/1000 mL.

Convert the strength of 1 mg/mL into a concentration ratio. Begin by setting up a ratio and solving for x, using the conversion factor 1000 mg = 1 g.

$$\frac{x \text{ mL}}{1000 \text{ mg}} = \frac{1 \text{ mL}}{1 \text{ mg}}$$

$$\frac{(1000 \text{ mg}) \, x \text{ mL}}{1000 \text{ mg}} = \frac{(1000 \text{ mg}) \, 1 \text{ mL}}{1 \text{ mg}}$$

$$x \text{ mL} = 1000 \text{ mL}$$

Therefore, x mL/1000 mg = 1000 mL/1000 mg, and 1000 mL/1000 mg = 1000 mL/1 g = 1 g/1000 mL, or a ratio of 1:1000. Thus, the 1:1000 injection should be chosen to fill this order. The label appears below.

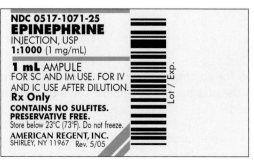

Quantity to Dispense

Every outpatient prescription order must indicate to the pharmacist what quantity to dispense. Sometimes, the indication is straightforward, as in Figure 3.1, where the physician has written the number of tablets to dispense next to "#" (used as a number sign). This number is often written as a Roman numeral or spelled out ("thirty" for #30) to hinder alteration. At other times, the physician will indicate the number of doses the patient is to take, or the number of days the therapy is to last, and the pharmacy staff will calculate the quantity to dispense from the information on the prescription.

When the quantity to dispense has been determined, the pharmacy technician selects the proper dispensing container. Commonly, amber ovals (bottles) are used for liquids and amber vials for tablets or capsules. Amber ovals are often marked with both fluid ounce and milliliter lines. Common practice uses the metric system, so the quantity indicated on the prescription drug label will be indicated in milliliters. When preparing tablets or

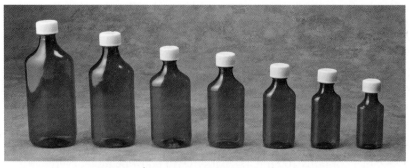

Amber medication bottles come in several sizes. The pharmacy technician will need to select the appropriate size to match the dispensed volume.

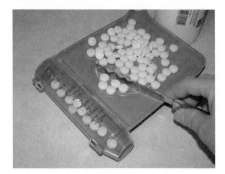

Tablets are frequently counted out by fives on a tray with a spatula and then placed in the dispensing container.

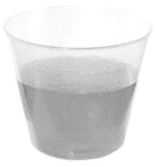

One fluid ounce is the size of most plastic dispensing cups.

capsules to fill a prescription, the tablets or capsules are generally counted out, using a specially designed tray and plastic or metal spatula, and placed in amber vials. Tablets and capsules are typically counted out by "fives."

The following examples show how the quantity to dispense is calculated.

Example 3.1.4

A prescription for an antacid reads "Take one ounce three times a day" and instructs the pharmacy to dispense a five-day supply. What volume is to be dispensed?

The patient takes one ounce three times a day, so first determine the number of ounces taken in one day. Note that the units cancel out, as shown below.

$$\frac{x \text{ oz}}{1 \text{ day}} = \frac{1 \text{ oz}}{1 \text{ dose}} \times \frac{3 \text{ doses}}{1 \text{ day}} = \frac{3 \text{ oz}}{1 \text{ day}}$$

You can determine the amount to dispense by multiplying the daily dose by the number of days.

$$x \text{ oz} = \frac{3 \text{ oz}}{1 \text{ day}} \times 5 \text{ days} = 15 \text{ oz}$$

Example 3.1.5

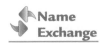
Name Exchange

Dificid is a brand name medication for the generic drug fidaxomicin. Both names appear on a medication label.

A prescription for Dificid reads "Take 200 mg every 12 hours" and instructs the pharmacy to dispense a one-week supply. The pharmacy has the following product in stock. How many tablets are dispensed?

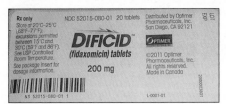

Because one tablet contains 200 mg, the patient will take one tablet every 12 hours, and there are 24 hours in a day. You can determine the number of tablets the patient will need in a single 24-hour period (a day) by setting up a ratio.

$$\frac{x \text{ tablets}}{24 \text{ hours}} = \frac{1 \text{ tablet}}{12 \text{ hours}}$$

$$\frac{(24 \text{ hours}) \, x \text{ tablets}}{24 \text{ hours}} = \frac{(24 \text{ hours}) \, 1 \text{ tablet}}{12 \text{ hours}}$$

$$x \text{ tablets} = 2 \text{ tablets}$$

A week is 7 days, so the pharmacist will dispense the following number of tablets.

$$\frac{x \text{ tablets}}{1 \text{ week}} = \frac{2 \text{ tablets}}{1 \text{ day}} \times \frac{7 \text{ days}}{1 \text{ week}} = \frac{14 \text{ tablets}}{1 \text{ week}}$$

Calculating Days' Supply

As each prescription is received in the pharmacy, personnel scan the prescription for completeness and validity, interpret the order, and then enter the information into the computer system. The electronic information becomes a part of the patient's permanent health record. Some information that must be entered into the computer is not always written on the prescription but must be calculated by the pharmacy technician or pharmacist. The pharmacist must verify the accuracy of the calculations and the data that is entered into the computer. Any calculation that the technician performs that requires written work should be available to the pharmacist when he or she verifies the accuracy of the prescription entry and calculations.

Prescriptions are often written for a specified number of doses or a specified duration of time. In either case, the technician will need to calculate the "**days' supply**." A prescription that is written for a specified number of doses such as #30 and with a dosing schedule of TID (or three times daily), will last 10 days. Another prescription may be written for a patient to use a medication TID for 10 days, and the physician has indicated the quantity as QS (or a sufficient quantity). You would calculate that the patient needs 30 doses to complete the therapy prescribed by the physician.

The most common information that requires a calculation is verifying that the days' supply and the quantity dispensed will meet the needs of the patient according to what the prescriber has indicated.

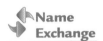

Name Exchange

The generic drug ibuprofen is commonly known as Motrin, one of several brand names for this medication.

Example 3.1.6

Calculate the days' supply for the following prescription.

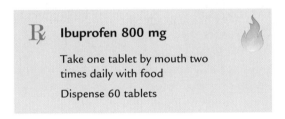

R℞   **Ibuprofen 800 mg**

Take one tablet by mouth two times daily with food

Dispense 60 tablets

$$\frac{x \text{ days}}{60 \text{ tablets}} = \frac{1 \text{ day}}{2 \text{ tablets}}$$

$$\frac{(60 \text{ tablets}) \, x \text{ days}}{60 \text{ tablets}} = \frac{1 \text{ day} \, (60 \text{ tablets})}{2 \text{ tablets}}$$

$$x = 30 \text{ days' supply}$$

Example 3.1.7

How many days' supply is this?

Acetaminophen/
codeine elixir is
the generic name
for the brand
name Tylenol
Elixir.

> R̸ **Acetaminophen 160 mg/**
> **codeine 8 mg per 5 mL elixir**
>
> Take 15 mL by mouth three times daily
>
> Dispense 270 mL

If the patient takes the medication three times daily, multiply 15 mL by 3 to
equal 45 mL for each day.

$$\frac{x \text{ days}}{270 \text{ mL}} = \frac{1 \text{ day}}{45 \text{ mL}}$$

$$\frac{(270 \text{ mL}) \; x \text{ days}}{270 \text{ mL}} = \frac{1 \text{ day } (270 \text{ mL})}{45 \text{ mL}}$$

$$x = 6 \text{ days' supply}$$

3.1 Problem Set

Which of the following DEA numbers meet the
standard validity test?

1. DEA number JC 2169870 for
   Dr. James Cardillo

2. DEA number MG 3081659 for
   nurse-midwife Laura Gonzales

3. DEA number BH 9998070 for
   Dr. Mai Hyuen

4. DEA number AL 6230618 for
   Dr. George Lewis

5. DEA number AD 7638224 for
   Dr. Daniel Lopez

6. DEA number BP 4412209 for
   Dr. Sarah Parker

7. DEA number AP 3051492 for
   Dr. Donna Perez

8. DEA number MW 2864228 for
   clinical nurse specialist Thomas Wright

Choose a drug product to fill the following orders.

9. acetic acid 1:400 irrigation

   a. glacial acetic acid

   b. 0.25% acetic acid

   c. 25% acetic acid

   d. 4% acetic acid

10. isoproterenol 5 mg/mL solution

    a. isoproterenol 5% solution

    b. isoproterenol 0.05% solution

    c. isoproterenol 1:200 solution

    d. isoproterenol 1:2 solution

Identify the information indicated for each provided drug label.

11. Brand/trade name: _____

    Generic name: _____

    Dosage form: _____

    Strength: _____

    Total quantity: _____

    Storage requirement(s): _____

    Manufacturer: _____

    NDC number: _____

NDC 52427-285-01   Rx Only   Store at controlled room temperature
100 mg   (59° to 86°F or 15° to 30°C).
                                   THIS IS A BULK CONTAINER AND NOT
Macrobid®   INTENDED FOR DISPENSING.
(nitrofurantoin monohydrate/   Dispense in a tight container.
macrocrystals)   DOSAGE: Adults: One 100-mg capsule
                                   every 12 hours with food. See package
URINARY TRACT   outsert for full prescribing information.
ANTIBACTERIAL   Mfg. by:
100 Capsules   Norwich Pharmaceuticals, Inc.
                                   Norwich, NY 13815 USA
Almatica ᶯ Pharma   Dist. by:
                                   Almatica Pharma, Inc.
                                   Pine Brook, NJ 07058 USA
                                   Rev 03/12 285-01-04   PKG01455

12. Brand/trade name: _____

    Generic name: _____

    Dosage form: _____

    Strength: _____

    Total quantity: _____

    Storage requirement(s): _____

    Manufacturer: _____

    NDC number: _____

NDC 0777-3105-02
100 PULVULES® No. 3105
PROZAC®
FLUOXETINE
CAPSULES, USP
Equiv. to
20 mg
Fluoxetine
Rx only
◇ DISTA
0777-3105-02
WIX 3381 DPX
Marketed by Lilly USA, LLC
Indianapolis, IN 46285, USA
Product of Switzerland
Expiration Date/Control No.
Medication Guide is to be dispensed to patients.
See accompanying literature for dosage.
Dispense in a tight, light-resistant container.
Keep Tightly Closed.
Store at Controlled Room Temperature 59° to
86°F (15° to 30°C)

13. Brand/trade name: _____

    Generic name: _____

    Dosage form: _____

    Strength: _____

    Total quantity: _____

    Storage requirement(s): _____

    Manufacturer: _____

    NDC number: _____

30 Capsules   NDC 0002-3238-30
               PU 3238
strattera®
atomoxetine HCl
Rx only   18 mg

               Each capsule equivalent
               to 18 mg atomoxetine
               Do not use if Lilly inner seal
               is missing or broken.
www.strattera.com   Lilly
WW 6715 AMX
Eli Lilly and Company
Indianapolis, IN 46285, USA
Product of Ireland
Expiration Date/Control No.
Store at 25°C (77°F); excursions permitted to 15°to
30°C (59° to 86°F) [see USP Controlled Room
temperature].
Medication Guide is to be dispensed to patients.
Keep tightly closed.
Keep out of the reach of children.
See accompanying literature for dosage information.
0002-3238-30

14. Brand/trade name: _____

    Generic name: _____

    Dosage form: _____

    Strength: _____

    Total quantity: _____

    Storage requirement(s): _____

    Manufacturer: _____

    NDC number: _____

Each film-coated tablet   ⦀⦀⦀**Mylan**®
contains:
Spironolactone, USP 50 mg   NDC 0378-0243-01
                               Spironolactone
0378-0243-01   Tablets, USP
                               50 mg   M
50 mg   243
Rx only   100 TABLETS
Dispense in a tight, light-resistant
container as defined in the USP
using a child-resistant closure.
Keep container tightly closed.
Keep this and all medication
out of the reach of children.
Store at 20° to 25°C (68° to 77°F).
[See USP Controlled Room
Temperature.]
Protect from light.
Usual Dosage: See accompanying
prescribing information.
Mylan Pharmaceuticals Inc.
Morgantown, WV 26505 U.S.A.
⦀⦀⦀**Mylan**®
www.mylan.com
RMO243A2

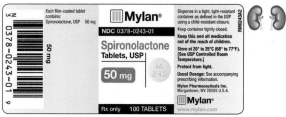

15. Brand/trade name:_____

    Generic name: _____

    Dosage form: _____

    Strength: _____

    Total quantity: _____

    Storage requirement(s): _____

    Manufacturer: _____

    NDC number: _____

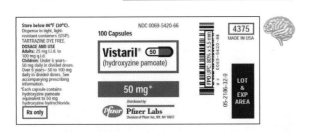

16. Brand/trade name: _____

    Generic name: _____

    Dosage form: _____

    Strength: _____

    Total quantity: _____

    Storage requirement(s): _____

    Manufacturer: _____

    NDC number: _____

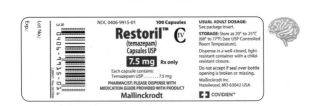

Applications

How much medication should be dispensed for the following prescriptions?

17.

℞ **Ibuprofen 400 mg tablet #XX**

Take one tablet by mouth four times daily with food.

18.

℞ **Amoxicillin capsule 500 mg**

Take one capsule three times daily for 10 days.

19.

℞ **Prednisone 5 mg tablet**

Take four tablets twice daily for two days,

then three tablets twice daily for two days,

then four tablets once daily for two days,

then three tablets once daily for two days,

then two tablets once daily for two days,

then one tablet once daily for two days.

20.
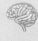

℞ **Milk of Magnesia**

Take one ounce every night at bedtime for one week.

21.

℞ **Phenytoin 100 mg capsule #CL**

Take three capsules every morning.

What is the days' supply for each of these prescriptions?

22.
> ℞ **Cephalexin**
> **500 mg capsules #28**
>
> Take one capsule by mouth every 12 hours.

23.
> ℞ **Bactrim DS Tablets #90**
>
> Take one tablet by mouth each morning.

24.
> ℞ **Norpace Capsules**
> **100 mg #120**
>
> Take one capsule by mouth every 6 hours.

25.
> ℞ **Advair HFA 45/21**
>
> Dispense one inhaler with 120 doses.
> Use inhaler two times daily.

Self-check your work in Appendix A.

3.2 Prescription Directions

Put Down Roots

The word *signa* comes from the Latin word *signāre*, meaning "to write, mark, or label." The signa, or sig, refers to the prescriber's instructions for the proper use of a medication.

A very important part of each prescription is the **signa (sig)**, a term that comes from the Latin word for "write." It consists of the prescriber's instructions for proper use of the medication and usually includes the following information:

- **Dose:** how much medication the patient will take at each administration. It is generally expressed as a number of units (e.g., tablets, capsules), an amount of drug (e.g., weight in milligrams or grains), or a volume of medication (e.g., ounces, teaspoonfuls).
- **Route of administration:** how the drug is to be administered. Routes of administration include oral (by mouth), injection (into veins, into muscles, under the skin), rectal, or topical (to the eye, ear, skin, or mucous membranes), among others.
- **Dosing schedule:** how often the drug is to be taken and, in some cases, how long therapy is to be continued.

Abbreviations

Healthcare professionals have developed their own shorthand for many aspects of patient care, and it is reflected in the abbreviations used in prescription directions. Many of the abbreviations used in prescriptions are derived from the initials of Latin or Greek words or phrases. Others come from medical terminology in English, and some even combine terms from multiple languages. Table 3.2 on the following page lists some of the most common abbreviations used in prescriptions. A more complete listing of abbreviations can be found in Appendix C.

When abbreviations are standardized (to have only one meaning) and are clearly written, they are useful because they save space and time. Abbreviations can cause problems, however, if they are misinterpreted. Sometimes this occurs when the same set of letters can have two different meanings. For example, "IVP" means "IV Push" or "administer by injection into the vein from a syringe" when used on a hospital medication order for an intravenous (IV) medication. In another context, however, "IVP" designates "intravenous pyelogram," an X-ray examination of the urinary tract.

TABLE 3.2 Common Prescription Abbreviations

Abbreviation	Translation	Abbreviation	Translation
ac	before meals	NKA	no known allergy
AD	right ear	NKDA	no known drug allergy
AS	left ear	npo	nothing by mouth
AU	both ears	OD	right eye
am	morning	OS	left eye
bid	twice daily	OU	both eyes
c̄	with	pc	after meals
cap	capsule	po	by mouth
DAW	dispense as written	prn	as needed
D/C	discontinue	q	every
g	gram	qh	every hour
gr	grain	q2 h	every 2 hours
gtt	drop	qid	four times a day
h or hr	hour	qs	a sufficient quantity
IM	intramuscular	stat	immediately
IV	intravenous	tab	tablet
L	liter	tid	three times daily
mcg	microgram	ud	as directed
mEq	milliequivalent	wk	week
mL	milliliter		

Note: Some prescribers may write abbreviations using capital letters or periods. However, periods should not be used with metric units or medical abbreviations as they can be a source of medication errors.

Safety in Numbers

Pharmacy personnel should exercise care when interpreting abbreviations on prescriptions.

Abbreviations are also problematic when they are not typed or written clearly. The abbreviation "q6 pm," for example, means "every evening at 6 p.m.," but if written hastily or printed on a fax machine low in toner, it may appear to say "q6 h," meaning every six hours. The abbreviation "qhs" means "nightly at bedtime" but could be misread as "qhr," meaning "every hour." Some abbreviations are so error-prone that the Joint Commission—an independent organization that evaluates and accredits practices in hospital systems—has declared that they are absolutely unacceptable for use in accredited institutions. To that end, the Joint Commission has published the Official "Do Not Use" List containing abbreviations that may lead to confusion among healthcare personnel and, consequently, may result in medication errors. This list can be found at www.paradigmcollege.net/pharmcalc5e/JointCommission. Another organization, the Institute for Safe Medication Practices (ISMP), has published an extensive list of dangerous abbreviations and symbols to avoid in the healthcare setting. This document, called the ISMP's Error-Prone Abbreviations, Symbols, and Dose Designations, can be found at www.paradigmcollege.net/pharmcalc5e/ISMP.

The common abbreviations should be committed to memory as they will become a part of the pharmacy technician's everyday language. The easiest ones to start with are the ones that indicate how many times per day a patient should take a medication: BID (twice daily), TID (three times daily), and QID (four times daily). The abbreviations are sometimes written in lowercase letters and sometimes written in uppercase letters. The letter "q" means "every" and is sometimes placed in front of other abbreviations.

Safety in Numbers

Instructions to patients on dispensed medications must be clear and should not include abbreviations.

Directions for Patients

Because most patients are not familiar with the abbreviations and shorthand used on prescriptions, directions must be "translated" from the sig and "written" on the label placed on the dispensing packaging. Sometimes, descriptive terms are added if appropriate. For example, a prescription for a fentanyl transdermal patch may have the sig "ī q 3d." The pharmacy label on the patient's package, however, will read "Apply one patch every 72 hours." Similarly, a prescription for hydrochlorothiazide 25 mg tablets may bear a sig of "12.5 mg po qam," but the patient's label must read "Take one-half tablet by mouth every morning." It is important that directions for patients be set forth in clear and unambiguous terms on the label, even if the doctor and the pharmacist explain verbally in great detail how the medication is to be used. It is easy for patients to misunderstand or forget what they were told days or weeks earlier, and having the label available for instructions at every dose is necessary for safe medication use.

3.2 Problem Set

Write out the meanings of these common abbreviations used in prescriptions.

1. bid

2. DAW

3. IM

4. IV

5. mL

6. NKA

7. npo

8. q3 h

9. qid

10. tid

Answer the following questions.

11. What is a route of administration?

12. Name four routes of administration.

13. Give one abbreviation for a route of administration and write out its meaning.

14. Give one abbreviation for a dosing schedule and write out its meaning.

15. Explain the difference between an IM administration and an IV administration of a medication.

Applications

Translate the following directions from a prescription order into wording that would be appropriate on a label for the patient's use.

16.
R̟ **Diphenhydramine capsules**

ii cap po qid prn itching

17.
R̟ **Nitroglycerin Transdermal Systems**

ī on qhs off qam

18.

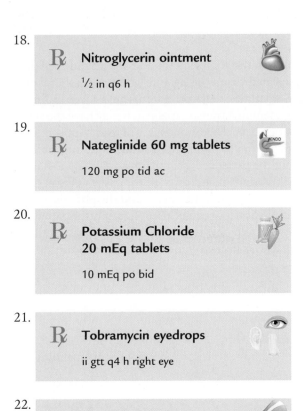

$\mathbb{R}$ **Nitroglycerin ointment**

½ in q6 h

19.

$\mathbb{R}$ **Nateglinide 60 mg tablets**

120 mg po tid ac

20.

$\mathbb{R}$ **Potassium Chloride 20 mEq tablets**

10 mEq po bid

21.

$\mathbb{R}$ **Tobramycin eyedrops**

ii gtt q4 h right eye

22.

$\mathbb{R}$ **Alendronate tablets**

i po q wk 30 minutes ac breakfast $\bar{c}$ H_2O

Determine the days' supply and quantity to dispense for the following prescriptions:

23.

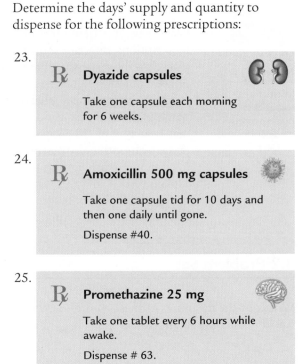

$\mathbb{R}$ **Dyazide capsules**

Take one capsule each morning for 6 weeks.

24.

$\mathbb{R}$ **Amoxicillin 500 mg capsules**

Take one capsule tid for 10 days and then one daily until gone.

Dispense #40.

25.

$\mathbb{R}$ **Promethazine 25 mg**

Take one tablet every 6 hours while awake.

Dispense # 63.

Self-check your work in Appendix A.

Chapter Summary

- Prescriptions can arrive at the pharmacy in many forms: handwritten, typed, faxed, or via telephone or voice mail.
- Prescriptions must be checked for validity before being filled.
- Patient information should be complete on the prescription to meet safety, legal, and insurance requirements.
- DEA numbers can be checked for validity by using a formula and performing a calculation.
- Drugs are identified on prescriptions using a brand and/or generic name.
- Drug labels contain standard information, including:
  - generic name of the drug (and brand name when there is one)
  - strength per unit
  - dosage form
  - quantity enclosed
  - manufacturer
  - special handling or storage requirements
  - National Drug Code (NDC)
- Some drug labels will display the strength per unit in several different manners.
- Quantity to dispense may need to be calculated if the prescriber does not indicate what should be dispensed on the prescription.
- Days' supply should be calculated to meet the need of the patient according to the duration of therapy indicated by the physician.
- Days' supply must be entered into the patient's record and submitted to insurance for every prescription.
- Prescriptions are written using shorthand that consists mainly of abbreviations derived from the initials of Latin or Greek phrases.
- Prescription instructions for the patient are called the signa (or sig).
- Route of administration for medications should always be specified on the prescription or medication order.
- Unacceptable abbreviations should be avoided.

Key Terms

brand name the name under which the manufacturer markets a drug; a registered trademark of the manufacturer; also known as the *trade name*

days' supply the number of days that a prescription or medication order will last a patient when taken as directed by the prescriber

DEA number a number issued by the Drug Enforcement Administration (DEA) to signify the authority of the holder to prescribe or handle controlled substances; made up of two letters followed by seven digits, the last of which is a checksum digit used to check the validity of the DEA number

dose on a prescription, the indication of how much medication the patient will take at each administration

dosing schedule on a prescription, the indication of how often the drug is to be taken

generic name the name under which a drug is approved by the Food and Drug Administration; sometimes denotes a drug that is not protected by a trademark; also referred to as a *USAN (United States Adopted Name)*

prescription an order for medication for a patient that is written by a physician or a qualified licensed practitioner to be filled by a pharmacist

route of administration on a prescription, the indication of how the medication is to be given

signa (sig) from the Latin word for "write"; the part of the prescription that provides instructions for proper use of the medication, including the dose, route of administration, and dosing schedule

Chapter Review

Assessing Comprehension

To check your comprehension of this chapter's key concepts, read the following multiple-choice questions and then record your answers on a separate sheet of paper. Write your answers as modeled in these examples: 1d; 2c; 3b; *etc.*

1. Prescriptions should be checked for completeness and validity
   a. to prevent medication from being erroneously dispensed.
   b. to verify that the physician has chosen the appropriate medication.
   c. to verify the patient's insurance coverage.
   d. to check if a generic is available for the patient.

2. What should always accompany the name of a drug on the prescription?
   a. the National Drug Code
   b. the handling instructions if kept in the refrigerator
   c. the dosage unit and form
   d. the physician's DEA number

3. The number of refills on a prescription
   a. should be filled in by the patient.
   b. is zero if left blank by the prescriber.
   c. is always one unless otherwise indicated.
   d. may be altered if the dose is not appropriate for the patient's weight.

4. A DEA number is issued to
   a. prescribers who are known to have abused controlled substances.
   b. prescribers who write orders for controlled substances.
   c. all physicians and nurses.
   d. emergency room physicians who need special privileges.

5. The checksum method of verifying a DEA number includes
   a. adding the digits together to get a total under 30.
   b. adding the digits together in a manner that compares the total to the last digit of the DEA number.
   c. doubling all even numbers and dividing by 2.
   d. multiplying the last two digits of the DEA number to equal the first two digits.

6. The name, address, and phone number of the patient should be complete on the prescription
   a. to more completely verify the patient's identity for security, safety, legal, and insurance requirements.
   b. to abide by HIPAA regulations.
   c. to double-check that the patient lives at the address on file with the pharmacy.
   d. to obtain full reimbursement from the patient's insurance company.

7. The quantity to dispense is
   a. determined only by calling or verifying the amount dispensed with the prescriber or his or her staff.
   b. calculated from information on the prescription that describes the daily dose and the duration of therapy.
   c. based on what the patient received on the previous prescription refill.
   d. calculated by what the insurance company will permit as the maximum number of doses.

8. Abbreviations on prescriptions are used
   a. to hide information on prescriptions from patients.
   b. to meet the guidelines set by the Joint Commission.
   c. to implement ambiguous Latin and Greek symbols.
   d. to provide a shorthand means of conveying the patient's instructions.

9. The directions for patients on a prescription are called the
   a. "dispense as written" instructions.
   b. signa.
   c. metric conversions.
   d. route of administration.

10. Days' supply is calculated to verify that
   a. the patient will have an adequate supply of medication to take for the duration of therapy.
   b. the prescriber's dosage form selection is accurate.
   c. the prescriber has selected the most appropriate therapy.
   d. the prescription complies with the guidelines of the Joint Commission.

Finding Solutions

To gain practice in handling challenging situations in the workplace, consider the following real-world scenarios and then use the guiding questions to help you formulate your responses.

Note: *To indicate your answers for Scenario C, Questions 9 and 10, ask your instructor for the handout depicting a dosing spoon and oral syringe and the handout depicting a dosing spoon and medicine cup.*

Scenario A: A prescription for a large quantity of narcotic pain medication has come into the pharmacy. Although the order is written on a hospital prescription blank, you are suspicious that the prescription may not be valid. The written directive is oddly worded, and the dose is not what is typically associated with the medication prescribed. A DEA number is handwritten at the bottom of the prescription.

1. Perform a checksum on the DEA number: AB 4423921. Is it valid?

2. The sig indicates that the patient should take 3 tabs q.i.d. or prn. What does this mean?

3. The drug name written is "Norco Hydrocodone APAP." What part of the drug name indicates the brand name and what part indicates the generic name?

Scenario B: An elderly patient with significant vision loss has asked you to write out instructions for her medication in very large print so that she can read them more easily. Write out the instructions (sig) for the following medications:

4. Lasix 20 mg; take 1 tab QD in AM for edema

5. ranitidine 150 mg; take 1 tab BID for stomach

6. acyclovir 800 mg; take 1 tab QID for 5 days for shingles

7. verapamil 80 mg; take 1 tablet TID for angina

8. diazepam 2 mg; take 1 tablet HS for sleep

Scenario C: Mrs. Zapata has three children with chicken pox, and the pediatrician's office has advised her to purchase OTC Benadryl for itching. Her oldest child can take capsules, but the two younger ones need liquid.

9. On the handout that you obtained from your instructor, select the most accurate measuring device (either the dosing spoon or the oral syringe) to administer a ½ tsp dose to a child. Fill in the correct volume on the measuring device.

10. On the handout that you obtained from your instructor, select the most accurate measuring device (either the dosing spoon or the medicine cup) to administer a 2 tsp dose to a child. Fill in the correct volume on the measuring device.

Sampling the Certification Exam

To provide you with practice for the Certification Exam, read the following questions that have been patterned after the test format and then record your answers on a separate sheet of paper. Write your answers as modeled in these examples: 1d; 2c; 3b; etc.

1. A prescription that is written with a sig of "2 tablets stat" should be dispensed
   a. immediately.
   b. at the next medication pass.
   c. as needed.
   d. when the patient is discharged.

2. A prescription for cefaclor 250 mg capsules contains the following sig: "1 capsule t.i.d. for 14 days." How many capsules should be dispensed?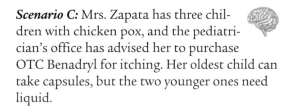
   a. 14
   b. 21
   c. 28
   d. 42

3. A prescription has a sig that instructs the patient to "place ii gtts OD b.i.d." Where will the patient use this medication?
   a. in the left ear
   b. in the right eye
   c. in the left eye
   d. in both eyes

4. A prescription that has a sig of "2 caps po t.i.d. ac" will be dispensed with the following patient instructions:
   a. Take 2 capsules twice daily with food.
   b. Take 2 capsules three times daily as needed.
   c. Take 2 capsules by mouth three times daily before meals.
   d. Take 2 capsules after each meal.

5. How many days will a prescription with a sig of "take 1 cap q.d. h.s." last if 45 capsules are dispensed?
   a. 11 days
   b. 14 days
   c. 22 days
   d. 45 days

To put your pharmacy calculation skills to the test, read the following questions and then record your answers on a separate sheet of paper.

Check the validity of the DEA numbers used by the following prescribers.

1. DEA number BK 4917186 for Albert King, MD

2. DEA number BA 4412209 for Norma Aborra, DO

3. DEA number MB 9231971 for Joanne Burgess, CRNP

4. DEA number AK 1521964 for Harold Kwong, DDS

Calculate the quantity to dispense for the following prescriptions.

5. #XC

   Sig: one tablet daily

6. 30 day supply

   Sig: one tablet daily

7. Sig: one cap TID × 10 days

8. Sig: one ounce TID × 10 days

9. Dispense 30 day supply

   Sig: 1½ tablets BID

10. Dispense 60 day supply

   Sig: 3 cap daily

Refer to the medication labels to complete questions 11 and 12.

11. Brand/trade name:_____

Generic name: _____

Dosage form: _____

Strength: _____

Total quantity: _____

Storage requirement(s): _____

Manufacturer: _____

NDC number: _____

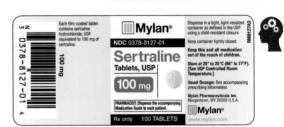

12. Brand/trade name: _____

Generic name: _____

Dosage form: _____

Strength: _____

Total quantity: _____

Storage requirement(s): _____

Manufacturer: _____

NDC number: _____

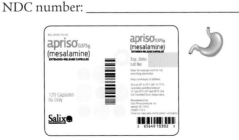

Write the meanings of the following abbreviations.

13. cap

14. DAW

15. gr

16. IM

17. IV

18. mL

19. NKA

20. po

21. q6 h

22. stat

Write the abbreviations that correspond to these phrases.

23. a sufficient quantity

24. as directed

25. discontinue

26. four times a day

27. gram

28. liter

29. milliequivalent

30. nothing by mouth

31. tablet

32. with

Translate the following directions from a prescription order into wording that would be appropriate on a label for the patient's use.

33. ĭ tab po q2 h prn

34. ĭĭ gtts o.d. bid

35. ĭ patch q wk

36. ĭ cap po tid ac ud

37. to rash prn itch

38. ĭ tablet qam c̄ food

What is missing from these prescriptions?

39.

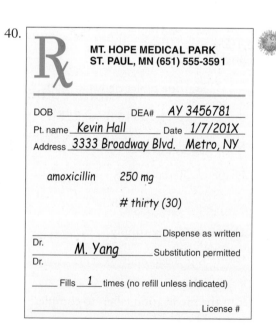

40.

Calculate the quantity and write out directions for the patient for each of the following prescriptions.

41.

℞ **Clonidine Transdermal System**

30 day supply

i̇ q3 days

42.

℞ **Ampicillin 250 mg cap**

500 mg po tid × 10 days

43.

℞ **Tobradex 5 mL**

i̇ gtt left eye bid × 7 days

44. Using the label below, how many bottles will be needed to provide the quantity ordered?

℞ **Zidovudine Syrup**

10 mL po q8 h × 10 days

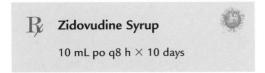

Each 5 mL (1 teaspoonful) contains zidovudine 50 mg and sodium benzoate 0.2% added as a preservative.

See package insert for Dosage and administration.

Store at 15° to 25°C (59° to 77°F).

NDC 0000-0000-00

Zidovudine Syrup

240 mL   Rx only

Answer the following questions.

45. What is a dosing schedule?

46. What are four routes of administration?

Applying Metric Measurements and Calculating Doses

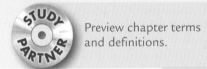

4

Learning Objectives

- Identify the basic units and prefixes of the metric system.

- Convert units within the metric system by moving the decimal point, using the ratio-proportion method, and using the dimensional analysis method.

- Calculate drug doses using the ratio-proportion and dimensional analysis methods.

- Calculate doses based on weight and body surface area.

- Calculate a pediatric dose using the patient's weight or age and the appropriate adult dose.

Preview chapter terms and definitions.

4.1 Basic Metric Units

 Put Down Roots

Three units of measure in the metric system have their roots in the Greek language. The word *meter* is from the Greek term *metron*, meaning "measure"; the word *gram* is from the Greek term *gramma*, meaning "small weight"; and the word *liter* is from the Greek term *litra*, meaning "pound."

Chapter 1 presented a brief overview of the decimal number system. Because of its accuracy, the decimal system is used in pharmacy measurements. Based on subdivisions and multiples of 10, the **metric system** uses decimals to indicate tenths, hundredths, and thousandths.

Identifying Metric Units of Measure

The metric system's three basic units of measure are the meter, the gram, and the liter (see Table 4.1). The **meter**, the unit for measuring length, has limited use in the pharmacy. A patient's height is often measured in feet and inches but could be measured in meters or centimeters. A meter is approximately three feet. The **gram**, the unit for measuring weight, is used in the pharmacy for measuring the amount of medication in solid form and for indicating the amount of solid medication in a

TABLE 4.1   Metric Units of Measure

Metric Unit	Measurement
meter (m)	length
gram (g)	weight
liter (L)	volume

solution. The gram is the weight of one cubic centimeter of water at 4 °C. The **liter** is the unit used for measuring the volume of liquid medications and liquids for solutions. One liter is equal to 1000 milliliters, and one milliliter is equal to the volume in one cubic centimeter.

TABLE 4.2 Metric System Prefixes

Prefix	Value
nano (n)	1/1,000,000,000 (one-billionth of the basic unit, or 0.000000001)
micro (mc)	1/1,000,000 (one-millionth of the basic unit, or 0.000001)
milli (m)	1/1000 (one-thousandth of the basic unit, or 0.001)
centi (c)	1/100 (one-hundredth of the basic unit, or 0.01)
deci (d)	1/10 (one-tenth of the basic unit, or 0.1)
kilo (k)	1000 (one thousand times the basic unit)

TABLE 4.3 Metric Abbreviations

Measurement	Metric Unit	Abbreviation
Weight	kilogram	kg
	gram	g
	milligram	mg
	microgram	mcg
Volume	kiloliter	kL
	liter	L
	milliliter	mL*
	microliter	mcL
Length	kilometer	km
	meter	m
	millimeter	mm
	micrometer	mcm†

* equivalent to cc, which stands for cubic centimeters, but cc is considered a dangerous abbreviation

† sometimes abbreviated as μm, but μm is considered a dangerous abbreviation

Using Metric Prefixes and Abbreviations

The set of prefixes shown in Table 4.2 is used to designate multiples of the basic metric units. The three prefixes most widely used in pharmaceutical calculations are kilo-, milli-, and micro-. The abbreviations shown in Table 4.3 are commonly used for metric measurements.

It is important to memorize the basic metric units along with their prefixes. All units in the metric system use the same prefixes. An example is the gram: The larger unit is the kilogram, whereas two of the smaller units are the milligram and microgram.

Most people can visualize an object that weighs a kilogram or a gram, and many can create a mental picture of a container that can hold a liter or milliliter of a liquid. However, it is impossible even to see something that weighs only a microgram.

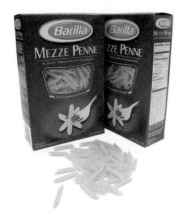

A kilogram is equivalent to a little more than two 1 lb boxes of pasta.

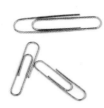

A single large paper clip, or two small paper clips, weighs about 1 g.

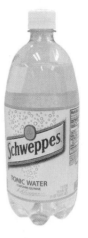

Remembering the amount of liquid that is contained in a standard, 1 L soda bottle will help you visualize the amount of liquid in a single liter.

Safety in Numbers

Pharmacy technicians should use the medication labels, not the color or shape of the pills, to confirm the amount of drug contained in a tablet or capsule.

Safety in Numbers

For a decimal value less than 1, use a leading zero to prevent errors.

Medications that contain micrograms, or even milligrams, of an active ingredient will almost always contain an inactive filler so that the dosage form becomes measurable. For example, a tablet with a weight of 300 micrograms would be hard to see and far too small to handle safely. The tablets shown in Figure 4.1 all contain different amounts of levothyroxine, but they are all the same size. Even though levothyroxine is available in a variety of doses, the tablet sizes remain the same. The colors of the tablets and the package labeling differentiate the amount of active ingredient.

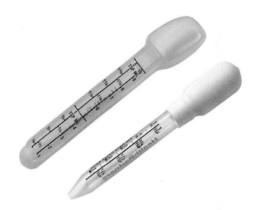

Dosing spoons and droppers are frequently marked with metric and household measures. Notice that 1 tsp is equivalent to 5 mL.

Parts of a unit are written as a decimal fraction. For example, two and a half milligrams is written as 2.5 mg. A leading zero is used if there is no whole number preceding the decimal point. For example, one-half liter is written as 0.5 L, and one-quarter gram is 0.25 g. These place-saving zeros help prevent medication errors.

When writing dosage strengths, unnecessary zeros after the decimal point are generally left off to reduce the chance of misreading the value. For example, 0.25 mL, 5 L, and 15.6 mL should not be written as 0.250 mL, 5.0 L, and 15.60 mL.

FIGURE 4.1 Levothyroxine

				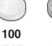							
25 mcg orange	50 mcg white	75 mcg violet	88 mcg olive	100 mcg yellow	112 mcg rose	125 mcg brown	137 mcg turquoise	150 mcg blue	175 mcg lilac	200 mcg pink	300 mcg green

4.1 Problem Set

State the abbreviation for each of the following metric units.

1. microgram

2. milligram

3. liter

4. gram

5. kilogram

6. meter

7. centimeter

8. milliliter

9. cubic centimeter

10. deciliter

Write the following numbers using an Arabic number with a decimal value and the appropriate abbreviation.

11. six-tenths of a gram

12. fifty kilograms

13. four-tenths of a milligram

14. four-hundredths of a liter

15. four and two-tenths of a gram

16. five-thousandths of a gram

17. six-hundredths of a gram

18. two and six-tenths liters

19. three-hundredths of a liter

20. two-hundredths of a milliliter

Applications

21. The Taro Pharmaceutical Company has donated a container labeled 5 kg of bulk Genocillin granules. The standard dose is 375 mg. How many single dose units can be obtained from the container?

22. The pharmacy receives the following prescription.

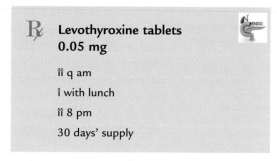

R℞ **Levothyroxine tablets 0.05 mg**

ii q am

i with lunch

ii 8 pm

30 days' supply

a. How many tablets will be dispensed?

b. How many milligrams will the patient take over the course of one month (30 days)?

23. If the total daily dose of a drug is 0.9 g and it is given tid, what is the amount of each dose in grams?

24. A patient is to receive 1.2 g of cimetidine per day in four divided doses.

a. How many grams will be in each dose?

b. If the available dosage forms are shown in the following labels, which will be chosen?

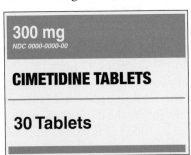

300 mg
NDC 0000-0000-00

CIMETIDINE TABLETS

30 Tablets

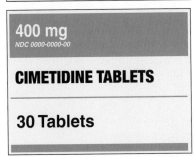

400 mg
NDC 0000-0000-00

CIMETIDINE TABLETS

30 Tablets

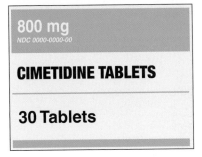

800 mg
NDC 0000-0000-00

CIMETIDINE TABLETS

30 Tablets

25. The following prescription for potassium permanganate has been brought into the compounding pharmacy.

℞ **Potassium permanganate**

1. Weigh out 1 g of potassium permanganate.

2. Add to a 1 L bottle of sterile water for irrigation. (Be sure to wear gloves, as this chemical stains.)

3. Replace cap on bottle and swirl to dissolve potassium permanganate.

The solution expires 30 days after mixing.

a. What is the percentage of potassium permanganate in this solution?

b. If today is August 1, 2015, what expiration date will you place on the bottle?

Self-check your work in Appendix A.

4.2 Conversions within the Metric System

This section will present three ways to convert units within the metric system: moving the decimal point, using the ratio-proportion method, and using the dimensional analysis method. Once you learn the three methods of conversion, you should select the method you are most comfortable with and stick to that method when making conversions. Before calculating a needed dose, you should be confident that the number you are working with is accurate and that the correct conversion has been made.

Moving the Decimal Point

To change the metric units of a number to smaller or larger units, you can multiply or divide by an appropriate multiple of 1000. (See Table 4.4 on the following page.) For

TABLE 4.4   Metric Unit Equivalents

Kilo	Base	Milli	Micro
0.001 kg	1 g	1000 mg	1,000,000 mcg
0.001 kL	1 L	1000 mL	1,000,000 mcL
0.001 km	1 m	1000 mm	1,000,000 mcm

instance, to convert 5 grams to milligrams, multiply by 1000 to get 5000 milligrams. (Move the decimal point three places to the right.) Multiplying 17 liters by 1,000,000 yields 17,000,000 microliters. (Move the decimal point six places to the right.) Conversely, changing to a larger unit requires division. So, to convert 25 meters to kilometers, divide by 1000 to get 0.025 kilometers. (Move the decimal point three places to the left.) Similarly, 3 microliters divided by 1000 yields 0.003 milliliters, and 22 milliliters divided by 1000 yields 0.022 liters. In each case, move the decimal point three places to the left.

The key to understanding the relationships in the metric system is to remember that the decimal point must be moved three places when converting from one unit to the next. Moving the decimal point three places is essentially equivalent to multiplying or dividing the number by 1000. The three "places" are representative of the three zeros in 1000.

Math Morsels

Moving the decimal point three spaces to the right is the same as multiplying by 1000. Moving the decimal point three places to the left is the same as dividing by 1000.

$$1 \text{ kg} = 1000 \text{ g}$$
$$1 \text{ g} = 1000 \text{ mg}$$
$$1 \text{ mg} = 1000 \text{ mcg}$$
$$1 \text{ L} = 1000 \text{ mL}$$

When converting from a smaller to a larger unit of measure, move the decimal point three places to the left.

$$4500 \text{ mL} = 4.500 \text{ L}$$
$$1287 \text{ mg} = 1.287 \text{ g}$$
$$480 \text{ mL} = 0.480 \text{ L}$$

When converting from a larger to a smaller unit of measure, move the decimal point three places to the right.

$$0.954 \text{ g} = 954 \text{ mg}$$
$$1.5 \text{ g} = 1500 \text{ mg}$$
$$0.238 \text{ g} = 238 \text{ mg}$$
$$0.621 \text{ mg} = 621 \text{ mcg}$$

Using the Ratio-Proportion Method

If you have difficulty remembering which way to move the decimal point when converting between units of measure in the metric system, the ratio-proportion method introduced in Chapter 2 is an effective alternative. This method is a "foolproof" way to convert metric units. Set up the conversion by placing the unknown and the value to be converted on one side of the equation and the conversion factor (the ratio of the desired unit to the given unit) on the other side.

When setting up proportions to solve for a variable, remember that the units in the numerators must match and so must the units in the denominators. Checking to make sure the units match before completing the calculation will ensure accuracy in the conversion. The next examples will demonstrate a conversion by moving the decimal point, followed by the same conversion using the ratio-proportion method.

Example 4.2.1

Change 2300 mg to grams.

One method is to divide by 1000 by moving the decimal point three places to the left.

$$2300 \text{ mg} = 2.300 \text{ g} = 2.3 \text{ g}$$

Another method is to use a proportion to solve for the unknown.

$$\frac{x \text{ g}}{2300 \text{ mg}} = \frac{1 \text{ g}}{1000 \text{ mg}}$$

$$\frac{(2300 \text{ mg}) \, x \text{ g}}{2300 \text{ mg}} = \frac{(2300 \text{ mg}) \, 1 \text{ g}}{1000 \text{ mg}}$$

$$x \text{ g} = \frac{2300 \text{ g}}{1000}$$

$$x \text{ g} = 2.3 \text{ g}$$

Example 4.2.2

Change 3.2 mg to micrograms.

You can multiply by 1000 by moving the decimal point three places to the right.

$$3.2 \text{ mg} = 3200. \text{ mcg} = 3200 \text{ mcg}$$

Alternatively, you can use a proportion.

$$\frac{x \text{ mcg}}{3.2 \text{ mg}} = \frac{1000 \text{ mcg}}{1 \text{ mg}}$$

$$\frac{(3.2 \text{ mg}) \, x \text{ mcg}}{3.2 \text{ mg}} = \frac{(3.2 \text{ mg}) \, 1000 \text{ mcg}}{1 \text{ mg}}$$

$$x \text{ mcg} = (3.2) \, 1000 \text{ mcg}$$

$$x \text{ mcg} = 3200 \text{ mcg}$$

Example 4.2.3

Change 3.785 L to milliliters.

Multiply by 1000 by moving the decimal point three places to the right.

$$3.785 \text{ L} = 3785. \text{ mL} = 3785 \text{ mL}$$

Or, alternatively,

$$\frac{x \text{ mL}}{3.785 \text{ L}} = \frac{1000 \text{ mL}}{1 \text{ L}}$$

$$\frac{(3.785 \text{ L}) \, x \text{ mL}}{3.785 \text{ L}} = \frac{(3.785 \text{ L}) \, 1000 \text{ mL}}{1 \text{ L}}$$

$$x \text{ mL} = (3.785) \, 1000 \text{ mL}$$

$$x \text{ mL} = 3785 \text{ mL}$$

Example 4.2.4

Change 454 g to kilograms.

Divide by 1000 by moving the decimal point three places to the left.

$$454 \text{ g} = 0.454 \text{ kg} = 0.454 \text{ kg}$$

Or set up a proportion.

$$\frac{x \text{ kg}}{454 \text{ g}} = \frac{1 \text{ kg}}{1000 \text{ g}}$$

$$\frac{(454 \text{ g}) \, x \text{ kg}}{454 \text{ g}} = \frac{(454 \text{ g}) \, 1 \text{ kg}}{1000 \text{ g}}$$

$$x \text{ kg} = \frac{454 \text{ kg}}{1000}$$

$$x \text{ kg} = 0.454 \text{ kg}$$

Using the Dimensional Analysis Method

The **dimensional analysis method** is based on the principle that multiplying a number by 1 does not change its value. In this method, the given number and unit are multiplied by the ratio of the desired unit to the given unit, which is equivalent to 1. The unit in the denominator will match the given unit, so the units will cancel each other out and the unit remaining in the numerator will be the unit to which you are converting.

For Good Measure

If 1 g = 1000 mg, then

$$\frac{1\,g}{1000\,mg} = 1$$

Multiplying a number by 1 does not change its value.

Example 4.2.5

Convert 486 mg to grams.

$$486\,\cancel{mg} \times \frac{1\,g}{1000\,\cancel{mg}} = 0.486\,g$$

Example 4.2.6

Convert 4.5 L to milliliters.

$$4.5\,\cancel{L} \times \frac{1000\,mL}{1\,\cancel{L}} = 4500\,mL$$

Example 4.2.7

Convert 240 mL to liters.

$$240\,\cancel{mL} \times \frac{1\,L}{1000\,\cancel{mL}} = 0.24\,L$$

Example 4.2.8

Convert 0.725 mg to micrograms.

$$0.725\,\cancel{mg} \times \frac{1000\,mcg}{1\,\cancel{mg}} = 725\,mcg$$

4.2 Problem Set

Convert the following units within the metric system by using the ratio-proportion method. Retain all significant figures and do not round the answers.

1. 1964 mcg = _____ mg

2. 418 mg = _____ g

3. 651 mg = _____ mcg

4. 0.84 mg = _____ mcg

5. 0.012 g = _____ mcg

6. 9,213,406 mcg = _____ g

7. 284 mg = _____ g

8. 9382.5 mcg = _____ mg

9. 12,321 mcg = _____ g

10. 184 g = _____ kg

Convert the following units within the metric system by using the dimensional analysis method. Retain all significant figures and do not round the answers.

11. 52 mL = _____ L

12. 2.06 g = _____ mg

13. 16 mg = _____ mcg

14. 256 mg = _____ g

15. 2,703,000 mcg = _____ g

16. 6.9 L = _____ mL

17. 62.5 mg = _____ g

18. 15 kg = _____ g

19. 2,785,000 mcg = _____ g

20. 8.234 mg = _____ mcg

Convert the following units by moving the decimal point, or by using the method that you prefer. Show all work. Retain all significant figures and do not round the answers.

21. 2 kg = _____ mg

22. 21 L = _____ mL

23. 576 mL = _____ L

24. 823 kg = _____ mg

25. 27 mcg = _____ mg

26. 5000 mcg = _____ mg

27. 20 mcg = _____ mg

28. 4.624 mg = _____ mcg

29. 3.19 g = _____ mg

30. 8736 mcg = _____ mg

31. 830 mL = _____ L

32. 0.94 L = _____ mL

33. 1.84 g = _____ mg

34. 560 mg = _____ g

35. 1200 mcg = _____ mg

36. 125 mcg = _____ mg

37. 0.275 mg = _____ mcg

38. 480 mL = _____ L

39. 239 mg = _____ g

40. 1500 mg = _____ g

Applications

41. The following prescription has come into the pharmacy.

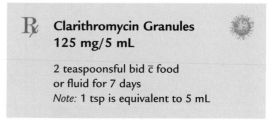

℞ **Clarithromycin Granules**
    125 mg/5 mL

2 teaspoonsful bid c̄ food
or fluid for 7 days
Note: 1 tsp is equivalent to 5 mL

a. How many milliliters will the patient take daily?

b. How many milliliters should be dispensed for the patient?

c. How many grams will the patient take daily?

d. Using the following drug label, how many bottles of clarithromycin will be needed to fill this prescription?

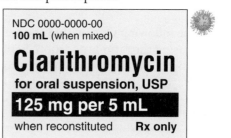

NDC 0000-0000-00
100 mL (when mixed)

Clarithromycin
for oral suspension, USP
125 mg per 5 mL
when reconstituted   **Rx only**

42. A patient is to take 1.5 g of amoxicillin before a dental procedure. The capsules available are shown in the following label. How many capsules will be dispensed to this patient?

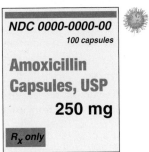

NDC 0000-0000-00

100 capsules

Amoxicillin Capsules, USP

250 mg

Rₓ only

43. A patient is to receive 1000 mg of vancomycin two times daily, diluted in IV solution. The following label shows the stock available.

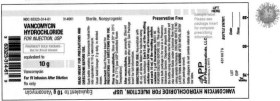

a. How many doses are available in one vial?

b. How many days will one unopened vial last?

Self-check your work in Appendix A.

4.3 Problem Solving in the Pharmacy

Many pharmacy calculations require problem solving. When faced with a "story problem" or other problem in which the calculation needed is not absolutely clear, it is important to begin by asking the question, "What am I looking for?" In dose calculations, this is usually a weight, expressed in milligrams, or a volume, expressed in milliliters.

Using the Ratio-Proportion Method to Solve Story Problems

In Chapter 2, you learned some basic calculations using the ratio-proportion method and applied that same method to converting between units of measure in the metric system. Now you will use ratios and proportions mathematically to compare a readily available product, consisting of an active ingredient and a **vehicle**, to a desired (prescribed) dosage. Like the available product, the desired dosage will consist of an active ingredient and a vehicle. A vehicle is an inert medium, such as syrup, in which a drug is administered.

For Good Measure

When setting up proportions, units in the numerators must match, and units in the denominators must match.

$$\frac{\text{active ingredient (desired)}}{\text{vehicle (desired)}} = \frac{\text{active ingredient (on hand)}}{\text{vehicle (on hand)}}$$

Keep in mind that the ratios on the two sides of the equation may be reversed, but the same units must appear in both numerators and the same units must appear in both denominators.

The steps outlined in Table 4.5 on the following page can be used as a basis for solving story problems or dose calculations using the ratio-proportion method. Usually, the following equation will be used to solve a story problem.

$$\frac{\text{desired amount of drug}}{\text{prescriber's order}} = \text{ratio of pharmacy stock}$$

Step 1. Read through the entire problem and identify what the question is asking for. This becomes the variable *x*, labeled with the unit you are looking for such as *x* mg or *x* mL.

Step 2. Identify the prescriber's order. Circle the dose ordered by the physician.

Step 3. Identify the appropriate stock available in the pharmacy. The ratio of pharmacy stock, such as 1 mg/tablet or 125 mg/5 mL, should be found on the labels of the drugs used in the pharmacy. Underline this information.

Step 4. Identify extraneous information. It is often helpful to draw a single pencil line through any information you identify as not needed. This prevents you from using that information in your setup.

Step 5. Estimate what your answer should be. Compare the ordered dose to what is on hand. Will the dose be larger or smaller than the dosage unit given?

Step 6. Use the ratio-proportion method to solve for *x*. When using the ratio-proportion method to solve your problem, place the physician-ordered dosage on the left side of the proportion and the pharmacy on-hand ratio on the right side.

Step 7. Round your answer to the appropriate number of significant figures. Weights are typically rounded to the nearest whole milligram, and volumes are typically rounded to the nearest tenth of a milliliter.

Example 4.3.1

A physician has ordered 370 mg of a drug, and you have a 10 mL vial of solution containing 250 mg/3 mL on hand. How many milliliters will you measure out?

Step 1. Identify the question being asked. You need to find out how many milliliters, so *x* mL is the unknown.

Step 2. Identify the prescribed amount and circle it. In this problem, the physician has ordered 370 mg.

Step 3. Identify the product available in the pharmacy and underline it. In this problem, the pharmacy has 250 mg/3 mL of the drug.

Step 4. Identify extraneous information and draw a line through it. In this problem, it is not important to know that the drug comes in a 10 mL vial.

Step 5. Estimate the answer. The ordered dose of 370 mg is larger than the dosage strength of 250 mg, so the dose volume should be more than 3 mL.

Step 6. Use the ratio-proportion method to solve for *x* mL.

$$\frac{\text{desired amount of drug}}{\text{prescriber's order}} = \text{ratio of pharmacy stock}$$

$$\frac{x \text{ mL}}{370 \text{ mg}} = \frac{3 \text{ mL}}{250 \text{ mg}}$$

$$x \text{ mL} = 4.44 \text{ mL}$$

Step 7. Since this is a liquid and volumes are typically rounded to the nearest tenth of a milliliter, round to 4.4 mL.

Example 4.3.2

A physician has ordered 100 mg of amoxicillin to be given to a child three times a day for 10 days. Amoxicillin is available in a 150 mL bottle with a dose strength of 125 mg/5 mL. How many milliliters will the child need at each dose?

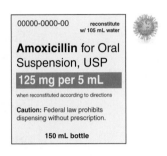

Step 1. Identify the question being asked. You need to find out how many milliliters, so x mL is the unknown.

Step 2. Identify the prescribed amount and circle it. In this problem, the physician has ordered 100 mg at each dose.

Step 3. Identify the product available in the pharmacy and underline it. In this problem, the pharmacy has 125 mg/5 mL of amoxicillin.

Step 4. Identify extraneous information and draw a line through it. In this problem, it is not important to know "three times a day for 10 days" and that the size of the amoxicillin bottle is 150 mL.

Step 5. Estimate the answer. The ordered dose of 100 mg is less than the dose strength of 125 mg, so the dose volume should be less than 5 mL.

Step 6. Use the ratio-proportion method to solve for x mL.

$$\frac{\text{desired amount of drug}}{\text{prescriber's order}} = \text{ratio of pharmacy stock}$$

$$\frac{x \text{ mL}}{100 \text{ mg}} = \frac{5 \text{ mL}}{125 \text{ mg}}$$

$$x \text{ mL} = 4 \text{ mL}$$

Step 7. No rounding is needed because the answer for this liquid measure does not extend beyond a tenth of a milliliter.

Some medications are ordered by a certain volume rather than by milligrams or weight. For example, a cough syrup may be ordered as 10 mL every four hours, and it may be necessary to calculate how much of the active ingredient is in this dose. The steps presented in Table 4.5 can also be used to solve this type of problem. In this case, however, the unknown will be the amount of the active ingredient instead of the overall volume.

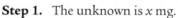

Example 4.3.3

A physician has ordered 10 mL of amoxicillin to be given to a child three times daily for 7 days. Amoxicillin is available in a 150 mL bottle with a dosage strength of 250 mg/5 mL. How many milligrams will the child get at each dose?

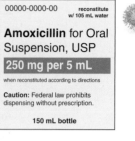

00000-0000-00   reconstitute
w/ 105 mL water

Amoxicillin for Oral
Suspension, USP

250 mg per 5 mL

when reconstituted according to directions

Caution: Federal law prohibits
dispensing without prescription.

150 mL bottle

Step 1. The unknown is x mg.

Step 2. The prescribed amount is 10 mL of amoxicillin.

Step 3. The pharmacy has 250 mg/5 mL of amoxicillin.

Step 4. The extraneous information includes "three times daily for 7 days" and that the size of the amoxicillin bottle is 150 mL.

Step 5. The answer will be more than 250 mg because 10 mL is larger than 5 mL.

Step 6. Use the ratio-proportion method to solve for x mg.

$$\frac{x \text{ mg}}{10 \text{ mL}} = \frac{250 \text{ mg}}{5 \text{ mL}}$$

$$x \text{ mg} = 500 \text{ mg}$$

Step 7. No rounding is needed because the answer for this weight does not have a decimal point and the significant figures are correct.

Example 4.3.4

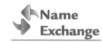

Name Exchange

Cefaclor is a generic drug name and is marketed under several brand names including Ceclor. Cefaclor is a cephalosporin antibiotic used to treat bacterial infections.

A physician has ordered cefaclor 375 mg/5 mL oral suspension. A 100 mL bottle is prepared and is labeled to administer 7.5 mL twice daily for 5 days. How many milligrams is the patient receiving at each dose?

NDC 0000-0000-00

CEFACLOR

for Oral Suspension, USP

375 mg per 5 mL

100 mL
Shake well before use.

R_x only

Step 1. The unknown is x mg.

Step 2. The prescribed amount is 7.5 mL suspension.

Step 3. Once the suspension is prepared, it contains 375 mg cefaclor/5 mL of suspension.

Step 4. The extraneous information includes "twice daily for 5 days" and that the size of the cefaclor bottle is 100 mL.

Step 5. The answer will be more than 375 mg because 7.5 mL is larger than 5 mL.

Step 6. Use the ratio-proportion method to solve for x mg.

$$\frac{x \text{ mg}}{7.5 \text{ mL}} = \frac{375 \text{ mg}}{5 \text{ mL}}$$

$$x \text{ mg} = 562.5 \text{ mg}$$

Step 7. The answer of 562.5 mg is rounded to the nearest whole milligram, or 563 mg.

Using Dimensional Analysis to Calculate a Drug Dose

Just as the dimensional analysis method was used to convert metric units earlier in this chapter, it can now be used to solve drug dosage problems by "converting" a dose from milligrams to tablets, or milligrams to milliliters. This is accomplished by multiplying the dose ordered by the ratio for the on-hand product. As in the metric conversions practiced earlier in the chapter, the ratio is set up so that the units of the given dose and the units in the denominator will cancel out. When the dimensional analysis method is used to solve drug dosage problems, the steps shown in Table 4.5 can still be used to analyze the information. The only difference is in the setup in Step 6.

The dimensional analysis method tends to be used most frequently for simple dosage calculations such as the number of tablets. For example, if a doctor has prescribed 100 mg of a drug and you have that drug on hand in 50 mg tablets, you can quickly determine that the patient will need two 50 mg tablets for the prescribed 100 mg dose. Although you may be able to do the calculations in the following exercises in your head, it is important to work through the steps to be sure you understand them.

Example 4.3.5

A physician has ordered a 25 mg dose of hydrochlorothiazide. You have a 100 count bottle of 50 mg tablets. What will you prepare to fill the order?

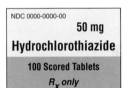
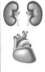

NDC 0000-0000-00
50 mg
Hydrochlorothiazide
100 Scored Tablets
R_x only

Step 1. The unknown is x tablets.
Step 2. The prescribed amount is 25 mg.
Step 3. The pharmacy has 50 mg tablets.
Step 4. The extraneous information includes "100 count bottle."
Step 5. The answer will be less than 1 tablet, as the requested dose is less than the amount of milligrams in 1 tablet.
Step 6. Convert the units using the dimensional analysis method.

$$25 \text{ mg} \times \frac{1 \text{ tablet}}{50 \text{ mg}} = 0.5 \text{ tablet}$$

Step 7. No rounding is required.

Example 4.3.6

A physician has ordered a 750 mg dose of amoxicillin. You have 150 mL of a 250 mg/5 mL suspension. What will you prepare to fill the order?

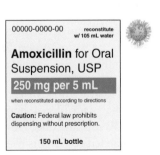

00000-0000-00   reconstitute
w/ 105 mL water
Amoxicillin for Oral
Suspension, USP
250 mg per 5 mL
when reconstituted according to directions
Caution: Federal law prohibits
dispensing without prescription.
150 mL bottle

Step 1. The unknown is x mL.
Step 2. The prescribed amount is 750 mg of amoxicillin.
Step 3. The pharmacy has 250 mg/5 mL.
Step 4. The extraneous information includes "150 mL suspension."
Step 5. The answer will be approximately three times as large as the unit given.

Step 6. Convert the units using the dimensional analysis method.

$$750 \text{ mg} \times \frac{5 \text{ mL}}{250 \text{ mg}} = 15 \text{ mL}$$

Step 7. No rounding is required.

4.3 Problem Set

Calculate the following doses using the ratio-proportion method.

1. A patient has a prescription order for 30 mg of a drug. The pharmacy has a partial container of 7.5 mg tablets. How many tablets will the patient need? *30 ÷ 7.5 = 4*

2. A prescription order is written for 20 mg of medication. The pharmacy has on hand a 10 mL vial of 25 mg/2 mL solution. How many milliliters will be prepared for this patient?

3. A patient is prescribed 125 mg of carbamazepine suspension. The label provided shows the drug that the pharmacy has in stock. How many milliliters will be prepared for this patient?

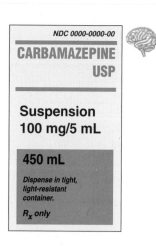

NDC 0000-0000-00

CARBAMAZEPINE USP

Suspension 100 mg/5 mL

450 mL

Dispense in tight, light-resistant container.

R$_x$ only

4. A patient is to receive 4 mg of haloperidol. The pharmacy has on hand a 1 mL vial of 5 mg/1 mL solution. How many milliliters are needed to fill this prescription?

5. A loading dose of 1750 mg is needed. The pharmacy has on hand a 500 count bottle of 250 mg capsules. How many capsules will be needed to fill this prescription?

6. A patient is to receive 40 mg of morphine sulfate. The pharmacy has the following medication available. How many milliliters will be prepared for this patient?

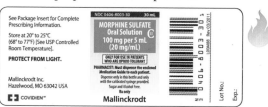

See Package Insert for Complete Prescribing Information.

Store at 20° to 25°C (68° to 77°F) [See USP Controlled Room Temperature].

PROTECT FROM LIGHT.

Mallinckrodt Inc.
Hazelwood, MO 63042 USA

COVIDIEN™

NDC 0406-8003-30   30 mL

MORPHINE SULFATE Oral Solution
100 mg per 5 mL
(20 mg/mL)

ONLY FOR USE IN PATIENTS WHO ARE OPIOID TOLERANT

PHARMACIST: Must dispense the enclosed Medication Guide to each patient.

Dispense only in this bottle and only with the calibrated syringe provided. Sugar and Alcohol Free.

Rx only

Mallinckrodt

7. A patient is to receive 400 mg of erythromycin ethylsuccinate three times daily. The available drug is shown in the label. How many milliliters will be prepared for the morning dose?

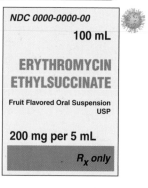

NDC 0000-0000-00

100 mL

ERYTHROMYCIN ETHYLSUCCINATE

Fruit Flavored Oral Suspension USP

200 mg per 5 mL

R$_x$ only

8. The following order is received by the pharmacy.

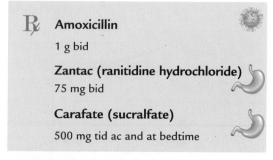

R$_x$ **Amoxicillin**

1 g bid

Zantac (ranitidine hydrochloride)

75 mg bid

Carafate (sucralfate)

500 mg tid ac and at bedtime

a. Amoxicillin is available as a 250 mg/5 mL suspension. How many milliliters of medication would you draw up in each oral syringe for the patient?

b. Zantac is available as 15 mg/mL. How many milliliters will you draw up in each oral syringe for the patient?

c. Carafate is available as 1 g tablets. How many tablets will be needed for one day?

9. A total regimen of therapy calls for 10 mg of a medication to be given to a patient over several days. In the pharmacy, a solution is available with 40 mcg/mL. How many milliliters must be dispensed to complete the regimen?

10. A patient was given 2 mL of gentamicin, shown in the label below. How many milligrams were given to the patient?

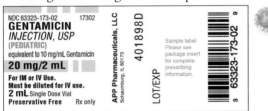

11. A patient receives 1 mg of atropine, shown in the label. How many milliliters is this?

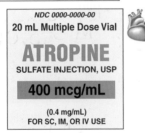

12. A patient receives 1.2 mL of the atropine solution shown in the preceding problem. How many micrograms is this?

13. A 0.63 mL dose of medication is to be given. The pharmacy stock solution contains 80 mg/15 mL. How many micrograms are in the dose?

14. A capsule contains 35 mg of an active ingredient. How many capsules would you need to accumulate 1.05 kg of ingredient?

15. A total regimen of a drug calls for 880 mg to be given. If two doses provide 80 mg, how many doses will have to be given?

16. You have 560 mL of a solution that contains 1600 mg. How many micrograms are in 4 mL of solution? (Round your answer to the nearest tenth.)

17. A total regimen of therapy calls for 10 mg of a medication to be given to a patient over several days. In the pharmacy, a solution is available with 40 mcg/mL. How many milliliters must be dispensed to complete the regimen?

18. A patient is to receive 2000 units of heparin. Use the following label to determine how many milliliters of heparin you will prepare.

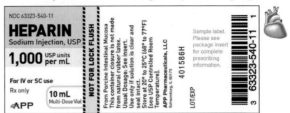

Use the following label to answer questions 19 and 20:

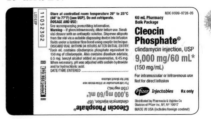

19. A medication order states that the patient is to take 900 mg of Cleocin. Use the medication label from the vial above to determine how many milliliters this will be.

20. A patient receives 4 mL of Cleocin. Use the medication label from the vial above to determine how many milligrams this will be.

Use the following label to answer questions 21 and 22:

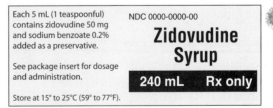

21. A patient is to take 12.5 mL of zidovudine syrup as shown. How many milligrams is this?

22. A patient is prescribed 100 mg of zidovudine syrup as shown. How many milliliters is this?

Use the following label to answer questions 23 and 24:

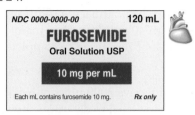

NDC 0000-0000-00   120 mL

FUROSEMIDE
Oral Solution USP

10 mg per mL

Each mL contains furosemide 10 mg.   **Rx only**

23. A pediatric patient is to take 0.5 mL of furosemide oral solution, and the medication shown in the label is to be used to fill the order. How many milligrams will the child take with each dose?

24. A pediatric patient is to take 0.8 mL of furosemide oral solution, and the medication shown in the label is to be used to fill the order. How many milligrams will the child take with each dose?

Use the adjacent label to answer questions 25 and 26:

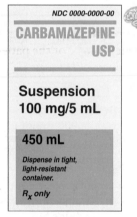

NDC 0000-0000-00

CARBAMAZEPINE
USP

Suspension
100 mg/5 mL

450 mL

Dispense in tight, light-resistant container.

R$_x$ only

25. A patient is to take 150 mg of carbamazepine every 12 hours, and the medication is available as presented in the label at right. How many milliliters will the patient take at each dose?

26. A patient is to take 0.5 g of carbamazepine. How many milliliters will be prepared?

Use the following label to answer questions 27 and 28:

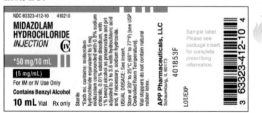

NDC 63323-412-10   410210
MIDAZOLAM
HYDROCHLORIDE
INJECTION (IV)

50 mg/10 mL
(5 mg/mL)
For IM or IV Use Only
Contains Benzyl Alcohol
10 mL Vial   Rx only

APP Pharmaceuticals, LLC
Schaumburg, IL 60173

Sample label. Please see package insert for complete prescribing information.

401853F

27. A patient is to receive 50 mg of midazolam intramuscularly (IM) every 4 to 6 hours as needed, and the medication shown in the label is to be used to fill the order. How many milliliters will the patient need for one dose?

28. A patient is to receive 0.8 mL of midazolam solution IM stat. How many milligrams is this?

Use the following label to answer questions 29 and 30:

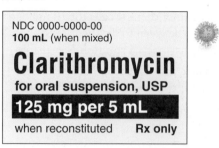

NDC 0000-0000-00
100 mL (when mixed)

Clarithromycin
for oral suspension, USP
125 mg per 5 mL
when reconstituted   **Rx only**

29. A patient is to take 100 mg of clarithromycin. How many milliliters will this be?

30. A patient is to take 7.5 mL of clarithromycin. How many milligrams will this be?

Use the following label to answer questions 31 and 32:

NDC 0000-0000-00   **4 fl oz**

Diphenhydramine
Hydrochloride Elixir USP

12.5 mg/5 mL
R$_x$ only

31. A pediatric patient is to receive 20 mg of diphenhydramine hydrochloride. How many milliliters of elixir will be administered?

32. An adult patient who has been stung by a wasp is to receive 50 mg of diphenhydramine hydrochloride immediately. How many milliliters of elixir will be administered?

33. A patient is to take 150 mg of nortriptyline per day. The pharmacy has on hand 25 mg, 50 mg, and 75 mg capsules.

   a. Select the product that will result in the patient taking the fewest number of capsules daily.

   b. How many capsules will need to be dispensed for a week's supply?

34. The following order has been received by the pharmacy.

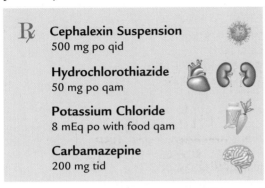

Cephalexin Suspension
500 mg po qid

Hydrochlorothiazide
50 mg po qam

Potassium Chloride
8 mEq po with food qam

Carbamazepine
200 mg tid

a. Cephalexin is available in a 200 mL bottle of 250 mg/5 mL suspension. How many milliliters will the patient need for the first day?

b. Hydrochlorothiazide is available from the pharmacy in a 1000 count bottle of 25 mg tablets. How many tablets will be needed for the first day of hospitalization?

c. Potassium chloride is available as a 20 mEq/15 mL sugar-free solution. It contains 5% alcohol. How many milliliters will be measured out for the patient's morning dose?

d. The pharmacy has a 450 mL bottle of 100 mg/5 mL carbamazepine solution. How many milliliters will be prepared for this patient for the first day?

Self-check your work in Appendix A.

4.4 Customized Doses

Most manufacturers offer dose ranges as prescribing guidelines. In some cases, the suggested dose may be based on the patient's weight or the patient's weight and height. Calculations to customize patient-specific doses are important in the pharmacy.

Calculating Doses Based on Weight

The patient's weight may be especially important when calculating a customized parenteral, pediatric, or geriatric dose of a medication. Medications that have a low margin of safety should have a customized dose. More commonly, children and elderly patients often need customized doses because they weigh significantly less than the "normal" adult patients the drugs are designed for. Also, their body systems may not metabolize or eliminate the drug as an adult's body might. In these cases, manufacturers will offer prescribing guidelines for medications based upon a therapeutic amount or range per unit of body weight. The most common unit used is milligram of a medication per kilogram of body weight.

The following examples will demonstrate calculations used to customize a dose. For the purposes of rounding when calculating weights and doses associated with a weight, round to the tenth, unless greater accuracy can be measured as indicated in the example or question provided.

Example 4.4.1

A patient weighs 60 kg, and she is to receive a medication of 15 mg/kg. What will her dose be? If the medication is available in a 300 mg capsule, how many capsules will be dispensed for one dose?

This problem has two parts. The first part asks for the dose, and the second part asks for the number of capsules to be dispensed for one dose. You can solve both parts of this problem using either the ratio-proportion method or the dimensional analysis method.

Part I.   Determine the dose.

Solution 1: Using the ratio-proportion method,

$$\frac{x \text{ mg}}{60 \text{ kg}} = \frac{15 \text{ mg}}{1 \text{ kg}}$$

$$\frac{(\cancel{60 \text{ kg}}) \, x \text{ mg}}{\cancel{60 \text{ kg}}} = \frac{(\cancel{60 \text{ kg}}) \, 15 \text{ mg}}{1 \, \cancel{\text{kg}}}$$

$$x \text{ mg} = (60) \, 15 \text{ mg}$$

$$x \text{ mg} = 900 \text{ mg}$$

Solution 2: Using the dimensional analysis method,

$$60 \, \cancel{\text{kg}} \times \frac{15 \text{ mg}}{1 \, \cancel{\text{kg}}} = 900 \text{ mg}$$

Part II.   Determine the number of capsules to be dispensed for one dose.

Solution 1: Using the ratio-proportion method,

$$\frac{x \text{ capsules}}{900 \text{ mg}} = \frac{1 \text{ capsule}}{300 \text{ mg}}$$

$$\frac{(\cancel{900 \text{ mg}}) \, x \text{ capsules}}{\cancel{900 \text{ mg}}} = \frac{(\cancel{900 \text{ mg}}) \, 1 \text{ capsule}}{300 \, \cancel{\text{mg}}}$$

$$x \text{ capsules} = \frac{900 \text{ capsules}}{300}$$

$$x \text{ capsules} = 3 \text{ capsules}$$

Solution 2: Using the dimensional analysis method,

$$900 \, \cancel{\text{mg}} \times \frac{1 \text{ capsule}}{300 \, \cancel{\text{mg}}} = 3 \text{ capsules}$$

Example 4.4.2

A patient weighs 74 kg, and he is to receive a medication of 0.4 mg/kg. What will his dose be? If the medication is available in a 15 mg/10 mL solution, how many milliliters of medication will the patient receive in a dose?

This problem has two parts. The first part asks for the dose, and the second part asks for the amount of milliliters to be dispensed. You can solve both parts of this problem using either the ratio-proportion method or the dimensional analysis method.

Part I.   Determine the dose.

Solution 1: Using the ratio-proportion method,

$$\frac{x \text{ mg}}{74 \text{ kg}} = \frac{0.4 \text{ mg}}{1 \text{ kg}}$$

$$\frac{(\cancel{74\ kg})\ x\ mg}{\cancel{74\ kg}} = \frac{(\cancel{74\ kg})\ 0.4\ mg}{1\ \cancel{kg}}$$

$$x\ mg = (74)\ 0.4\ mg$$

$$x\ mg = 29.6\ mg$$

Solution 2: Using the dimensional analysis method,

$$74\ \cancel{kg} \times \frac{0.4\ mg}{1\ \cancel{kg}} = 29.6\ mg$$

Part II. Determine the number of milliliters to be dispensed for one dose.
Solution 1: Using the ratio-proportion method,

$$\frac{x\ mL}{29.6\ mg} = \frac{10\ mL}{15\ mg}$$

$$\frac{(\cancel{29.6\ mg})\ x\ mL}{\cancel{29.6\ mg}} = \frac{(\cancel{29.6\ mg})\ 10\ mL}{15\ \cancel{mg}}$$

$$x\ mL = \frac{296\ mL}{15}$$

$$x\ mL = 19.733\ mL,\ \text{rounded to } 19.7\ mL$$

Solution 2: Using the dimensional analysis method,

$$29.6\ \cancel{mg} \times \frac{10\ mL}{15\ \cancel{mg}} = 19.733\ mL,\ \text{rounded to } 19.7\ mL$$

Calculating Doses Based on Body Surface Area

Body surface area (BSA) is a measurement that is based on weight and height variables and expressed as meters squared (m^2). BSA is usually estimated using a nomogram. Table 4.6 outlines the steps for using a nomogram, and Figures 4.2 and 4.3 are nomograms used for estimating BSA for children and adults. Some medications, such as chemotherapy drugs, require BSA to calculate a patient-specific dose.

TABLE 4.6   Steps for Reading a Nomogram for Estimating BSA

Step 1. Mark the patient's height on the left column.

Step 2. Mark the patient's weight on the right column.

Step 3. Draw a line or place a straight-edge ruler on the two marks.

Step 4. Read the BSA by noting where the straight edge crosses the center column. When the straight edge crosses between two numbers, the BSA should be estimated to the nearest one-half unit.

FIGURE 4.2   **Nomogram for Estimating Body Surface Area of Children**

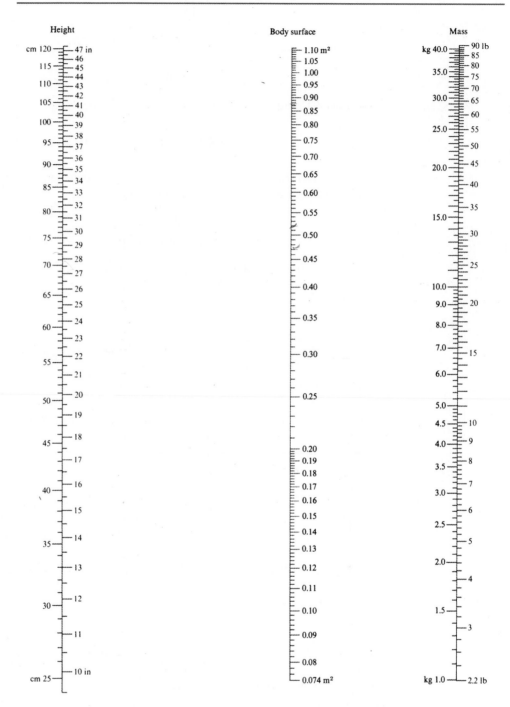

Height

Body surface

Mass

FIGURE 4.3 Nomogram for Estimating Body Surface Area of Adults

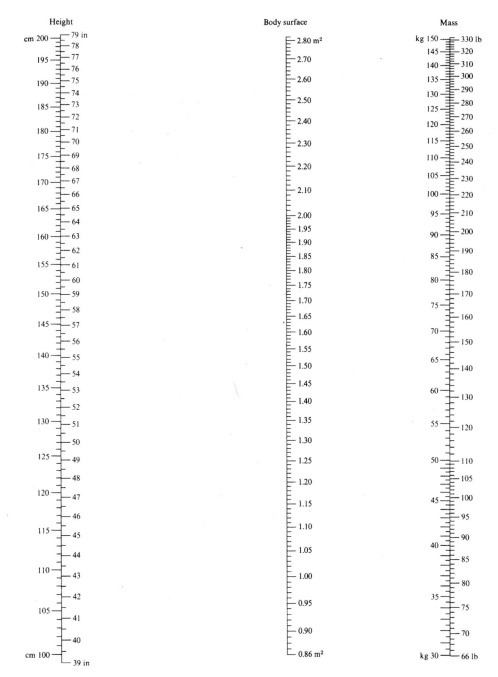

Example 4.4.3

A patient is to receive a medication with the dose based on 50 mg/m². If the patient has a BSA of 0.90 m², what will the dose be? If the medication is available only in 15 mg tablets, how many will be dispensed for one dose?

Part I. Since the dose is to be based on 50 mg/m², multiply by the number of square meters of the BSA, in this case 0.90.

$$0.90 \, \text{m}^2 \times \frac{50 \, \text{mg}}{\text{m}^2} = 45 \, \text{mg}$$

Part II. Use the dose to determine the number of tablets to dispense.

$$45 \, \text{mg} \times \frac{1 \, \text{tablet}}{15 \, \text{mg}} = 3 \, \text{tablets}$$

Example 4.4.4

A patient with a BSA of 1.30 m² is to receive a medication with the dose based on 0.80 mg/m². The prescription is to be divided into three equal doses. How much will each dose be? If the medication is available only as 50 mcg tablets, how many will be dispensed?

Part I. Multiply the number of mg/m² by the number of m², which is the BSA.

$$1.30 \, \text{m}^2 \times \frac{0.80 \, \text{mg}}{\text{m}^2} = 1.04 \, \text{mg}$$

$$1.04 \, \text{mg} \div 3 \, \text{doses} = 0.35 \, \text{mg/dose}$$

Part II. Convert the dose in milligrams to micrograms, the units of the tablets, by using the equivalency 1 mg = 1000 mcg.

$$0.35 \, \text{mg} \times \frac{1000 \, \text{mcg}}{1 \, \text{mg}} = 350 \, \text{mcg}$$

Therefore, a dose is 350 mcg. Since the tablets are 50 mcg each,

$$350 \, \text{mcg} \times \frac{1 \, \text{tablet}}{50 \, \text{mcg}} = 7 \, \text{tablets}$$

Calculating Pediatric Doses

If a manufacturer does not suggest an exact pediatric dose for a medication, such as a dose based on body weight or BSA, an appropriate dose may be calculated using the normal adult dose and one of several formulas. **Young's Rule** bases the suggested dose on a child's age in years, and **Clark's Rule** bases the suggested dose on a child's weight. Both formulas include the usual adult dose, but because the manufacturer

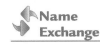

For Good Measure

The formula for Young's Rule is: age in years/(age in years + 12 years) × adult dose = pediatric dose.

The formula for Clark's Rule is: weight in lb/150 lb × adult dose = pediatric dose.

often provides this as a range (such as 20–30 mg), the physician or pharmacist must determine the "usual dose" for purposes of the formula. Many medications have a broad dose range, and the patient's response and adverse reactions can vary widely, even in adults. For this reason, many physicians prefer to prescribe to children only those medications that have a known suggested pediatric dose. Consequently, Young's and Clark's Rules are used infrequently. A more common method for determining pediatric doses, using dosing tables, will be presented in Chapter 5. In addition, for pediatric doses, it is also common practice to round down to the nearest whole number or down to the most accurate, measurable amount. The pharmacy technician should verify the common practice used in his or her pharmacy workplace.

Young's Rule

$$\frac{\text{age (in years)}}{\text{age} + 12\ \text{years}} \times \text{adult dose} = \text{pediatric dose}$$

Clark's Rule

$$\frac{\text{weight (in lb)}}{150\ \text{lb}} \times \text{adult dose} = \text{pediatric dose}$$

Example 4.4.5

A 6-year-old child needs a dose of a medication that has a suggested adult dose of 500 mg. Using Young's Rule, what is the appropriate pediatric dose?

$$\frac{6\ \text{years}}{6\ \text{years} + 12\ \text{years}} \times 500\ \text{mg} = 166.66\ \text{mg}$$

Example 4.4.6

An 80 lb child needs a dose of a medication that has a suggested adult dose of 250 mg. Using Clark's Rule, what is the appropriate pediatric dose?

$$\frac{80\ \text{lb}}{150\ \text{lb}} \times 250\ \text{mg} = 133.33\ \text{mg}$$

Example 4.4.7

Name Exchange

The generic drug acetaminophen is commonly known among pharmacy staff members as APAP or Tylenol.

Calculate the dose of acetaminophen for a 5-year-old child who weighs 44 lb (20 kg). The normal adult dose is 650 mg every 4 to 6 hours as needed. Determine the child's dose based on Young's Rule and Clark's Rule.

Young's Rule: $\dfrac{5\ \text{years}}{5\ \text{years} + 12\ \text{years}} \times 650\ \text{mg} = 191.18\ \text{mg}$

Clark's Rule: $\dfrac{44\ \text{lb}}{150\ \text{lb}} \times 650\ \text{mg} = 190.67\ \text{mg}$

Example 4.4.8

The manufacturer in Example 4.4.7 recommends a dosage range of 10–15 mg/kg for a child age 4–5 years. What is the dosage range for the 5-year-old child who weighs 20 kg?

$$20 \text{ kg} \times \frac{10 \text{ mg}}{\text{kg}} = 200 \text{ mg}$$

$$20 \text{ kg} \times \frac{15 \text{ mg}}{\text{kg}} = 300 \text{ mg}$$

Thus, the manufacturer's suggested dosage range for this child is 200–300 mg. This is a little more than the dose determined by the formulas in Example 4.4.7. For this medication, in fact, the manufacturer specifically recommends a dose of 240 mg per dose for a child between the ages of 4 and 5 years.

4.4 Problem Set

Use the nomogram to determine the following BSA values. (For homework purposes, round to the hundredths place.)

1. Child of normal height and weight: 28 inches, 20 lb

2. Child of normal height and weight: 34 inches, 32 lb

3. Child of normal height and weight: 48 inches, 51 lb (approximate your answer)

4. Child of normal height and weight: 95 cm, 21 kg

5. Young adult of normal height and weight: 141 cm, 42.5 kg

6. Adult: 60 inches, 78 kg

7. Adult: 66 inches, 64 kg

8. Adult: 71 inches, 76 kg

9. Adult: 58 inches, 57 kg

10. Adult: 200 cm, 80 kg

Applications

Calculate the following weight-based doses based on the provided recommended dose. (For homework purposes, round to the hundredths place.)

11. Cortisone is dosed at 0.5 mg/kg per day. If the patient weighs 56 kg, what is the dose?

12. A postsurgical patient is to receive 125 mg/kg per day of cephalosporin divided into six doses daily. What will each dose be for a patient weighing 87 kg?

13. A premature infant is to receive 4 mL/kg of a medication. If the infant weighs 1.4 kg, how much medication will be administered?

14. A drug is to be given at a dose of 0.625 mg/kg.

    a. If a patient weighs 80 kg, what is the proper dose?

    b. The dose determined above is to be divided and given three times over the course of 24 hours. What is the size of each dose, to the nearest hundredth of a milligram?

15. A newborn weighs 6 kg and is to be given medication at 5 mg/kg per day in two divided doses. How much will each dose be?

16. A patient weighs 68.64 kg and is to be dosed at 125 mg/kg per day. How many milligrams is this?

17. A child weighs 10 kg and is to be dosed at 10 mg/kg per day. The medication should be administered in equal doses every 12 hours. How many milligrams are in each dose?

Calculate the following BSA-based doses based on the provided recommended dose.

18. A patient is to receive medication with the dose based on 25 mg/m² per day, divided into two equal doses. This patient has a BSA of 1.1 m². How much will each dose be?

19. A patient is to receive medication with the dose based on 0.75 mg/m². This patient has a BSA of 0.67 m². How much of the medication will you prepare? (Round to the nearest tenth.)

20. The medication order for a patient says that the dose is to be based on 100 mg/m². If this patient has a BSA of 0.85 m², how much will be prepared?

21. A child is to receive acyclovir at 250 mg/m². The child's BSA is 0.71 m². What will the dose be?

22. Methotrexate is to be given at 3.3 mg/m². The patient has a BSA of 0.83 m². What will the dose be?

Determine if the following doses are safe according to the manufacturer's recommended doses.

23. A pediatric patient weighs 40 lb and is 43 inches in height. The manufacturer of vincristine has a recommended dose of 2 mg/m². The physician has ordered 1.9 mg of vincristine. Is the physician's order safe according to the recommended dose?

24. A pediatric patient weighs 27 lb and is 30 inches in height. The manufacturer of methotrexate has a recommended dose of 3.3 mg/m². The physician has ordered 2.5 mg of methotrexate. Is the physician's order safe according to the recommended dose?

25. A pediatric patient weighs 23 lb and is 32 inches in height. The manufacturer of acyclovir has a recommended dose of 250 mg/m² every 8 hours. The physician has ordered 200 mg of acyclovir tid. Is the physician's order safe according to the recommended dose?

26. A patient weighs 40.9 kg and is 58 inches in height. The manufacturer of erythromycin has a recommended dose of 50 mg/kg per day. The physician has ordered 300 mg of erythromycin tid. Is the physician's order safe according to the recommended dose?

Calculate dosage ranges for the following and determine whether the prescribed dose is in the recommended safe range.

27. A pediatric patient weighs 36.4 kg and is 48 inches in height. The manufacturer of cefazolin has a recommended dose of 50 to 100 mg/kg per day. The physician has prescribed 250 mg tid.

    a. Calculate the minimum daily dose for this pediatric patient.

    b. Calculate the maximum daily dose for this pediatric patient.

    c. Is the physician's dose within the recommended safe range?

    d. How many milliliters will be prepared for one prescribed dose if the product is available as a 500 mg/50 mL solution?

28. A pediatric patient weighs 5.45 kg and has a length of 21 inches. The manufacturer of amoxicillin has a recommended dose of 20 to 40 mg/kg per day. The physician has ordered 125 mg tid.

    a. Calculate the minimum daily dose for this pediatric patient.

    b. Calculate the maximum daily dose for this pediatric patient.

    c. Is the physician's dose within the recommended safe range?

    d. How many milliliters will be prepared for one prescribed dose if the product is available as a 125 mg/5 mL suspension?

29. A pediatric patient weighs 11.8 kg and is 31 inches in height. The physician has ordered acetaminophen with codeine, and safe dosing of acetaminophen with codeine is based on the amount of codeine. The manufacturer of codeine has a recommended dose of 0.5 to 1 mg/kg per dose. The physician has ordered 10 mL of 12 mg codeine/5 mL oral elixir.

    a. Calculate the minimum daily dose for this pediatric patient.

    b. Calculate the maximum daily dose for this pediatric patient.

    c. How many milligrams of codeine are in the 10 mL of oral elixir?

    d. Is the physician's dose within the recommended safe range?

30. A pediatric patient weighs 9.32 kg and is 28 inches in length. The manufacturer of ibuprofen has a recommended dose of 5 to 10 mg/kg every 6 to 8 hours. The physician has ordered 125 mg q8 h.

    a. Calculate the minimum daily dose for this pediatric patient.

    b. Calculate the maximum daily dose for this pediatric patient.

    c. Is the physician's dose within the recommended safe range?

    d. How many milliliters will be prepared for one prescribed dose if the product is available as a 100 mg/5 mL suspension?

31. A pediatric patient weighs 50 kg and is 65 inches in height. The manufacturer of cephalexin has a recommended dose of 25 to 50 mg/kg per day in two or four equal doses. The physician has ordered 500 mg bid.

    a. Calculate the minimum daily dose for this pediatric patient.

    b. Calculate the maximum daily dose for this pediatric patient.

    c. Is the physician's dose within the recommended safe range?

    d. How many milliliters will be prepared for one prescribed dose if the product is available as a 250 mg/5 mL suspension?

32. A pediatric patient weighs 28.6 kg and is 50 inches in height. The manufacturer of acetaminophen has a recommended dose of 10 to 15 mg/kg per day. The physician has ordered 325 mg/day.

    a. Calculate the minimum daily dose for this pediatric patient.

    b. Calculate the maximum daily dose for this pediatric patient.

    c. Is the physician's dose within the recommended safe range?

    d. How many milliliters will be prepared for one dose if the product is available as a 160 mg/5 mL suspension?

33. An 8-year-old child weighs 68 lb (30.9 kg) and is to take acyclovir, which has a normal adult dose of 600 mg.

    a. Using Young's Rule, what is the appropriate pediatric dose?

    b. Using Clark's Rule, what is the appropriate pediatric dose?

    Self-check your work in Appendix A.

Chapter Summary

- The basic units of measure in the metric system are meter (length), gram (weight), and liter (volume).
- The metric system uses prefixes that describe the value of the unit by multiples of 10, 100, or 1000.
- The milligram and microgram are the two most common units of weight measure in the pharmacy.
- A gram weighs about the same as a large paper clip.
- The liter and milliliter are the two most common units of volumetric measure in the pharmacy.
- Many beverages are measured in 1-, 2-, and 3-liter bottles.
- The meter and centimeter are the two most common units of measure used to describe lengths and heights in a healthcare setting.
- A meter is about the same length as a yard, or three feet.
- Converting units in the metric system often requires multiplying or dividing by 1000, *or* moving the decimal point three places when changing the unit of measure.
- Use the ratio-proportion method to convert the unit if you need a foolproof way to perform the conversion—especially if you get confused as to which direction you should move the decimal point.

- The dimensional analysis method can be used to convert units of measure.
- When solving a story problem, remember to identify what the question is asking for, then designate this unknown variable with the letter x when writing your calculations.
- Always double-check that units in the numerator positions match on both sides of your ratio-proportion; the units in the denominator positions should match as well.
- When solving for x, cross out (cancel) your units to verify that you are left with the correct unit.
- You should always check your answer by multiplying the two means and the two extremes in your ratio.
- Pediatric patients often need a dose customized for them based on their weight.
- Body surface area is used to calculate some patients' doses, especially chemotherapy agents for pediatric patients.
- Clark's Rule and Young's Rule are older methods of calculating a pediatric dose based on what is normal for an adult dose.

Formulas for Success

Young's Rule	$\dfrac{\text{age (in years)}}{\text{age} + 12 \text{ years}} \times \text{adult dose} = \text{pediatric dose}$
Clark's Rule	$\dfrac{\text{weight (in lb)}}{150 \text{ lb}} \times \text{adult dose} = \text{pediatric dose}$

Important Equivalencies

TABLE 4.4 Metric Unit Equivalents

Kilo	Base	Milli	Micro
0.001 kg	1 g	1000 mg	1,000,000 mcg
0.001 kL	1 L	1000 mL	1,000,000 mcL
0.001 km	1 m	1000 mm	1,000,000 mcm

TABLE 4.5 Steps for Using the Ratio-Proportion Method for Solving Story Problems

Step 1. Read through the entire problem and identify what the question is asking for. This becomes the variable x, labeled with the unit you are looking for such as x mg or x mL.

Step 2. Identify the prescriber's order. Circle the dose ordered by the physician.

Step 3. Identify the appropriate stock available in the pharmacy. The ratio of pharmacy stock, such as 1 mg/tablet or 125 mg/5 mL, should be found on the labels of the drugs used in the pharmacy. Underline this information.

Step 4. Identify extraneous information. It is often helpful to draw a single pencil line through any information you identify as not needed. This prevents you from using that information in your setup.

Step 5. Estimate what your answer should be. Compare the ordered dose to what is on hand. Will the dose be larger or smaller than the dosage unit given?

Step 6. Use the ratio-proportion method to solve for x. When using the ratio-proportion method to solve your problem, place the physician-ordered dosage on the left side of the proportion and the pharmacy on-hand ratio on the right side.

Step 7. Round your answer to the appropriate number of significant figures. Weights are typically rounded to the nearest whole milligram, and volumes are typically rounded to the nearest tenth of a milliliter.

Key Terms

body surface area (BSA) a measurement related to a patient's weight and height, expressed in meters squared (m²), and used to calculate patient-specific doses of medications

Clark's Rule a formula used to determine an appropriate pediatric dose by using the child's weight in pounds and the normal adult dose; weight in lb/150 lb × adult dose = pediatric dose

dimensional analysis method a conversion method in which the given number and unit are multiplied by the ratio of the desired unit to the given unit, which is equivalent to 1

gram the basic unit for measuring weight in the metric system

liter the basic unit for measuring volume in the metric system

meter the basic unit for measuring length in the metric system

metric system a measurement system based on subdivisions and multiples of 10; made up of three basic units: meter, gram, and liter

vehicle an inert medium, such as a syrup, in which a drug is administered

Young's Rule a formula used to determine an appropriate pediatric dose by using the child's age in years and the normal adult dose; age in years/(age in years + 12 years) × adult dose = pediatric dose

Chapter Review

Assessing Comprehension

To check your comprehension of this chapter's key concepts, read the following multiple-choice questions and then record your answers on a separate sheet of paper. Write your answers as modeled in these examples: 1d; 2c; 3b; etc.

1. The metric system unit of measure for weight is the
   a. meter.
   b. liter.
   c. milliliter.
   d. gram.

2. When converting from a larger unit (liter) to a smaller unit (milliliter), move the decimal point
   a. two places to the left.
   b. two places to the right.
   c. three places to the left.
   d. three places to the right.

3. A foolproof way to convert metric units is to use
   a. the dimensional analysis method.
   b. Clark's Rule.
   c. the ratio-proportion method.
   d. Young's Rule.

4. Why are leading zeros used in pharmacy calculations?
   a. to ensure the decimal point is in the correct place
   b. to avoid medication errors resulting from incorrect interpretation of numbers
   c. to improve the accuracy of the calculations
   d. to verify that the correct conversion has been made

5. Which units should match when using the ratio-proportion method?
   a. the numerators only
   b. the denominators only
   c. both the numerators and denominators
   d. the BSA and the conversion factor

6. The dimensional analysis method uses the principle of
   a. moving the decimal point three places to the right or left.
   b. matching the numerators and denominators on both sides of an equation.
   c. multiplying by an equivalent of "1" to obtain a conversion of units or cancellation of units.
   d. converting all units to the metric system.

7. The first step to solve a story problem is to
   a. determine the unknown variable x.
   b. convert metric units to grams.
   c. match the numerators on both sides of the equation.
   d. round the dose to the nearest tenth.

8. The *vehicle* is the
   a. inert medium, such as a syrup, that is used in drug administration.
   b. conversion factor used in pharmacy calculations.
   c. math formula used in the dimensional analysis method.
   d. method used to interpret a nomogram.

9. A pediatric patient often needs
   a. half of the adult dose.
   b. a customized patient-specific dose.
   c. a standardized dose.
   d. a geriatric dose.

10. What units do manufacturers commonly use when providing prescribing guidelines for medications?
    a. milliliters of medication per kilograms of body weight
    b. grams of medication per kilograms of body weight
    c. milligrams of medication per kilograms of body weight
    d. millimeters of medication per pounds of body weight

Finding Solutions

To gain practice in handling challenging situations in the workplace, consider the following real-world scenarios and then use the guiding questions to help you formulate your responses.

Scenario A: A mother approaches you and hands you a prescription for thioridazine for her son, who weighs 15 kg and is 41 inches tall. The manufacturer of thioridazine recommends a dose between 0.5 mg/kg to a maximum of 3 mg/kg per day for children, to be given in divided doses. The boy's physician has prescribed 15 mg every 12 hours.

1. Calculate the minimum daily dose for this pediatric patient.

2. Calculate the maximum daily dose for this pediatric patient.

3. Is the physician's dose within the recommended safe range?

4. How many milliliters of 5 mg/mL strength thioridizine suspension will be given at each prescribed dose?

Scenario B: Your pharmacy just received a prescription from a pediatrician for acetaminophen 325 mg. Her pediatric patient weighs 21.8 kg and is 52 inches in height. The manufacturer of acetaminophen has a recommended dose of 10 to 15 mg/kg per day.

5. Calculate the minimum daily dose for this pediatric patient.

6. Calculate the maximum daily dose for this pediatric patient.

7. Is the physician's dose within the recommended safe range?

8. How many milliliters will be prepared for one prescribed dose if the product is available as a 160 mg/5 mL suspension?

Scenario C: A 12-year-old child, who weighs 80 lb (36.36 kg), has been prescribed zidovudine. The normal adult dose is 600 mg.

9. Using Young's Rule, what is the appropriate pediatric dose?

10. Using Clark's Rule, what is the appropriate pediatric dose?

Scenario D: An e-prescription for Flumadine arrived at your pharmacy for a 9-year-old child who weighs 62 lb (28.2 kg). Flumadine has a normal adult dose of 100 mg twice daily for 7 days.

11. Using Young's Rule, what is the appropriate pediatric dose?

12. Using Clark's Rule, what is the appropriate pediatric dose?

Sampling the Certification Exam

To provide you with practice for the Certification Exam, read the following questions that have been patterned after the test format and then record your answers on a separate sheet of paper. Write your answers as modeled in these examples: 1d; 2c; 3b; etc.

1. Which amount indicates the correct conversion of 125 micrograms to milligrams?
   a. 0.125 mg
   b. 1.25 mg
   c. 12.5 mg
   d. 125,000 mg

2. A patient is to receive 6.25 mg of diphenhydramine. If the available dosage strength is 12.5 mg/5 mL, how many milliliters would be needed?
   a. 2 mL
   b. 2.5 mL
   c. 5 mL
   d. 7.5 mL

3. A patient weighs 9.4 kg and is to receive Levaquin at 8 mg/kg two times daily. How many milligrams per dose will the patient receive?
   a. 9.4 mg
   b. 18.75 mg
   c. 75 mg
   d. 363 mg

4. A patient is taking 0.6 g oxcarbazepine daily in a divided dose: one dose in the morning and one dose at night. The label reads 300 mg/5 mL. How many milliliters does the patient take each morning?
   a. 2.5 mL
   b. 5 mL
   c. 6 mL
   d. 12 mL

5. A patient is to receive 14,000 units of heparin *stat.* The vial on hand is a 10 mL bottle of 5,000 units/mL. How many milliliters will this be?
   a. 2.8 mL
   b. 3.5 mL
   c. 5 mL
   d. 5.6 mL

To put your pharmacy calculation skills to the test, read the following questions and then record your answers on a separate sheet of paper.

Note: *Questions 8, 10, 14, 15, and 16 have accompanying handouts that must be obtained from your instructor.*

Convert the following units within the metric system.

1. 1821 mcg = _____ mg

2. 6864 mg = _____ g

3. 34.5 mg = _____ mcg

4. 186 g = _____ kg

Calculate the following.

5. A patient is to take 2.25 g of amoxicillin before a dental procedure. The capsules available are 250 mg per capsule. How many capsules will be dispensed to this patient?

6. A dose of an antacid is 30 mL. How many doses can be prepared from a 360 mL bottle?

7. A patient has a prescription order for 15 mg of a medication to be taken at bedtime on the night prior to hospitalization. The pharmacy has a partial container of 2.5 mg tablets. How many tablets will the patient need?

8. A patient is to receive 4 mg of haloperidol. The pharmacy has on hand a 1 mL vial of 5 mg/mL solution. How many milliliters are needed to fill this prescription? On the handout that you obtained from your instructor, indicate the correct volume on the correct measuring device.

9. A total regimen of therapy calls for 70 mg of a medication to be given to a patient over several days. In the pharmacy, a solution is available with 100 mcg/mL. How many milliliters must be dispensed to complete the regimen?

10. A patient receives 1.2 mg of atropine, shown in the label. How many milliliters is this? On the handout that you

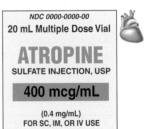

obtained from your instructor, indicate the correct volume on the correct measuring device.

11. A patient receives 2.8 mL of the atropine solution shown in the label. How many micrograms is this?

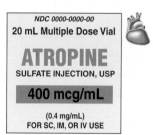

NDC 0000-0000-00
20 mL Multiple Dose Vial
ATROPINE
SULFATE INJECTION, USP
400 mcg/mL
(0.4 mg/mL)
FOR SC, IM, OR IV USE

12. A total regimen of a drug calls for 720 mg to be given. If two doses equal 80 mg, how many doses will have to be given?

13. You have 480 mL of a solution that contains 8 g. How many micrograms are in 4 mL of solution? (Round your answer to the nearest tens place.)

14. A patient is to receive 7000 units of heparin. Heparin is available as 5,000 units/mL. How many milliliters do you prepare? On the handout that you obtained from your instructor, indicate the correct volume on the correct measuring device.

15. A pediatric patient is to take 45 mcg of digoxin each morning. The pediatric elixir is available in a 60 mL dropper bottle with the concentration 0.05 mg/mL. How many milliliters will the patient take with each dose? On the handout that you obtained from your instructor, indicate the correct volume on the correct measuring device.

16. A patient is to take 200 mcg of a drug each morning. The medication is available in a 0.4 mg/5 mL solution. How many milliliters will the patient take each morning? On the handout that you obtained from your instructor, indicate the correct volume on the correct measuring device.

Calculate the following weight-based BSA doses based on the provided recommended dose. (Use the nomograms in Figures 4.2 and 4.3 to determine the BSA values when necessary.)

17. A medication is dosed at 8 mg/kg divided into three equal doses daily. The adult patient is 67 inches in height and weighs 63 kg. How many milligrams will be given at each dose?

18. A medication is dosed at 0.5 mg/m^2 per day. The pediatric patient is 34 inches in height and weighs 32 lb. What is the recommended dose for this patient?

19. A newborn weighs 3.86 kg and is to be given medication at 5 mg/kg per day divided into two doses. How much will each dose be?

20. A patient weighs 73 kg and is 67 inches in height. He is to be dosed at 125 mg/m^2 per day. How many milligrams is this?

Using Household Measure in Pharmacy Calculations

5

Learning Objectives

- Identify units of household measure and convert between them.
- Solve medication problems by using household measure and the metric system.
- Convert body weight between kilograms and pounds.
- Determine pediatric doses using dosing tables.
- Calculate the amount of medication to be dispensed.
- Calculate temperature conversions between Celsius and Fahrenheit.

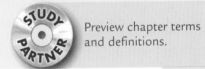

Preview chapter terms and definitions.

5.1 Household Measure

Household measure is a system of measure used in homes, particularly in kitchens, in the United States. The units of household measure for volume include teaspoonful, tablespoonful, cup, pint, quart, and gallon. The units of household measure for weight are pounds and ounces. Table 5.1 lists the household measure equivalents and their abbreviations. Figure 5.1 on the following page illustrates the more often used equivalents in household measure.

Safety in Numbers

To avoid misreading c for c̄ or 0, do not abbreviate *cup*.

TABLE 5.1 Household Measure Equivalents

Volume		Weight	
3 teaspoonsful (tsp)	= 1 tablespoonful (tbsp)	1 pound (lb)	= 16 ounces (oz)
2 tablespoonsful (tbsp)	= 1 fluid ounce (fl oz)		
8 fluid ounces (fl oz)	= 1 cup		
2 cups	= 1 pint (pt)		
2 pints (pt)	= 1 quart (qt)		
4 quarts (qt)	= 1 gallon (gal)		

FIGURE 5.1
Household Measure Equivalents

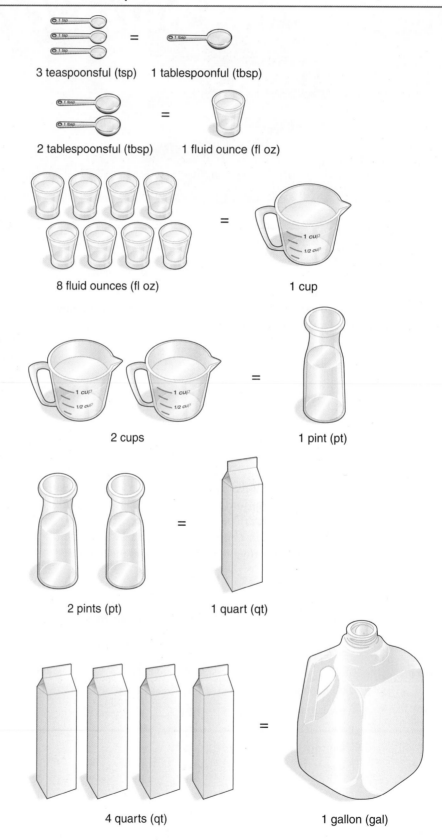

3 teaspoonsful (tsp)　　1 tablespoonful (tbsp)

2 tablespoonsful (tbsp)　　1 fluid ounce (fl oz)

8 fluid ounces (fl oz)　　　　1 cup

2 cups　　　　1 pint (pt)

2 pints (pt)　　1 quart (qt)

4 quarts (qt)　　　　1 gallon (gal)

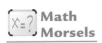

Measuring volume using the household measure is less accurate than using other systems because the measuring utensils can vary in size. Nevertheless, household volume measure may be used in community pharmacy practice when dispensing drugs that will be administered in the patient's home because patients may not have other measuring devices at their disposal. Labels instructing patients on how to take a medication often use household measure units for this reason.

However, there is a growing trend among prescribers and pharmacies to use the preferred metric system for medication dosage. To that end, dosage spoons marked with both metric and household measurements are commonly provided to patients at minimal or no cost.

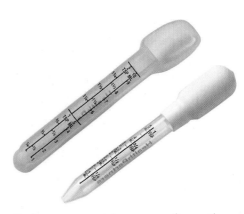

Dosing spoons and droppers are frequently marked with metric and household measures.

Converting Household Volume Measures

Like all systems, units of household volume measures can be converted to larger or smaller units. The following examples will demonstrate this type of conversion.

Example 5.1.1

How many teaspoonfuls are in two tablespoonfuls?

Begin the solution by noting the appropriate equivalents indicated in Table 5.1 and Figure 5.1.

$$3 \text{ tsp} = 1 \text{ tbsp}$$

Using these equivalents, the solution can be determined in two ways.

Solution 1: Using the ratio-proportion method:

$$\frac{x \text{ tsp}}{2 \text{ tbsp}} = \frac{3 \text{ tsp}}{1 \text{ tbsp}}$$

$$\frac{(2 \text{ tbsp}) \, x \text{ tsp}}{2 \text{ tbsp}} = \frac{(2 \text{ tbsp}) \, 3 \text{ tsp}}{1 \text{ tbsp}}$$

$$x = 6 \text{ tsp}$$

Solution 2: Using the dimensional analysis method:

$$2 \text{ tbsp} \times \frac{3 \text{ tsp}}{1 \text{ tbsp}} = 6 \text{ tsp}$$

Example 5.1.2

How many tablespoonsful are in 2 cups of medication?

Begin the solution by noting the appropriate equivalents indicated in Table 5.1 and Figure 5.1.

$$2 \text{ tbsp} = 1 \text{ fl oz}$$
$$1 \text{ cup} = 8 \text{ fl oz}$$

Using these equivalents, the solution can be determined in two ways.

Solution 1: Using the ratio-proportion method, first determine the number of fluid ounces in 2 cups.

$$\frac{x \text{ fl oz}}{2 \text{ cups}} = \frac{8 \text{ fl oz}}{1 \text{ cup}}$$

$$\frac{(2 \text{ cups}) \, x \text{ fl oz}}{2 \text{ cups}} = \frac{(2 \text{ cups}) \, 8 \text{ fl oz}}{1 \text{ cup}}$$

$$x \text{ fl oz} = 16 \text{ fl oz}$$

Second, determine the number of tablespoonsful in 16 fl oz.

$$\frac{x \text{ tbsp}}{16 \text{ fl oz}} = \frac{2 \text{ tbsp}}{1 \text{ fl oz}}$$

$$\frac{(16 \text{ fl oz}) \, x \text{ tbsp}}{16 \text{ fl oz}} = \frac{(16 \text{ fl oz}) \, 2 \text{ tbsp}}{1 \text{ fl oz}}$$

$$x \text{ tbsp} = 32 \text{ tbsp}$$

Solution 2: Using the dimensional analysis method,

$$x \text{ tbsp} = 2 \text{ cups} \times \frac{8 \text{ fl oz}}{1 \text{ cup}} \times \frac{2 \text{ tbsp}}{1 \text{ fl oz}} = 32 \text{ tbsp}$$

Note that the cup units cancel, the fluid ounce units cancel, and the tablespoonsful unit remains.

Example 5.1.3

How many 1 tsp doses are in 3 cups of liquid medication?

Begin the solution by noting the appropriate equivalents indicated in Table 5.1.

$$3 \text{ tsp} = 1 \text{ tbsp}$$
$$2 \text{ tbsp} = 1 \text{ fl oz}$$
$$8 \text{ fl oz} = 1 \text{ cup}$$

Using these equivalents, the solution can be determined in two ways.

Solution 1: Using the ratio-proportion method, first determine the number of fluid ounces in 3 cups.

$$\frac{x \text{ fl oz}}{3 \text{ cups}} = \frac{8 \text{ fl oz}}{1 \text{ cup}}$$

$$\frac{(3 \text{ cups}) \, x \text{ fl oz}}{3 \text{ cups}} = \frac{(3 \text{ cups}) \, 8 \text{ fl oz}}{1 \text{ cup}}$$

$$x \text{ fl oz} = 24 \text{ fl oz}$$

Second, calculate the number of tablespoonful in 24 fl oz.

$$\frac{x \text{ tbsp}}{24 \text{ fl oz}} = \frac{2 \text{ tbsp}}{1 \text{ fl oz}}$$

$$\frac{(24 \text{ fl oz}) \, x \text{ tbsp}}{24 \text{ fl oz}} = \frac{(24 \text{ fl oz}) \, 2 \text{ tbsp}}{1 \text{ fl oz}}$$

$$x \text{ tbsp} = 48 \text{ tbsp}$$

Third, determine the number of teaspoonful in 48 tbsp.

$$\frac{x \text{ tsp}}{48 \text{ tbsp}} = \frac{3 \text{ tsp}}{1 \text{ tbsp}}$$

$$\frac{(48 \text{ tbsp}) \, x \text{ tsp}}{48 \text{ tbsp}} = \frac{(48 \text{ tbsp}) \, 3 \text{ tsp}}{1 \text{ tbsp}}$$

$$x \text{ tsp} = 144 \text{ tsp}$$

Solution 2: Using the dimensional analysis method,

$$x \text{ tsp} = 3 \text{ cups} \times \frac{8 \text{ fl oz}}{1 \text{ cup}} \times \frac{2 \text{ tbsp}}{1 \text{ fl oz}} \times \frac{3 \text{ tsp}}{1 \text{ tbsp}} = 144 \text{ tsp}$$

Note that the cup units cancel, the fluid ounce units cancel, the tablespoonful units cancel, and the teaspoonful unit remains.

Example 5.1.4

How many 1 fl oz doses are in 3 pt of liquid medication?

Begin the solution by noting the appropriate equivalents indicated in Table 5.1.

$$8 \text{ fl oz} = 1 \text{ cup}$$
$$2 \text{ cups} = 1 \text{ pt}$$
$$2 \text{ pt} = 1 \text{ qt}$$

Using these equivalents, the solution can be determined in two ways.

Solution 1: Using the ratio-proportion method, first determine the number of cups in 3 pt.

2 cups   1 pt

$$\frac{x \text{ cups}}{3 \text{ pt}} = \frac{2 \text{ cups}}{1 \text{ pt}}$$

$$x \text{ cups} = 6 \text{ cups}$$

Second, calculate the number of fluid ounces in 6 cups.

$$\frac{x \text{ fl oz}}{6 \text{ cups}} = \frac{8 \text{ fl oz}}{1 \text{ cup}}$$

$$x \text{ fl oz} = 48 \text{ fl oz}$$

8 fl oz   1 cup

Solution 2: Using the dimensional analysis method,

$$x \text{ fl oz} = 3 \text{ pt} \times \frac{2 \text{ cups}}{1 \text{ pt}} \times \frac{8 \text{ fl oz}}{1 \text{ cup}} = 48 \text{ fl oz}$$

Example 5.1.5

How many 1 fl oz doses are in 2 qt of liquid medication?

Begin the solution by noting the appropriate equivalents indicated in Table 5.1.

$$8 \text{ fl oz} = 1 \text{ cup}$$
$$2 \text{ cups} = 1 \text{ pt}$$
$$2 \text{ pt} = 1 \text{ qt}$$

Using these equivalents, the solution can be determined in two ways:

Solution 1: Using the ratio-proportion method, first determine the number of pints in 2 qt.

2 pt   1 qt

$$\frac{x \text{ pt}}{2 \text{ qt}} = \frac{2 \text{ pt}}{1 \text{ qt}}$$

$$x \text{ pt} = 4 \text{ pt}$$

Second, calculate the number of cups in 4 pt.

2 cups   1 pt

$$\frac{x \text{ cup}}{4 \text{ pt}} = \frac{2 \text{ cups}}{1 \text{ pt}}$$

$$x \text{ cup} = 8 \text{ cups}$$

Third, determine the number of fluid ounces in 8 cups.

$$\frac{x \text{ fl oz}}{8 \text{ cups}} = \frac{8 \text{ fl oz}}{1 \text{ cup}}$$

$$x \text{ fl oz} = 64 \text{ fl oz}$$

8 fl oz   1 cup

Solution 2: Using the dimensional analysis method,

$$x \text{ fl oz} = 2 \cancel{\text{qt}} \times \frac{2 \cancel{\text{pt}}}{1 \cancel{\text{qt}}} \times \frac{2 \cancel{\text{cups}}}{1 \cancel{\text{pt}}} \times \frac{8 \text{ fl oz}}{1 \cancel{\text{cup}}} = 64 \text{ fl oz}$$

Converting between Household Measure and the Metric System

Because of the inaccuracy of the measuring tools used in household measure, it is often preferable to convert all quantities into the metric system. These conversions may seem like additional work for some problems, but using the metric system will serve you better than relying on the household system, which is declining in use.

Prescriptions that are interpreted and entered into a computer as part of the patient's record will need to be converted to the metric system. Typically, such computer programs are set up to accept quantity measurements using milliliters for liquid prescriptions and grams for solid prescriptions such as for creams or ointments. When a prescription is written for a liquid, the volume to be dispensed and the quantity to be given at each dose will be used to calculate the amount of medication needed for 24 hours, or one day. Calculating the volume to be dispensed and days' supply are important steps in the processing of each prescription. These calculations provide the pharmacist information that is needed to accurately fill the prescription, ensuring that the patient is getting the prescribed therapy.

Although some references list exact values for conversions between the household measure and the metric system, the equivalents shown in Table 5.2 and Figure 5.2 on the following page are generally accepted for use for these conversions in daily pharmacy practice. All of these conversion values should be committed to memory.

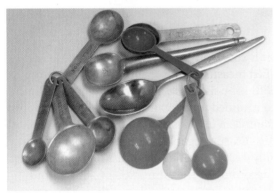

The volume held by a household teaspoon may vary, but a true teaspoon equals 5 mL.

TABLE 5.2   Household Measure and Metric System Conversion Values

Volume		Weight	
1 tsp	= 5 mL	1 oz	= 30 g[†]
1 tbsp	= 15 mL	1 lb	= 454 g[†]
1 fl oz	= 30 mL*	2.2 lb	= 1 kg
1 cup	= 240 mL		
1 pt	= 480 mL*		
1 qt	= 960 mL		
1 gal	= 3840 mL		

* There are actually 29.57 mL in 1 fl oz, but 30 mL is usually used. When packaging a pint, companies will typically include 473 mL, rather than the full 480 mL. Additionally, 1 gal is actually equivalent to 3785 mL.

[†] There are actually 28.34952 g in an avoirdupois ounce; however, pharmacy personnel often round up to 30 g. It is common practice to use 454 g as the equivalent for a pound (28.35 g × 16 oz/lb = 453.6 g/lb, rounded to 454 g/lb).

FIGURE 5.2
Household Measure and Metric System Conversion Volume Values

Most common household measure and metric system equivalents for volume

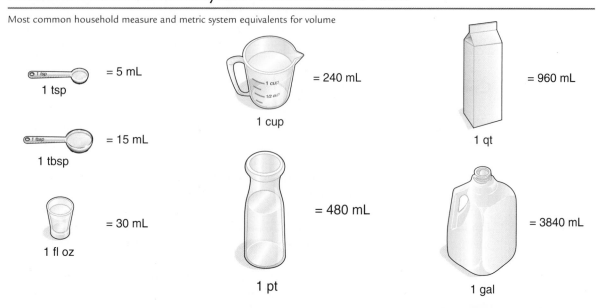

As seen in Table 5.2 and Figure 5.2, it is common practice to round a household fluid ounce (29.57 mL) up to 30 mL. When measuring this amount, this estimation is often appropriate because the volume differs by such a small amount. When measuring multiple fluid ounces that have been rounded up to 30 mL, however, the discrepancy becomes far more apparent. For example, if asked to measure a pint (16 fl oz), you would measure roughly 480 mL. This measurement becomes problematic because 29.57 mL multiplied by 16 is equal to only 473.12 mL, not 480 mL. Most stock bottles are labeled 473 mL, yet pharmacies bill according to the estimation of 480 mL and measure out fluid ounces in 30 mL increments. For the purposes of this chapter, use the rounded 30 mL and 480 mL values.

The following examples show some typical conversion problems the pharmacy technician must be able to solve.

Example 5.1.6

You are to dispense 300 mL of hydrocodone bitartrate/APAP 7.5 mg/500 mg per 15 mL solution. The prescription states the patient is to take 2 tsp BID. How many doses will the dispensed volume contain?

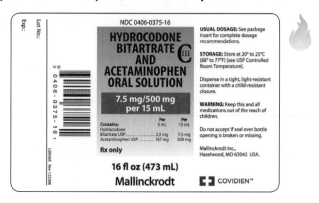

2 tsp = 10 mL

Begin solving this problem by converting to a common unit of measure using the conversion values in Table 5.2 and Figure 5.2.

$$1 \text{ dose} = 2 \text{ tsp} = 2 \times 5 \text{ mL} = 10 \text{ mL}$$

Using these converted measurements, the solution can be determined in two ways:

Solution 1: Using the ratio-proportion method and the metric system,

$$\frac{x \text{ doses}}{300 \text{ mL}} = \frac{1 \text{ dose}}{10 \text{ mL}}$$

$$\frac{(300 \text{ mL}) \, x \text{ doses}}{300 \text{ mL}} = \frac{(300 \text{ mL}) \, 1 \text{ dose}}{10 \text{ mL}}$$

$$x \text{ doses} = 30 \text{ doses}$$

Solution 2: Using the dimensional analysis method,

$$300 \text{ mL} \times \frac{1 \text{ dose}}{10 \text{ mL}} = 30 \text{ doses}$$

Example 5.1.7

Using the medication and dosing instructions in Example 5.1.6, how many days will the 300 mL last?

The patient is to take 1 dose twice daily (BID), and, as calculated in Example 5.1.6, there are 30 doses in the dispensed volume.

$$\frac{x \text{ days}}{30 \text{ doses}} = \frac{1 \text{ day}}{2 \text{ doses}}$$

$$x = 15 \text{ days}$$

$$30 \text{ doses} \times \frac{1 \text{ day}}{2 \text{ doses}} = 15 \text{ days}$$

Example 5.1.8

A patient is to purchase a 12 fl oz bottle of antacid. The patient is to take 15 mL before each meal and at bedtime. How many doses does the bottle contain?

1 fl oz = 30 mL

Begin solving this problem by converting to a common unit of measure using the conversion values in Table 5.2 and Figure 5.2. Using the conversion values in the table will become easier with practice and with writing out the conversions or saying them out loud.

1 fl oz = 30 mL, so 0.5 fl oz = 15 mL, and 12 fl oz = 360 mL

Using these converted measurements, the solution can be determined in three ways:

Solution 1: Using the ratio-proportion method and the metric system,

$$\frac{x \text{ doses}}{360 \text{ mL}} = \frac{1 \text{ dose}}{15 \text{ mL}}$$

$$x \text{ dose} = 24 \text{ doses}$$

Solution 2: Using the dimensional analysis method and the metric system,

$$360 \text{ mL} \times \frac{1 \text{ dose}}{15 \text{ mL}} = 24 \text{ doses}$$

Solution 3: Using the dimensional analysis method and the household system,

$$12 \text{ fl oz} \times \frac{1 \text{ dose}}{0.5 \text{ fl oz}} = 24 \text{ doses}$$

Example 5.1.9

Using the medication and dosing instructions in Example 5.1.8 , if the patient eats three times a day, how many days will the 12 fl oz bottle last?

The patient is to take 1 dose with every meal and at bedtime, so a daily dose is

$$\frac{1 \text{ dose}}{\text{meal}} \times \frac{3 \text{ meals}}{\text{day}} + 1 \text{ dose at bedtime} = \frac{4 \text{ doses}}{\text{day}}$$

If 24 doses are dispensed, as calculated in Example 5.1.7,

$$24 \text{ doses} \times \frac{1 \text{ day}}{4 \text{ doses}} = 6 \text{ days}$$

Example 5.1.10

How many 2 tbsp doses are in 480 mL?

1 tbsp = 15 mL

Using the conversion values in Table 5.2 and Figure 5.2, 1 tbsp = 15 mL. Because 1 dose equals 2 tbsp,

$$1 \text{ dose} = 2 \text{ tbsp} = 2 \times 15 \text{ mL} = 30 \text{ mL}$$

Using these converted measurements, this problem can be solved in two ways.

Solution 1: Using the ratio-proportion method,

$$\frac{x \text{ doses}}{480 \text{ mL}} = \frac{1 \text{ dose}}{30 \text{ mL}}$$

$$x \text{ dose} = 16 \text{ doses}$$

Solution 2: Using the dimensional analysis method,

$$480 \ \cancel{mL} \times \frac{1 \ \text{dose}}{30 \ \cancel{mL}} = 16 \ \text{doses}$$

Example 5.1.11

Theophylline elixir contains 80 mg/15 mL. A dose is 2 tbsp. How many milligrams are in 1 dose of the theophylline elixir?

Using the conversion values in Table 5.2 and Figure 5.2,

$$1 \ \text{dose} = 2 \ \text{tbsp} = 2 \times 15 \ \text{mL} = 30 \ \text{mL}$$

This problem can be solved in two ways:

Solution 1: Using the ratio-proportion method,

$$\frac{x \ \text{mg}}{30 \ \text{mL}} = \frac{80 \ \text{mg}}{15 \ \text{mL}}$$

$$x \ \text{mg} = 160 \ \text{mg}$$

NDC 0000-0000-00
THEOPHYLLINE ELIXIR
Contains 80 mg/15 mL
480 mL
Dispense in tight, light-resistant container.
R$_x$ only

Solution 2: Using the dimensional analysis method,

$$30 \ \cancel{mL} \times \frac{80 \ \text{mg}}{15 \ \cancel{mL}} = 160 \ \text{mg}$$

Like volumes, weights can be converted between household measure and metric measure. The most common conversions are between the household measurements of pounds and ounces and the metric measurements of kilograms and grams. These conversions were presented in Table 5.2.

Example 5.1.12

A physician has written a prescription for a 1.5 oz tube of ointment. How many grams is this?

Since 1 oz equals 30 g, this problem can be solved in two ways:

Solution 1: Using the ratio-proportion method,

$$\frac{x \ \text{g}}{1.5 \ \text{oz}} = \frac{30 \ \text{g}}{1 \ \text{oz}}$$

$$x \ \text{g} = 45 \ \text{g}$$

Solution 2: Using the dimensional analysis method,

$$1.5 \ \cancel{oz} \times \frac{30 \ \text{g}}{1 \ \cancel{oz}} = 45 \ \text{g}$$

Example 5.1.13

You have a 1 lb jar of ointment available. You are instructed to use this stock to fill smaller jars with 20 g of ointment each. How many jars can you fill?

Because 1 lb equals 454 g, this problem can be solved in two ways.

Solution 1: Using the ratio-proportion method,

$$\frac{x \text{ jars}}{454 \text{ g}} = \frac{1 \text{ jar}}{20 \text{ g}}$$

$$x \text{ jar} = 22.7 \text{ jars, or 22 full jars}$$

Solution 2: Using the dimensional analysis method,

$$454 \text{ g} \times \frac{1 \text{ jar}}{20 \text{ g}} = 22.7 \text{ jars, or 22 full jars}$$

In both solutions, there is 0.7 jar of ointment remaining. You can determine how many grams of ointment are left over with the following calculation:

$$\frac{20 \text{ g}}{\text{jar}} \times 0.7 \text{ jar leftover ointment} = 14 \text{ g leftover ointment}$$

Converting Body Weight

As discussed in the previous chapter, drugs are sometimes dosed based on the weight of the patient. Increasingly, drug manufacturers are providing a recommended dose based on a specific dose in milligrams per kilogram of the patient's weight. Because most drugs are dosed on the basis of kilograms, if a patient's weight is documented in pounds, the weight will have to be converted to kilograms before calculating the appropriate dose.

Example 5.1.14

 Math Morsels

Pharmacy technicians should remember the following conversion: 2.2 lb = 1 kg

A patient weighs 134 lb. What is this patient's weight in kilograms?

Since 1 kg equals 2.2 lb, this problem can be solved in two ways:

Solution 1: Using the ratio-proportion method,

$$\frac{x \text{ kg}}{134 \text{ lb}} = \frac{1 \text{ kg}}{2.2 \text{ lb}}$$

$$x \text{ kg} = 60.909 \text{ kg, rounded to } 60.9 \text{ kg}$$

Solution 2: Using the dimensional analysis method,

$$134 \text{ lb} \times \frac{1 \text{ kg}}{2.2 \text{ lb}} = 60.909 \text{ kg, rounded to } 60.9 \text{ kg}$$

Example 5.1.15

A patient weighs 76 lb. What is this patient's weight in kilograms?

Because 1 kg equals 2.2 lb, this problem can be solved in two ways:

Solution 1: Using the ratio-proportion method,

$$\frac{x \, \text{kg}}{76 \, \text{lb}} = \frac{1 \, \text{kg}}{2.2 \, \text{lb}}$$

$$x \, \text{kg} = 34.545 \, \text{kg}, \text{ rounded to } 34.5 \, \text{kg}$$

Solution 2: Using the dimensional analysis method,

$$76 \, \cancel{\text{lb}} \times \frac{1 \, \text{kg}}{2.2 \, \cancel{\text{lb}}} = 34.545 \, \text{kg}, \text{ rounded to } 34.5 \, \text{kg}$$

A kilogram is equal to 2.2 lb, which is slightly more than two boxes of pasta.

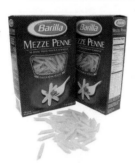

Although it is important to understand the conversion using both the ratio-proportion and the dimensional analysis methods, a shorthand method for converting a patient's weight from pounds to kilograms is to divide the amount by 2.2 lb/1 kg. Similarly, you can convert a patient's weight from kilograms to pounds by multiplying it by 2.2 lb/1 kg.

Example 5.1.16

A patient weighs 58 kg. What is this patient's weight in pounds?

$$58 \, \text{kg} \times 2.2 \, \text{lb}/1 \, \text{kg} = 127.6 \, \text{lb}$$

Check this answer by converting the answer from pounds back to kilograms.

$$127.6 \, \text{lb} \times 1 \, \text{kg}/2.2 \, \text{lb} = 58 \, \text{kg}$$

Example 5.1.17

A patient in the neonatal ICU weighs 1250 g. How many pounds is this?

First, convert the grams to kilograms.

$$1250 \, \text{g} = 1.25 \, \text{kg}$$

Second, convert kilograms to pounds.

$$1.25 \, \text{kg} \times 2.2 \, \text{lb}/1 \, \text{kg} = 2.75 \, \text{lb}$$

Check the answer by converting the answer from pounds back to kilograms.

$$2.75 \, \text{lb} \times 1 \, \text{kg}/2.2 \, \text{lb} = 1.25 \, \text{kg}$$

5.1 Problem Set

Convert the given volumes within the household measure system. Round your answer to the nearest tenth unless otherwise indicated.

1. 8 cups = _____ pt

2. 3 pt = _____ fl oz

3. 1 pt = _____ tbsp

4. 3 qt = _____ fl oz

5. 28 tsp = _____ fl oz

6. 1 pt = _____ qt

7. 6 cups = _____ tsp

Convert the given volumes between the household measure and metric systems. Round your answer to the nearest tenth unless otherwise indicated.

8. 80 mL = _____ tbsp

9. 6 fl oz = _____ mL

10. 90 mL = _____ fl oz

11. 800 mL = _____ pt

12. 53 mL = _____ tsp

13. 35 mL = _____ tsp

14. 10 L = _____ gal

15. 4 tbsp = _____ mL

16. 15 mL = _____ tsp

17. 720 mL = _____ pt

18. 30 tsp = _____ mL

19. 120 mL = _____ fl oz

20. ½ gal = _____ mL

21. 2 L = _____ pt

Convert the following commonly used volumes to milliliters. Round your answer to the nearest tenth unless otherwise indicated.

22. 3 tbsp = _____ mL

23. 1 fl oz = _____ mL

24. 2 fl oz = _____ mL

25. 3 fl oz = _____ mL

26. 4 fl oz = _____ mL

27. 5 fl oz = _____ mL

28. 6 fl oz = _____ mL

29. 7 fl oz = _____ mL

30. 8 fl oz = _____ mL

31. 12 fl oz = _____ mL

32. 16 fl oz = _____ mL

Convert the following weights between the household measure and metric systems. Round your answer to the nearest tenth unless otherwise indicated.

33. 2 oz = _____ g

34. 1.5 oz = _____ g

35. 8 oz = _____ g

36. 906 g = _____ lb

37. 30 g = _____ lb

38. 0.8 oz = _____ g

Convert the following patient weights from pounds to kilograms. Round your answer to the nearest tenth unless otherwise indicated.

39. 3.5 lb

40. 14 lb

41. 42 lb

42. 97 lb

43. 112 lb

44. 165 lb

45. 178 lb

46. 247 lb

Applications

In solving these problems, convert all quantities into the metric system, even when the problem could be solved using only the household measure. Round your answer to the nearest tenth unless otherwise indicated.

47. How many 1 tsp doses are in 2 pt, 6 fl oz?

48. How many 2 tsp doses are in 3 cups?

49. How many 1 tbsp doses are in 12 bottles containing 16 fl oz each?

50. How many 5 mL doses are in a 5 fl oz bottle?

51. How many 3 tsp doses are in 1 pt?

52. A dose of 1.5 fl oz is to be given three times daily. How many milliliters will be given in one day?

53. How many 1½ tsp doses are in an 8 fl oz bottle of cough syrup?

Use the following label to answer questions 54 and 55. Round your answer to the nearest tenth unless otherwise indicated.

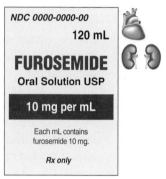

NDC 0000-0000-00

120 mL

FUROSEMIDE

Oral Solution USP

10 mg per mL

Each mL contains furosemide 10 mg.

Rx only

54. A prescription states that a patient is to take ½ tsp of furosemide oral solution daily. Using the furosemide label shown above, how many milligrams are in a dose?

55. Using the furosemide label shown above, how many days will a 4 fl oz bottle last a patient taking 20 mg daily?

Use the following label to answer questions 56 and 57. Round your answer to the nearest tenth unless otherwise indicated.

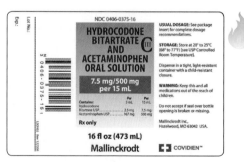

NDC 0406-0375-16

HYDROCODONE BITARTRATE AND ACETAMINOPHEN ORAL SOLUTION

7.5 mg/500 mg per 15 mL

	Per 5 mL	Per 15 mL
Contains: Hydrocodone Bitartrate USP	2.5 mg	7.5 mg
Acetaminophen USP	167 mg	500 mg

Rx only

16 fl oz (473 mL)

Mallinckrodt

USUAL DOSAGE: See package insert for complete dosage recommendations.

STORAGE: Store at 20° to 25°C (68° to 77°F) (see USP Controlled Room Temperature).

Dispense in a tight, light-resistant container with a child-resistant closure.

WARNING: Keep this and all medications out of the reach of children.

Do not accept if seal over bottle opening is broken or missing.

Mallinckrodt Inc. Hazelwood, MO 63042 USA.

COVIDIEN™

56. A prescription states that a patient is to take 20 mL hydrocodone bitartrate/APAP daily. Using the provided label, calculate the equivalent dose measured in teaspoonsful.

57. How many days will the bottle of hydrocodone bitartrate/APAP 7.5 mg/500 mg per 15 mL last a patient if the patient is taking 3 tsp daily?

58. A medication is prescribed as 2 tsp/68 kg/day for an adult patient. How many doses would you get in a 300 mL bottle for a patient who weighs 180 lb?

59. A medication is prescribed as 1 tsp/20 kg/day for a pediatric patient. How many doses will a 4 fl oz bottle provide for a 52 lb patient?

60. A laxative medication is prescribed as 2 tbsp/50 kg. How many doses will a 12 fl oz bottle last for a patient who weighs 172 lb?

Self-check your work in Appendix A.

5.2 Oral Doses

It is important that pharmacy technicians be able to perform calculations involving oral dosing of medications. Oral medications are prescribed over other dosage forms whenever possible and appropriate because oral medications typically are safe and cost-effective. Most prescriptions taken orally come in tablet or capsule form, but liquid forms are also common. Liquid medications are used most commonly by children and by adults with a disease that impairs swallowing. For all dosing calculations, accuracy of conversions from the metric to the household system, dosing amounts, and dispensing amounts need to be checked for safety as well as billing purposes.

Determining Pediatric Doses Using Dosing Tables

Not all drugs that are safe and effective for adult use are appropriate for the pediatric population. In the past, formulas using the child's weight or age were used to reduce the normal adult dose to a smaller amount appropriate for the pediatric patient. Today, prescribers are reluctant to use a medication for a child unless the pharmaceutical manufacturer indicates the proper dose. A manufacturer will provide specific age- and/or weight-related prescribing guidelines for pediatric-appropriate doses of a medication as soon as its safety and effectiveness for the pediatric population have been established. These guidelines are provided in dosing tables as a dose range that is a function of the patient's weight and/or age. When a recommended dose is not provided, often the reason is that the Food and Drug Administration has not approved the particular drug for use in children. The dosing tables are satisfactory for many purposes, but when a more accurate calculation is needed, either the weight-based dosing method or the body surface area (BSA) dosing method, which were discussed in Chapter 4, must be used.

A typical **dosing table** includes an age range and/or a weight range with corresponding doses. Dosing tables are used for both oral liquids and solid dosage forms, but oral liquids are easier for young patients to take and thus are more common.

Dosing tables often appear on over-the-counter (OTC) packaging for products used for children older than age two. For medications used for children under age two, the instruction "Consult your physician" appears. The table for children under age two is available to healthcare providers in pharmacies and physicians' offices. Physicians often instruct parents to purchase OTC medications for small children, so appropriate dosing instructions must be provided for these patients. Dosing may need to be translated from metric units to household measure units. The dosing information listed in Table 5.3 and Table 5.4 will be used to complete the following examples.

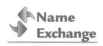
TABLE 5.3   Acetaminophen Dosing

Age	Dose
0–3 mo	40 mg
4–11 mo	80 mg
1–2 yr	120 mg
2–3 yr	160 mg
4–5 yr	240 mg
6–8 yr	320 mg
9–10 yr	400 mg
11 yr to adult	480 mg
adult	325–650 mg q4–6 h or 1000 mg 3–4 times daily
adult maximum	4000 mg daily

TABLE 5.4   Ibuprofen Dosing

Age	Weight	Dose
6–11 mo	12–17 lb	50 mg
12–23 mo	18–23 lb	75 mg
2–3 yr	24–35 lb	100 mg
4–5 yr	36–47 lb	150 mg
6–8 yr	48–59 lb	200 mg
9–10 yr	60–71 lb	250 mg
11 yr	72–95 lb	300 mg

Example 5.2.1

A 12-month-old child weighing 22 lb is to receive one dose of acetaminophen. According to the dosing information in Table 5.3, what is an appropriate dose?

Because the acetaminophen dosing is by age, not weight, use dosing for the age category 1–2 yr. The appropriate dose would be 120 mg.

Example 5.2.2

A parent wants to give her 15-month-old child who weighs 21 lb an appropriate dose of OTC ibuprofen. The package provides the dosing information in Table 5.4. What is the appropriate dose?

The dose can be determined by either age or weight, and for this child, the dosing would be the same. The appropriate dose would be 75 mg.

Dispensing Liquid Medications

Many oral liquid medications are actually solids, suspended in a liquid. These suspensions are often indicated by the number of milligrams per milliliter. For example, amoxicillin is available as a 125 mg/5 mL oral liquid. In other words, 5 mL of the liquid contains 125 mg of amoxicillin.

Oral liquid medications are most often dosed by teaspoonsful, tablespoonsful, fluid ounces, or now—in the metric system—milliliters. Being able to convert accurately between household measure and the metric measure system is a necessary skill for the pharmacy technician. When calculating volumes of oral medication, it is best to convert everything into the same units. The preferred method is to use the metric system. Patient instructions will usually indicate teaspoonsful if the amount is an even half or full teaspoon. However, the instructions should indicate milliliters if the dose is not easily measured using the household system. An oral syringe, as shown in Figure 5.3, is helpful to patients dosing oral liquids using the metric or household systems.

Usually, an oral liquid medication's written prescription includes a specific volume to be given at each dose, as well as the total volume to be dispensed. It is important to have a working knowledge of the volumes of oral liquid medications that are commonly prescribed. Most frequently, the dosage amount is between 2 mL and 60 mL, or roughly ½ tsp to 2 fl oz. Oral doses are often verified in the pharmacy by means of reference and established protocols.

FIGURE 5.3
Oral Syringe

This oral syringe is marked with both household and metric units of measure.

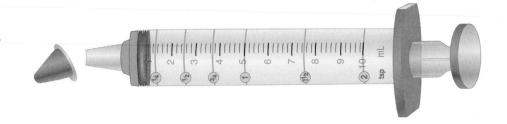

Example 5.2.3

The pharmacy receives a prescription for 100 mg of amoxicillin to be taken three times daily for 10 days. The pharmacy has a 150 mL bottle of 125 mg/5 mL amoxicillin. How many milliliters of the suspension will be dispensed, and what will the patient's dosing instructions on the label state?

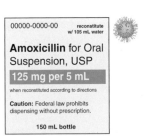

Determine what quantity of suspension contains 100 mg amoxicillin. This can be solved in two ways:

Solution 1: Using the ratio-proportion method,

$$\frac{x \text{ mL}}{100 \text{ mg}} = \frac{5 \text{ mL}}{125 \text{ mg}}$$

$$x \text{ mL} = 4 \text{ mL}$$

Solution 2: Using the dimensional analysis method,

$$100 \ \cancel{mg} \times \frac{5 \ mL}{125 \ \cancel{mg}} = 4 \ mL$$

Using the amount determined for a single dose, calculate the total amount of suspension to be dispensed for 10 days.

$$4 \ mL \times 3 \ doses/day \times 10 \ days = 120 \ mL$$

The patient's instructions will state, "Take 4 mL three times daily for 10 days." The patient will need a dosing syringe to dispense the required amount of medication.

Example 5.2.4

If a 12 fl oz bottle of mouthwash contains 0.75 g of the active ingredient, how many milligrams will be in a 1 tbsp dose?

Begin the problem by converting all of the household measure units to metric units.

$$12 \ fl \ oz = 360 \ mL$$
$$1 \ tbsp = 15 \ mL$$

Also, convert 0.75 g to 750 mg. Using these converted values, this problem can be solved in two ways:

Solution 1: Using the ratio-proportion method,

$$\frac{x \ mg}{15 \ mL} = \frac{750 \ mg}{360 \ mL}$$

$$x \ mg = 31.25 \ mg$$

Solution 2: Using the dimensional analysis method,

$$15 \ \cancel{mL} \times \frac{750 \ mg}{360 \ \cancel{mL}} = 31.25 \ mg$$

Example 5.2.5

The pharmacy receives a prescription for amoxicillin suspension 1 g bid. The pharmacy has a supply of amoxicillin 250 mg/5 mL. How many milliliters are in one dose? What will the patient's dosing instructions on the bottle label indicate?

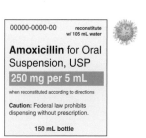

First, determine how many milligrams are needed for one dose.

$$1 \ g = 1000 \ mg$$

Then calculate what quantity of suspension contains 1000 mg.

Solution 1: Using the ratio-proportion method,

$$\frac{x \text{ mL}}{1000 \text{ mg}} = \frac{5 \text{ mL}}{250 \text{ mg}}$$

$$x \text{ mL} = 20 \text{ mL}$$

Solution 2: Using the dimensional analysis method,

$$1000 \text{ mg} \times \frac{5 \text{ mL}}{250 \text{ mg}} = 20 \text{ mL}$$

Convert the amount in milliliters to teaspoonsful: 5 mL = 1 tsp, so 20 mL = 4 tsp. The patient's instructions will state, "Take 20 mL (or 4 teaspoonsful) two times daily."

Example 5.2.6

A patient is to take 7 mL of amoxicillin 250 mg/5 mL. How many milligrams are present in one dose?

Solution 1: Using the ratio-proportion method,

$$\frac{x \text{ mg}}{7 \text{ mL}} = \frac{250 \text{ mg}}{5 \text{ mL}}$$

$$x \text{ mg} = 350 \text{ mg}$$

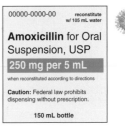

Solution 2: Using the dimensional analysis method,

$$7 \text{ mL} \times \frac{250 \text{ mg}}{5 \text{ mL}} = 350 \text{ mg}$$

Example 5.2.7

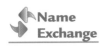
Name Exchange

Diphenhydramine elixir is commonly known by the brand name Benadryl.

A patient is taking 4 tsp of diphenhydramine elixir at bedtime. He wishes to take oral capsules instead of the elixir. The 12.5 mg/5 mL elixir comes in a 4 fl oz bottle and is 14% alcohol. The 25 mg capsules come in a 100 count bottle. How many capsules will he need to take to equal the dose in the 4 tsp of elixir?

Begin by determining the milligrams per dose of the oral liquid using one of the following methods:

Solution 1: Using the ratio-proportion method,

$$\frac{x \text{ mg}}{20 \text{ mL}} = \frac{12.5 \text{ mg}}{5 \text{ mL}}$$

$$x \text{ mg} = 50 \text{ mg}$$

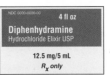

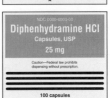

Solution 2: Using the dimensional analysis method,

$$20 \ \cancel{mL} \times \frac{12.5 \ mg}{5 \ \cancel{mL}} = 50 \ mg$$

Now, compare the milligrams to the alternative capsule product.

Solution 1: Using the ratio-proportion method,

$$\frac{x \ capsules}{50 \ mg} = \frac{1 \ capsule}{25 \ mg}$$

$$x \ capsule = 2 \ capsules$$

Solution 2: Using the dimensional analysis method,

$$50 \ \cancel{mg} \times \frac{1 \ capsule}{25 \ \cancel{mg}} = 2 \ capsules$$

Because the patient's dose is 50 mg, and the capsules come in 25 mg, he will need to take two capsules to provide the proper amount of the drug.

Example 5.2.8

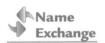

Name Exchange

Biaxin is a brand name for the generic drug clarithromycin.

1 tbsp = 15 mL

1 tsp = 5 mL

How many milligrams of medication are in 1 tbsp of clarithromycin that contains 125 mg/tsp?

Convert both volumes to the metric system using the following values from Table 5.2.

| |
NDC 0000-0000-00
100 mL (when mixed)

Clarithromycin
for oral suspension, USP

125 mg per 5 mL

when reconstituted   Rx only

$$1 \ tbsp = 15 \ mL$$
$$1 \ tsp = 5 \ mL$$

Using these equivalents, this problem can be solved in two ways.

Solution 1: Using the ratio-proportion method,

$$\frac{x \ mg}{15 \ mL} = \frac{125 \ mg}{5 \ mL}$$

$$x \ mg = 375 \ mg$$

Solution 2: Using the dimensional analysis method,

$$15 \ \cancel{mL} \times \frac{125 \ mg}{5 \ \cancel{mL}} = 375 \ mg$$

Calculating the Volume to Dispense

How long the volume of medication dispensed will last the patient must be determined when the prescription is entered into the patient's computerized record. Pharmacies typically bill liquid medications by the milliliter and solid medications by the unit, such as a tablet. Insurance companies require claims for reimbursement for prescription drugs to include the volume of drug dispensed as well as the number of days that the dispensed volume should last. The volume dispensed is usually indicated by the prescriber; however, if it is not indicated, the volume to be dispensed is calculated by multiplying the volume of drug needed for a single day by the number of days of treatment. Not only is the dispensed volume needed for insurance purposes, but the pharmacy also needs to ensure that the patient is receiving enough medication to last for the duration of treatment, whether the medication is in liquid or solid form.

Example 5.2.9

A patient is taking 2 tsp of medication every 8 hours. He has a 6 fl oz bottle of medication. How much medication will the patient take in one day, and how many days will the medication last?

1 tsp = 5 mL

1 fl oz = 30 mL

Begin by converting all of the stated volumes to the metric system using the conversion values in Table 5.2.

$$1 \text{ tsp} = 5 \text{ mL; therefore, 2 tsp/dose} = 10 \text{ mL/dose}$$
$$1 \text{ fl oz} = 30 \text{ mL; therefore, 6 fl oz/bottle} = 180 \text{ mL/bottle}$$

Next, determine how much medication is needed for one day of treatment. The dose is every 8 hours, and there are 24 hours in a day, so

$$24 \text{ hours/day} \times 1 \text{ dose/8 hours} = 3 \text{ doses/day}$$
$$3 \text{ doses/day} \times 10 \text{ mL/dose} = 30 \text{ mL/day}$$

Finally, calculate the number of days the medication will last.

$$180 \text{ mL/bottle} \times 1 \text{ day/30 mL} = 6 \text{ days/bottle}$$

Example 5.2.10

A patient is to take 1 tsp of a medication twice daily, and she has a 4 fl oz bottle of medication. How much medication will the patient take in a day, and how many days will the medication last?

1 tsp = 5 mL

1 fl oz = 30 mL

Begin by converting all of the stated volumes to the metric system using the conversion values in Table 5.2.

$$1 \text{ tsp} = 5 \text{ mL; therefore, 1 tsp/dose} = 5 \text{ mL/dose}$$
$$1 \text{ fl oz} = 30 \text{ mL; therefore, 4 fl oz/bottle} = 120 \text{ mL/bottle}$$

Next, determine how much medication is needed for one day.

The dose is taken twice daily, so there are 2 doses/day.

$$2 \text{ doses/day} \times 5 \text{ mL/dose} = 10 \text{ mL/day}$$

Finally, calculate the number of days the medication will last.

$$120 \text{ mL/bottle} \times 1 \text{ day/10 mL} = 12 \text{ days/bottle}$$

Example 5.2.11

1 tsp = 5 mL

1 fl oz = 30 mL

Safety in Numbers

The professional judgment of the pharmacist must be used in assigning a days' supply to a prescription with a *prn* or "as needed" instruction.

A patient has a prescription that states the following: "Take Magic Cough Syrup 1–2 tsp every 4–6 hours prn cough. Disp: 8 fl oz." How many days will the cough syrup last?

Begin by converting all of the stated volumes to the metric system using the conversion values in Table 5.2.

1 tsp = 5 mL; therefore, 1–2 tsp/dose = 5–10 mL/dose

1 fl oz = 30 mL; therefore, for this prescription calculation,
8 fl oz/bottle = 240 mL/bottle

Next, determine how much medication is needed for one day. Assume that the patient will take medication every 4–6 hours during the waking hours. This will give the minimum number of days the medication will last.

A patient will most likely take the medication upon awakening, midday, and before bedtime.

3 doses/day × 10 mL/dose = 30 mL/day

Finally, determine the number of days the medication will last.

240 mL/bottle × 1 day/30 mL = 8 days/bottle

Note that the bottle will run out sooner if the patient takes 1 tsp every four hours, increasing the doses per day to more than the 3 doses assumed in the calculation.

Some prescriptions do not come with explicit instructions as to how much medication is to be dispensed. The prescription may state, "Take 2 tsp every morning for 10 days." The quantity indicated on the prescription may also state, "QS," which means to dispense a "quantity sufficient" to meet the needs of the patient with the instructions given. When the duration of treatment is indicated, the volume of medication needed for a single day and the total volume to be dispensed can be calculated as demonstrated in the following examples.

Example 5.2.12

A patient comes to the pharmacy with a prescription that does not indicate a quantity. It states, "Amoxicillin 125 mg/5 mL, 1 tsp tid for 10 days." What is the total volume of medication to be dispensed?

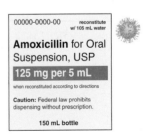

00000-0000-00   reconstitute w/ 105 mL water

Amoxicillin for Oral Suspension, USP

125 mg per 5 mL

when reconstituted according to directions

Caution: Federal law prohibits dispensing without prescription.

150 mL bottle

Begin by converting all of the dosage volumes to the metric system using the conversion values in Table 5.2.

1 tsp = 5 mL; therefore, 1 tsp/dose = 5 mL/dose

Next, calculate how much medication is needed for one day. Because "tid" means three times daily,

$$5 \text{ mL/dose} \times 3 \text{ doses/day} = 15 \text{ mL/day}$$

Finally, determine the volume of medication to dispense.

$$15 \text{ mL/day} \times 10 \text{ days} = 150 \text{ mL}$$

Example 5.2.13

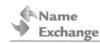

Name Exchange

Fluoxetine, a generic drug, is widely known as the brand name Prozac and is used to treat depression.

A patient is to take 2 tsp of fluoxetine each morning for 30 days. How many milliliters will be needed? How many bottles with the label shown here will be required to fill this prescription?

Begin by converting all of the dosage volumes to the metric system using the conversion values in Table 5.2 and Figure 5.2.

Since 1 tsp = 5 mL, 2 tsp/dose = 10 mL/dose.

NDC 0000-0000-00

120 mL

FLUOXETINE

Fluoxetine
Hydrochloride
Oral Solution

Equivalent to

20 mg per 5 mL

Base

Rx only

Next, determine how many milliliters are needed for 30 days.

$$10 \text{ mL/day} \times 30 \text{ days} = 300 \text{ mL}$$

Finally, calculate the number of bottles of medication needed. The label indicates that each bottle contains 120 mL. Therefore,

$$2 \text{ bottles} \times 120 \text{ mL/bottle} = 240 \text{ mL}$$
$$3 \text{ bottles} \times 120 \text{ mL/bottle} = 360 \text{ mL}$$

So, two full bottles and part of a third bottle will be needed to fill this prescription. (There will be 60 mL left over.)

The same procedure is used when calculating the number of tablets needed to fill a prescription or the number of days a given prescription will last.

Example 5.2.14

A patient has brought in a prescription for an antidiabetic drug. The prescription states, "Take 2 tablets before breakfast, 1 before lunch and supper, and 1 at bedtime." Determine the quantity needed for 30 days.

Begin by determining the number of tablets required for one day.

2 before breakfast + 1 before lunch + 1 before supper + 1 at bedtime = 5

The patient will take 5 tablets/day, so a 30-day supply will be

5 tablets/day × 30 days = 150 tablets

Example 5.2.15

A patient is to take a prescription for prednisone that uses a tapered dosing schedule. Determine the number of 5 mg tablets needed.

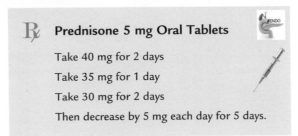

R̸ **Prednisone 5 mg Oral Tablets**

Take 40 mg for 2 days

Take 35 mg for 1 day

Take 30 mg for 2 days

Then decrease by 5 mg each day for 5 days.

In this problem, the number of tablets taken each day changes, so the most straightforward way to determine the number of tablets needed is to make a list of how many tablets the patient will take each day of treatment.

Day 1: 40 mg/day ÷ 5 mg/tablet = 8 tablets

Day 2: 40 mg/day ÷ 5 mg/tablet = 8 tablets

Day 3: 35 mg/day ÷ 5 mg/tablet = 7 tablets

Day 4: 30 mg/day ÷ 5 mg/tablet = 6 tablets

Day 5: 30 mg/day ÷ 5 mg/tablet = 6 tablets

Day 6: 25 mg/day ÷ 5 mg/tablet = 5 tablets

Day 7: 20 mg/day ÷ 5 mg/tablet = 4 tablets

Day 8: 15 mg/day ÷ 5 mg/tablet = 3 tablets

Day 9: 10 mg/day ÷ 5 mg/tablet = 2 tablets

Day 10: 5 mg/day ÷ 5 mg/tablet = 1 tablet

The sum of the daily totals is 50 tablets for a 10-day regimen.

Aspirin is typically contraindicated in children. If a child is unable to take acetaminophen or ibuprofen, however, aspirin may be used. Additionally, aspirin is indicated for some conditions in children such as antiplatelet therapy and antirheumatic therapy. Items 1–4 show the age of a child. For each child, determine the milligram dose of aspirin every 4 hours using the dosing table provided.

Safety in Numbers

Some manufacturers provide a normal range of dosage to account for overweight or underweight patients.

Aspirin			
Age (years)	Weight		Dose (mg every 4 hr)
	lb	kg	
2–3	24–35	10.6–15.9	162
4–5	36–47	16–21.4	243
6–8	48–59	21.5–26.8	324
9–10	60–71	26.9–32.3	405
11	72–95	32.4–43.2	486
12–14	≥96	≥43.3	648

1. 4 years

2. 7 years

3. 10 years

4. 14 years

Levothyroxine is indicated for children with hypothyroidism. Many states require infants to be tested for hypothyroidism shortly after birth so that therapy can begin immediately if needed. In adult patients, the dose is adjusted up or down based on blood titers and clinical signs and symptoms. Newborn patients are more difficult to assess, so a standard dosing table based on kilograms has been developed. For items 5–8, determine the daily dose of levothyroxine for each child using the dosing table provided.

Levothyroxine	
Age	Daily dose per kg (mcg)
0–3 mo	10–15
3–6 mo	8–10
6–12 mo	6–8
1–5 yr	5–6
6–12 yr	4–5
>12 yr	2–3

5. newborn (6 lb)

6. newborn (7 lb, 12 oz)

7. 11-month-old (23 lb)

8. 15-month-old (18 lb)

Applications

Calculate the following using either the dimensional analysis method or the ratio-proportion method.

9. A patient takes 1 tsp daily of a medication with the concentration 80 mg/15 mL. How many milligrams are in one dose?

10. A patient needs to have 60 mg of medication, and the drug has the concentration 120 mg/5 mL. How many teaspoonsful will the patient take?

11. If there are 24 mg in a teaspoonful of liquid medication, how many grams are in 8 fl oz?

12. How many milligrams are in 4 fl oz of liquid medication with the concentration of 65 mg/tbsp?

13. How many milligrams are in a 2 tsp dose of liquid medication if there are 2.5 g in 2 fl oz?

14. How many milligrams are in a 1 tbsp dose of liquid medication if there are 260 mg in 600 mL?

15. A prescription is received for Drug YXZ to be taken 2 tsp bid. The required strength of the drug is 25 mg/tsp. How many grams are needed to prepare 20 fl oz?

16. A prescription is received for Drug YXZ to be taken 1 tbsp qam. The required strength of the drug is 30 mg/5 mL. How many milligrams are in a 1 tbsp dose?

17. A prescription is received for Drug YXZ to be taken 1 tbsp bid. The required strength of the drug is 40 mg/mL. How many grams of medication are needed to prepare 1 pint?

18. A patient is taking ¾ tsp of an antibiotic suspension three times a day.

    a. How long will a 150 mL bottle of antibiotic suspension last this patient?

    b. How many milliliters will be left after 10 days?

19. An antibiotic suspension is available in 80 mL, 150 mL, and 200 mL bottles.

    a. What size bottle of antibiotic suspension will a patient need in order to take 1 tsp twice daily for 14 days?

    b. How much antibiotic suspension will remain after 14 days?

20. How many days will a 12 fl oz bottle last if a patient takes 1 tbsp tid?

21. A patient is on an alternate-day therapy consisting of 2 tsp of a medication one day and 1 tbsp the next. How long will a 300 mL bottle last?

22. If there are 25 mg in a tablespoonful of liquid medication, how many grams are in 20 fl oz?

23. A patient uses an antacid 1 fl oz tid and hs. How many 12 fl oz bottles will this patient need to last 14 days?

24. How many prednisone 5 mg tablets are needed to fill the following prescription?

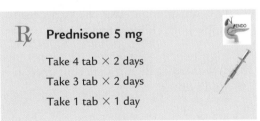

℞ **Prednisone 5 mg**

Take 4 tab × 2 days
Take 3 tab × 2 days
Take 1 tab × 1 day

25. How many milliliters of nystatin must be dispensed for the following prescription?

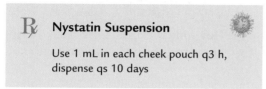

℞ **Nystatin Suspension**

Use 1 mL in each cheek pouch q3 h, dispense qs 10 days

26. There are 25 mg in a teaspoonful of medication. You are dispensing 12 fl oz.

a. How many milligrams will be in the bottle?

b. If the patient is to get a total of 9 g for a full therapy program, how many refills will be needed?

27. For the prescription below, how many fluid ounces of nystatin must be dispensed?

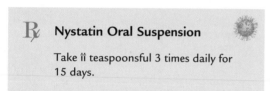

℞ **Nystatin Oral Suspension**

Take ii teaspoonsful 3 times daily for 15 days.

28. A prescription states, "Take 2 tbsp of an oral elixir three times daily for 20 days." How many milliliters should be dispensed?

Use the label below to answer questions 29 and 30.

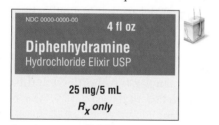

NDC 0000-0000-00

4 fl oz

Diphenhydramine
Hydrochloride Elixir USP

25 mg/5 mL

R_x *only*

29. A mother has two children with poison ivy. One child takes 1 tsp tid, and the other child takes 2 tsp tid. How many bottles of diphenhydramine elixir will be needed to supply both children for 4 days?

30. How many milligrams are contained in each child's dose?

Use the label below to answer questions 31–34.

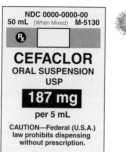

NDC 0000-0000-00
50 mL (When Mixed) M-5130

℞

CEFACLOR
ORAL SUSPENSION
USP

187 mg

per 5 mL

CAUTION—Federal (U.S.A.) law prohibits dispensing without prescription.

31. How many milligrams are in ¾ tsp?

32. How many milligrams are in 1½ tsp?

33. How many milliliters are needed to provide 125 mg?

34. How many milliliters are needed to provide 500 mg?

35. The following prescription for buttocks cream has been brought into the compounding pharmacy for compounding on January 3, 201X.

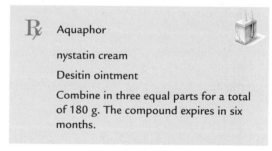

℞ Aquaphor

nystatin cream

Desitin ointment

Combine in three equal parts for a total of 180 g. The compound expires in six months.

a. How much of each ingredient will you use?

b. What size of ointment jar (ounces) will you use to store the compound?

c. What expiration date will you put on the compound?

36. The following order for absolute (dehydrated) alcohol has been brought into the compounding pharmacy. How many syringes will be sent to the floor?

R
1. Obtain a 12 fl oz bottle of absolute alcohol from the narcotics cabinet.
2. Filter through a 0.2 micron filter.
3. Send to the floor in 60 mL syringes.

Self-check your work in Appendix A.

5.3 Temperature Measurement

Temperature is a factor in dealing with chemical compounds. Two temperature scales are used to measure temperatures: the **Celsius** system and the **Fahrenheit** system. Both were developed almost 300 years ago.

 ## Understanding Temperature Measurement Systems

Daniel Fahrenheit, a German physicist, invented an alcohol thermometer in 1709, a mercury thermometer in 1714, and a temperature scale in 1724. This temperature scale was based on ice water and salt as a low point (0 °F) and the human body temperature as the high point (100 °F). Fahrenheit used his own body temperature as the standard, but in the years that followed, scientists learned that body temperature varied. Therefore, the Fahrenheit scale was keyed to water for both the low point and the high point. The freezing point of water at sea level was set at 32 °F, and the boiling point of water at sea level was set at 212 °F.

About 1742, Anders Celsius, a Swedish astronomer, developed what became the Celsius or centigrade thermometer. In Celsius measurement, water freezes at 0 °C and boils at 100 °C.

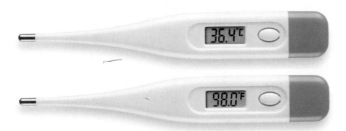

Pharmacy technicians may be asked to help patients convert between temperature readings in degrees Celsius and Fahrenheit. As with all conversions, this calculation must be done accurately.

Converting Celsius and Fahrenheit Temperatures

Both measurement systems are in common use today. Pharmacy personnel must know the two systems and be able to convert back and forth between them. The formulas for converting from one temperature measuring system to another are based on the fact that each Celsius degree equals 1.8 or ⁹⁄₅ of each Fahrenheit degree. Below are the conversion formulas. Note that temperatures should be rounded to the nearest tenth.

degrees Celsius to degrees Fahrenheit:

$$°F = \left(\frac{9 \times °C}{5} \right) + 32°$$

or

$$°F = (1.8 \times °C) + 32°$$

degrees Fahrenheit to degrees Celsius:

$$°C = (°F - 32°) \times \frac{5}{9}$$

or

$$°C = \frac{°F - 32°}{1.8}$$

Example 5.3.1

Convert 40 °C to its equivalent in the Fahrenheit scale.

Solution 1:

$$°F = \left(\frac{9 \times °C}{5} \right) + 32°$$

$$= \left(\frac{9 \times 40°}{5} \right) + 32°$$

$$= \frac{360°}{5} + 32°$$

$$= 72° + 32°$$

$$= 104 \, °F$$

Solution 2:

$$°F = (1.8 \times °C) + 32°$$

$$= (1.8 \times 40°) + 32°$$

$$= 72° + 32°$$

$$= 104 \, °F$$

Example 5.3.2

Convert 82 °F to its equivalent in the Celsius scale.

Solution 1:

$$°C = (°F - 32°) \times \frac{5}{9}$$

$$= (82° - 32°) \times \frac{5}{9}$$

$$= 50° \times \frac{5}{9}$$

$$= 27.777 \text{ °C, rounded to } 27.8 \text{ °C}$$

Solution 2:

$$°C = \frac{(°F - 32°)}{1.8}$$

$$= \frac{(82° - 32°)}{1.8}$$

$$= \frac{50°}{1.8}$$

$$= 27.777 \text{ °C, rounded to } 27.8 \text{ °C}$$

Completing a Temperature Chart

Often medication comes with specific instructions regarding refrigeration. To store medication under "refrigerated" conditions means to store it between 2 °C and 5 °C (35.6 °F and 41 °F). It is important that temperatures of refrigerators for storing medications be monitored daily.

Most pharmacies have specific charts for recording temperatures of refrigerators and freezers used for storage. See Figure 5.4 and Figure 5.5 on the following page for examples of these charts.

FIGURE 5.4
Refrigerator Temperature Chart (Celsius)

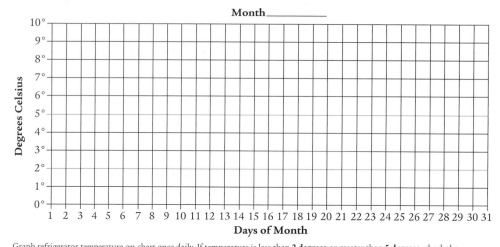

Graph refrigerator temperature on chart once daily. If temperature is less than **2 degrees** or greater than **5 degrees,** check the thermostat setting and correct as necessary. Recheck temperature in one hour, and if temperature is out of stated range, contact maintenance for evaluation and repair. Contact the appropriate area for storage of supplies.

Documentation of Repairs: _____   Documentation of Cleaning: _____

FIGURE 5.5
Refrigerator Temperature Chart (Fahrenheit)

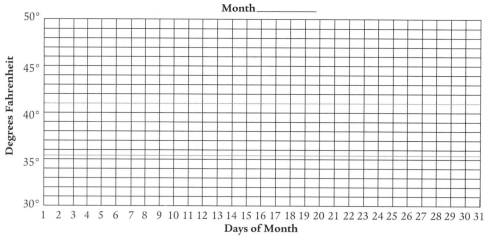

Graph refrigerator temperature on chart once daily. If temperature is less than **35.6 degrees** or greater than **41 degrees,** check the thermostat setting and correct as necessary. Recheck temperature in one hour, and if temperature is out of stated range, contact maintenance for evaluation and repair. Contact the appropriate area for storage of supplies.

Documentation of Repairs: _____   Documentation of Cleaning: _____

5.3 Problem Set

Convert the following Fahrenheit temperatures to Celsius. Round the temperatures to the nearest tenth.

1. 0 °F

2. 23 °F

3. 36 °F

4. 40 °F

5. 64 °F

6. 72 °F

7. 98.6 °F

8. 100.5 °F

9. 102.8 °F

10. 105 °F

Convert the following Celsius temperatures to Fahrenheit. Round the temperatures to the nearest tenth.

11. −15 °C

12. 18 °C

13. 27 °C

14. 31 °C

15. 38 °C

16. 40 °C

17. 49 °C

18. 63 °C

19. 99.8 °C

20. 101.4 °C

Applications

21. When making a mixture, you are instructed to heat the mixture to 130 °C. You have only a Fahrenheit thermometer. What is the equivalent temperature on the Fahrenheit scale?

22. The following prescription is sent to the hospital pharmacy:

R_x **Alteplase in a Syringe**

alteplase, 2 mg/mL 50 mg

sterile water for injection (SWFI) 25 mL

1. Reconstitute the alteplase with SWFI.

2. Draw up 5 mL in 10 mL syringes.

3. Label syringes with contents, concentration, and date of preparation.

4. Place syringes in freezer. They should be frozen with the premixed piggybacks.

The syringes are stable for six months, or 180 days, −20° C.

a. What is the Fahrenheit temperature at which you should store this product?

b. What expiration date should you put on this compound if today is February 1, 2015?

23. A prescription is sent to the hospital pharmacy requesting a substance to be heated in a 300 °F oven for 12–18 hours. At what Celsius temperature does the oven need to be set?

24. Convert the following refrigerator temperatures and log them on the Celsius chart. Round the temperatures to the nearest tenth, and note any temperatures out of the safe range.

Date	Degrees F	Degrees C
5/5	36.1°	a. _____
5/6	37.7°	b. _____
5/7	39.0°	c. _____
5/8	35.7°	d. _____
5/9	36.9°	e. _____
5/10	34.9°	f. _____
5/11	36.4°	g. _____
5/12	36.8°	h. _____
5/13	35.5°	i. _____
5/14	38.8°	j. _____

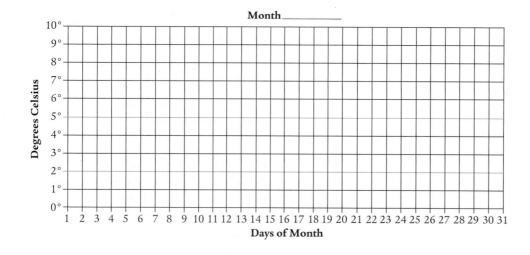

Month_____

Degrees Celsius

Days of Month

25. Convert the following refrigerator temperatures and log them on the Fahrenheit chart. Round the temperatures to the nearest tenth, and note any temperatures out of the safe range.

Date	Degrees C	Degrees F
7/12	1.8°	a. _____
7/13	3.1°	b. _____
7/14	2.8°	c. _____
7/15	3.0°	d. _____
7/16	4.5°	e. _____
7/17	3.2°	f. _____
7/18	3.9°	g. _____
7/19	2.5°	h. _____
7/20	4.1°	i. _____
7/21	4.7°	j. _____

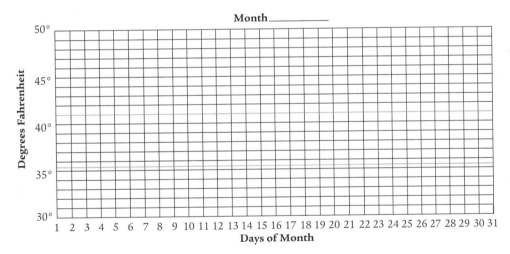

Month_____

Days of Month

Degrees Fahrenheit

Self-check your work in Appendix A.

Chapter Summary

- Patients are most familiar with household measurements such as teaspoons and cups.
- Household measuring devices are often less accurate than the measuring devices used in the pharmacy.
- Household measurements may be easily converted to metric using either the ratio-proportion method or the dimensional analysis method.
- Some drugs are dosed based on a patient's weight in kilograms.
- Weights measured in pounds may be converted to kilograms by dividing the pounds by 2.2.

- The preferred measurement for liquid oral doses is milliliters.
- Most oral doses are between 2 mL and 60 mL (or roughly ½ tsp to 2 fluid ounces).
- Teaspoon and fluid ounce conversions should be memorized: 1 tsp = 5 mL and 1 fl oz = 30 mL.
- Celsius uses a measurement system in which 0° is freezing and 100° is boiling.
- Fahrenheit uses a measurement system in which 32° is freezing and 212° is boiling.
- Temperatures in pharmacy refrigerators and freezers must be checked daily to ensure medications are being stored at the appropriate temperature.

Formulas for Success

3 teaspoonsful (tsp) = 1 tablespoonful (tbsp)	2 cups = 1 pint (pt)
2 tablespoonsful (tbsp) = 1 fluid ounce (fl oz)	2 pints (pt) = 1 quart (qt)
8 fluid ounces (fl oz) = 1 cup	4 quarts (qt) = 1 gallon (gal)

Key Terms

Celsius a thermometric scale in which 100° is the boiling point of water and 0° is the freezing point of water

dosing table a table providing dose recommendations based on the age and/or the weight of the patient; often used for determining the safe dose for a pediatric patient

Fahrenheit a thermometric scale in which 212° is the boiling point of water and 32° is the freezing point of water

household measure a system of measure used in homes, particularly in kitchens, in the United States; units of measure for volume include teaspoonful, tablespoonful, cup, pint, quart, and gallon; units for weight are pound and ounce

Chapter Review

Assessing Comprehension

To check your comprehension of this chapter's key concepts, read the following multiple-choice questions and then record your answers on a separate sheet of paper. Write your answers as modeled in these examples: 1d; 2c; 3b; etc.

1. Which of the following equivalents is correct?
   a. 2 cups = ½ pint
   b. 2 cups = 1 pint
   c. 2 cups = 1 quart
   d. 2 cups = ½ gallon

2. Which of the following equivalents is correct?
   a. 3 tsp = 1 tbsp
   b. 3 tsp = 1 fl oz
   c. 3 tsp = ½ cup
   d. 3 tsp = 1 cup

3. Which of the following equivalents is correct?
   a. 1 tsp = 1 mL
   b. 1 tsp = 1 fl oz
   c. 1 tsp = 5 mL
   d. 1 tsp = 15 mL

4. Which of the following instructions is preferable for a patient?
   a. Take 2 ⅓ tsp by mouth daily.
   b. Take 1 fluid ounce by mouth daily.
   c. Take ½ tbsp by mouth daily.
   d. Take 10 mL by mouth daily.

5. Most medications that are dosed based on a patient's weight use _____ as the unit of weight for the patient.
   a. pounds
   b. pounds and ounces
   c. kilograms
   d. grams

6. What unit of measure is used when weighing creams and ointments in the pharmacy?
   a. pounds
   b. ounces
   c. grams
   d. kilograms

7. Common OTC medication doses for children are determined by
   a. a manufacturer-provided dosing table or instructions on the packaging.
   b. contacting the primary care physician to identify an appropriate dose.
   c. calculating the dose based on the child's age.
   d. using a standard dose for all children over age 2.

8. Prescription instructions that direct a patient to take a range of medication on an as-needed basis should have the days' supply determined by
   a. calculating the maximum number of doses a patient could take each day.
   b. calculating the minimum number of doses a patient could take each day.
   c. asking the patient how frequently he or she intends to use the medication.
   d. relying on the pharmacist's professional judgment based on common and safe practice.

9. Temperature that is recorded in Fahrenheit may be converted to Celsius by
   a. subtracting 32° from the Fahrenheit temperature.
   b. adding 32° to the Fahrenheit temperature.
   c. using a formula to convert the temperature.
   d. multiplying the Fahrenheit temperature by 1.8.

10. Temperature is checked daily in the pharmacy's refrigerator and freezer to
    a. ensure that medications are kept at the lowest temperature possible.
    b. verify that medications are stored in the appropriate temperature range.
    c. prevent refrigeration malfunction.
    d. monitor temperature change trends to determine when the refrigerator needs to be replaced.

Finding Solutions

To gain practice in handling challenging situations in the workplace, consider the following real-world scenarios and then use the guiding questions to help you formulate your responses.

> **Note:** *To indicate your answer for Scenario A, Question 4, ask your instructor for the handout depicting an oral syringe; for Scenario B, Question 8, ask your instructor for the handout depicting a medicine cup.*

Scenario A: Lucy Ramirez, a 14-month-old patient in the pediatric unit, weighs 22 pounds. She has just been diagnosed with gastroesophageal reflux disease (GERD). Her physician has prescribed Pepcid Oral Suspension, which is dosed at 1 mg/kg per day, divided into two doses. Pepcid Oral Suspension is available in a 40 mg/5 mL strength.

1. How many kilograms does Lucy weigh?

2. How many milligrams should Lucy be taking each day?

3. How many milligrams will be given at each dose?

4. How many milliliters will be given at each dose? On the handout that you obtained from your instructor, indicate on the measuring device the amount of medication that should be administered to the child.

5. Is this dose more or less than a teaspoon?

6. How will this volume of medication be measured accurately?

Scenario B: Tamara Rigoni has a severe skin infection that her physician wants to treat with cephalexin, an oral antibiotic. The physician wants her patient to receive a liquid suspension of cephalexin at a dosage of 4 g per day, in four divided doses. Cephalexin is available in a 250 mg/5 mL suspension.

7. How many milligrams will be given at each dose?

8. How many milliliters will be given at each dose? On the handout that you obtained from your instructor, indicate on the measuring device the amount of medication that should be administered to the patient.

9. How many teaspoons are in each dose?

10. How many milliliters will the patient need to complete a 10-day course of therapy?

Sampling the Certification Exam

To provide you with practice for the Certification Exam, read the following questions that have been patterned after the test format and then record your answers on a separate sheet of paper. Write your answers as modeled in these examples: 1d; 2c; 3b; *etc.*

1. Convert 1 pint of Bactrim Suspension to fluid ounces.
   a. 64 fluid ounces
   b. 32 fluid ounces
   c. 16 fluid ounces
   d. 4 fluid ounces

2. If a patient takes 1 tsp tid, how many milliliters will be needed for a 7-day course of therapy?
   a. 50 mL
   b. 100 mL
   c. 105 mL
   d. 150 mL

3. How many tablespoonful doses are in 1 pint?
   a. 64 tbsp
   b. 32 tbsp
   c. 16 tbsp
   d. 4 tbsp

4. You have dispensed a 250 mL bottle of Trileptal. How many doses are in the bottle if the patient takes 1½ tsp at each dose?
   a. 25
   b. 30
   c. 33
   d. 40

5. A patient has been prescribed prednisone with the following instructions:

   Prednisone 5 mg
   Take 5 tablets for 2 days.
   Take 4 tablets for 1 day.
   Take 3 tablets for 2 days.
   Take 2 tablets for 1 day.
   Take 1 tablet for 2 days.

   How many tablets will the patient need to complete the therapy?
   a. 21 tablets
   b. 23 tablets
   c. 24 tablets
   d. 33 tablets

To put your pharmacy calculation skills to the test, read the following questions and then record your answers on a separate sheet of paper.

Note: *Questions 11, 12, 18, and 19 have accompanying handouts that must be obtained from your instructor.*

Convert the given volumes within the household measure system.

1. 3 tsp = _____ fl oz

2. 8 fl oz = _____ tsp

Convert the given volumes between the household measure and metric systems.

3. 8 mL = _____ tsp

4. 8 fl oz = _____ mL

Answer the following questions.

5. How many kilograms does a 192 lb patient weigh?

6. How many 5 mL doses are in a 5 fl oz bottle of antibiotic preparation?

7. How many 3 tsp doses are in 500 mL?

Determine the dose of acetaminophen for each of the following children using the dosing table provided.

Acetaminophen			
Age	Dose (mg)	Age	Dose (mg)
0–3 mo	40	6–8 yr	320
4–11 mo	80	9–10 yr	400
1–<2 yr	120	11 yr	480
2–3 yr	160	12–14 yr	640
4–5 yr	240	>14 yr	650

8. 11-month-old (22 lb)

9. 15-month-old (21 lb)

Calculate the following using either the dimensional analysis or the ratio-proportion method.

10. Using the following label, how many grams of amoxicillin are in the bottle?

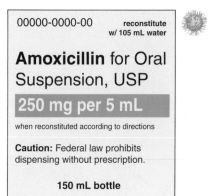

00000-0000-00   reconstitute
w/ 105 mL water

Amoxicillin for Oral
Suspension, USP

250 mg per 5 mL

when reconstituted according to directions

Caution: Federal law prohibits
dispensing without prescription.

150 mL bottle

11. Using the following label, how many milligrams of theophylline are in 3 tbsp? On the handout that you obtained from your instructor, indicate the correct volume on the correct measuring device.

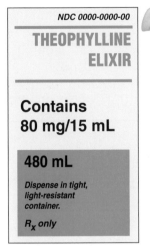

NDC 0000-0000-00

THEOPHYLLINE ELIXIR

Contains 80 mg/15 mL

480 mL

Dispense in tight, light-resistant container.

R$_X$ only

12. Using the following label, how many milligrams of furosemide are contained in 3 mL? On the handout that you obtained from your instructor, indicate the correct volume on the correct size of oral syringe.

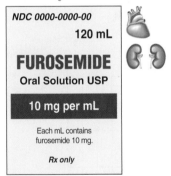

NDC 0000-0000-00

120 mL

FUROSEMIDE

Oral Solution USP

10 mg per mL

Each mL contains furosemide 10 mg.

Rx only

13. Using the following label, how many milligrams of clarithromycin are contained in 2½ tsp?

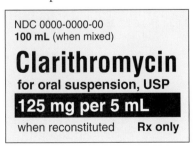

NDC 0000-0000-00
100 mL (when mixed)

Clarithromycin

for oral suspension, USP

125 mg per 5 mL

when reconstituted   **Rx only**

14. Using the label shown for question 13, determine how many days a bottle of clarithromycin will last if a patient is taking 3 tsp every 12 hours.

15. How many prednisone 10 mg tablets are needed to fill the following prescription?

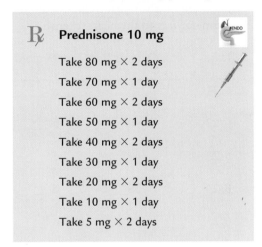

R̶ **Prednisone 10 mg**

Take 80 mg × 2 days

Take 70 mg × 1 day

Take 60 mg × 2 days

Take 50 mg × 1 day

Take 40 mg × 2 days

Take 30 mg × 1 day

Take 20 mg × 2 days

Take 10 mg × 1 day

Take 5 mg × 2 days

Use the label to answer the following questions.

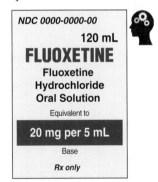

NDC 0000-0000-00

120 mL

FLUOXETINE

Fluoxetine Hydrochloride Oral Solution

Equivalent to

20 mg per 5 mL

Base

Rx only

16. How many milligrams are in ½ tsp?

17. How many milligrams are in ¾ tsp?

18. How many milliliters are needed to provide 40 mg? On the handout that you obtained from your instructor, indicate the correct volume on the correct size of oral syringe.

19. How many milliliters are needed to provide 5 mg? On the handout that you obtained from your instructor, indicate the correct volume on the correct size of oral syringe.

20. Convert the following temperatures and log them on the Celsius chart. Round all temperatures to the nearest tenth.

Date	Degrees F	Degrees C
6/21	43°	a. _____
6/22	40°	b. _____
6/23	41°	c. _____
6/24	38°	d. _____
6/25	39°	e. _____
6/26	40.5°	f. _____
6/27	37°	g. _____

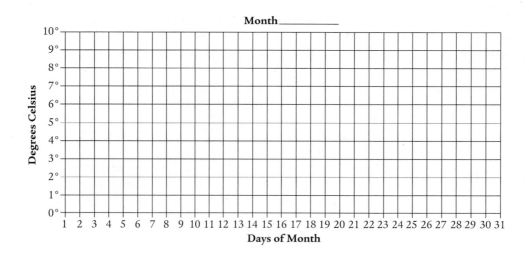

Preparing Injectable Medications

6

Learning Objectives

- Calculate the volume to be measured when given a specific dose.

- Calculate the amount of drug in a given volume.

- Identify drugs that use units as a dose designation.

- Calculate the volume of a substance that has an electrolyte as its primary ingredient.

- Determine the quantity of units in a given concentration and dose.

- Calculate the volume of insulin to be administered.

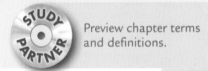

Preview chapter terms and definitions.

6.1 Parenteral Injections and Infusions

Put Down Roots

The word *subcutaneous* has Latin roots: *sub* meaning "under" and *cutis* meaning "skin." Thus, *subcutaneous* is defined as "under the skin." The term *intramuscular*, meaning "within the muscle," also has Latin roots: *intra*, meaning "inward," and *musculus*, meaning "little mouse." The latter meaning stems from comparisons between the shape and movement of the biceps to a mouse.

An **injection** is a method of administering medications in which a syringe with a needle or cannula is used to penetrate through the skin or membrane into the tissue below. An **infusion** is a type of injection in which a large volume of fluid is administered over a long period through a needle or catheter, usually into a vein. Medications given as injections or infusions are considered **parenteral**, which literally means occurring outside the intestines. In other words, the medications do not pass through the gastrointestinal (GI) system.

There are three main types of injections: subcutaneous injections, intramuscular injections, and intravenous infusions. All three types of injections are given by healthcare professionals on a regular basis. A **subcutaneous (SC) injection** is given into the vascular, fatty layer of tissue under the layers of skin. Most medications given by this route are quickly absorbed. Patients can self-administer medications such as insulin by this route. An **intramuscular (IM) injection** is given into the aqueous muscle tissue. Water-soluble medications are absorbed rapidly when given intramuscularly, whereas oil-based medications are absorbed slowly. With proper training, patients can self-administer medications by IM injection, but this route requires more skill and coordination than the subcutaneous route and is often more painful as well. An **intravenous (IV) infusion** is given into a vein. Large-volume IV infusions, such as 500–1000 mL, may be administered over a period of hours. IV infusions of 50–100 mL are often given over a period of 30–60 minutes. Smaller volumes, such as 5–30 mL, may be given via a syringe as an "IV push medication" over a few minutes. Most IV infusions are administered to inpatients, although the trend of home and office administration of IVs is on the rise.

Medications given by injection are often ordered by milligrams, and the pharmacy or nursing staff must select and prepare an appropriate concentration of medication from available stock. The amount of medication is determined using the same methods for calculating liquid oral solutions.

When calculating the dose, personnel should choose a syringe size based on the volume needed. In most institutional pharmacies, syringes with barrel sizes that will hold a total volume of 1 mL, 3 mL, 5 mL, 10 mL, 20 mL, and 50 mL are available. The syringes are marked to indicate volume using tenths or twentieths of a milliliter. Become familiar with these demarcations before using any syringe to measure a volume.

Ideally, the syringe chosen is one that will provide the most accurate volume measurement. Typically, the smaller the syringe, the more accurate its measure. Therefore, the total volume to be prepared should generally fill at least half of the syringe barrel. For example, when measuring 2.8 mL of medication, the selection of the 3 mL or 5 mL syringe would be appropriate because the 2.8 mL would fill half or more of either syringe. If the 10 mL syringe were chosen for dispensing 2.8 mL, the volume of fluid might not be measured as accurately as it would be in the smaller syringes.

Calculating the Volume of an Injectable Solution

The volume of medication to be administered is calculated by both the pharmacy staff and the nursing staff who will administer the medication. Some facilities prepare syringes ahead of time for the nursing staff, but others provide the vial and syringe for the nursing staff to draw up just before administration.

The following examples will demonstrate how to calculate the volume using the ratio-proportion and dimensional analysis methods. When a small volume (less than 20 mL) is to be administered, it is rounded off to the nearest tenth or hundredth, depending on the size of the syringe barrel and its degree of accuracy. Larger volumes are rounded to the tenth or whole milliliter.

Example 6.1.1

How many milliliters of the medication shown in the label below must be prepared to provide 12.5 mg to a patient?

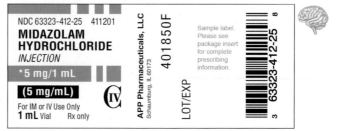

NDC 63323-412-25   411201
MIDAZOLAM HYDROCHLORIDE
INJECTION
5 mg/1 mL
(5 mg/mL)
For IM or IV Use Only
1 mL Vial   Rx only

APP Pharmaceuticals, LLC
Schaumburg, IL 60173

401850F

LOT/EXP

Sample label. Please see package insert for complete prescribing information.

3 63323-412-25 8

Solution 1: Using the ratio-proportion method,

$$\frac{x \text{ mL}}{12.5 \text{ mg}} = \frac{1 \text{ mL}}{5 \text{ mg}}$$

$$x \text{ mL} = \frac{(12.5 \text{ mg}) \times 1 \text{ mL}}{5 \text{ mg}} = 2.5 \text{ mL}$$

Solution 2: Using the dimensional analysis method,

$$12.5 \text{ mg} \times \frac{1 \text{ mL}}{5 \text{ mg}} = 2.5 \text{ mL}$$

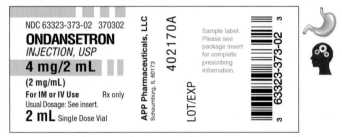

2.5 mL of medication in a 3 mL syringe.

Example 6.1.2

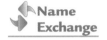

Name Exchange

The generic drug ondansetron is commonly known by the brand name Zofran.

How many milliliters of the medication shown in the label below must be prepared to provide 8 mg of ondansetron to a patient?

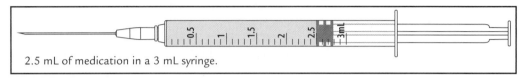

NDC 63323-373-02 370302
ONDANSETRON
INJECTION, USP
4 mg/2 mL
(2 mg/mL)
For IM or IV Use   Rx only
Usual Dosage: See insert.
2 mL Single Dose Vial

APP Pharmaceuticals, LLC
Schaumburg, IL 60173

402170A

LOT/EXP

Sample label.
Please see
package insert
for complete
prescribing
information.

63323-373-02

Solution 1: Using the ratio-proportion method,

$$\frac{x \text{ mL}}{8 \text{ mg}} = \frac{2 \text{ mL}}{4 \text{ mg}}$$

$$x \text{ mL} = \frac{(8 \text{ mg}) \times 2 \text{ mL}}{4 \text{ mg}} = 4 \text{ mL}$$

Solution 2: Using the dimensional analysis method,

$$8 \text{ mg} \times \frac{2 \text{ mL}}{4 \text{ mg}} = 4 \text{ mL}$$

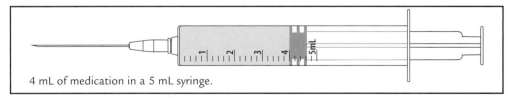

4 mL of medication in a 5 mL syringe.

Example 6.1.3

How many milliliters of medication shown in the label below must be prepared to provide 10 mg of adenosine?

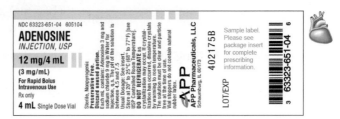

Solution 1: Using the ratio-proportion method,

$$\frac{x \text{ mL}}{10 \text{ mg}} = \frac{4 \text{ mL}}{12 \text{ mg}}$$

$$x \text{ mL} = \frac{(10 \text{ mg}) \times 4 \text{ mL}}{12 \text{ mg}} = 3.333 \text{ mL, rounded to } 3.3 \text{ mL}$$

Solution 2: Using the dimensional analysis method,

$$10 \text{ mg} \times \frac{4 \text{ mL}}{12 \text{ mg}} = 3.333 \text{ mL, rounded to } 3.3 \text{ mL}$$

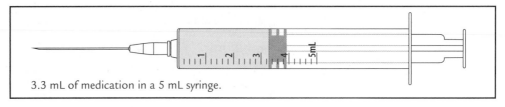

3.3 mL of medication in a 5 mL syringe.

Calculating the Quantity of Drug in an Injectable Solution

The ratio-proportion and dimensional analysis methods can also be used to determine the amount of drug in an injectable solution. The following examples will demonstrate these calculations.

Example 6.1.4

How many milligrams are in 2 mL of the solution shown in the label below?

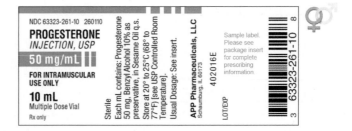

Solution 1: Using the ratio-proportion method,

$$\frac{x \text{ mg}}{2 \text{ mL}} = \frac{50 \text{ mg}}{1 \text{ mL}}$$

$$x \text{ mg} = \frac{(2 \text{ mL}) \times 50 \text{ mg}}{1 \text{ mL}} = 100 \text{ mg}$$

Solution 2: Using the dimensional analysis method,

$$2 \text{ mL} \times \frac{50 \text{ mg}}{1 \text{ mL}} = 100 \text{ mg}$$

Example 6.1.5

How many milligrams of carboplatin are in 30 mL of the solution shown in the label below?

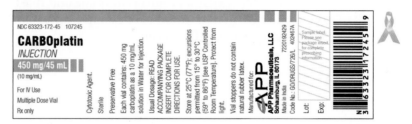

Solution 1: Using the ratio-proportion method,

$$\frac{x \text{ mg}}{30 \text{ mL}} = \frac{450 \text{ mg}}{45 \text{ mL}}$$

$$x \text{ mg} = \frac{(30 \text{ mL}) \times 450 \text{ mg}}{45 \text{ mL}} = 300 \text{ mg}$$

Solution 2: Using the dimensional analysis method,

$$30 \text{ mL} \times \frac{450 \text{ mg}}{45 \text{ mL}} = 300 \text{ mg}$$

Example 6.1.6

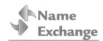
Name Exchange

Lasix, the brand name for the generic drug furosemide, is a commonly dispensed medication in pharmacy practice.

How many milligrams of furosemide are in 6 mL of the solution shown in the label below?

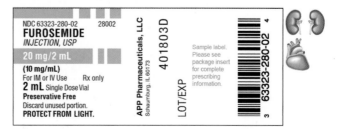

Solution 1: Using the ratio-proportion method,

$$\frac{x \text{ mg}}{6 \text{ mL}} = \frac{20 \text{ mg}}{2 \text{ mL}}$$

$$x \text{ mg} = \frac{(6 \text{ mL}) \times 20 \text{ mg}}{2 \text{ mL}} = 60 \text{ mg}$$

Solution 2: Using the dimensional analysis method,

$$6 \text{ mL} \times \frac{20 \text{ mg}}{2 \text{ mL}} = 60 \text{ mg}$$

Calculating Ratio Strength

The **ratio strength** *a:b* (read as "*a* to *b*") means there are *a* parts of a pure drug in *b* parts of a liquid solution. The units indicated in a ratio strength are *a* grams:*b* milliliters. This formula is the same unit rule that is used to indicate the percent strength of medications. For example, a 1% solution could be written as 1:100, and the units would be 1 g:100 mL.

Example 6.1.7

How many grams of pure drug are in 500 mL of a 1:200 solution?

Solution 1: Using the ratio-proportion method,

$$\frac{x \text{ g}}{500 \text{ mL}} = \frac{1 \text{ g}}{200 \text{ mL}}$$

$$x \text{ g} = \frac{(500 \text{ mL}) \times 1 \text{ g}}{200 \text{ mL}} = 2.5 \text{ g}$$

Solution 2: Using the dimensional analysis method,

$$500 \text{ mL} \times \frac{1 \text{ g}}{200 \text{ mL}} = 2.5 \text{ g}$$

Example 6.1.8

How many grams of pure drug are in 500 mL of a 1:3000 solution?

Solution 1: Using the ratio-proportion method,

$$\frac{x \text{ g}}{500 \text{ mL}} = \frac{1 \text{ g}}{3000 \text{ mL}}$$

$$x \text{ g} = \frac{(500 \text{ mL}) \times 1 \text{ g}}{3000 \text{ mL}} = 0.1666 \text{ g, rounded to } 0.17 \text{ g}$$

Solution 2: Using the dimensional analysis method,

$$500 \text{ mL} \times \frac{1 \text{ g}}{3000 \text{ mL}} = 0.1666 \text{ g, rounded to } 0.17 \text{ g}$$

Example 6.1.9

How many milligrams of pure drug are in 1.5 mL of a 1:1000 solution of epinephrine?

Solution 1: Using the ratio-proportion method,

$$\frac{x \text{ g}}{1.5 \text{ mL}} = \frac{1 \text{ g}}{1000 \text{ mL}}$$

$$x \text{ g} = \frac{(1.5 \text{ mL}) \times 1 \text{ g}}{1000 \text{ mL}} = 0.0015 \text{ g} = 1.5 \text{ mg}$$

Solution 2: Using the dimensional analysis method,

$$1.5 \text{ mL} \times \frac{1 \text{ g}}{1000 \text{ mL}} = 0.0015 \text{ g} = 1.5 \text{ mg}$$

Example 6.1.10

How many milliliters are needed to provide 20 mg of a drug if the solution available is 1:500?

Begin by converting 20 mg to 0.02 g.

Solution 1: Using the ratio-proportion method,

$$\frac{x \text{ mL}}{0.02 \text{ g}} = \frac{500 \text{ mL}}{1 \text{ g}}$$

$$x \text{ mL} = \frac{(0.02 \text{ g}) \times 500 \text{ mL}}{1 \text{ g}} = 10 \text{ mL}$$

Solution 2: Using the dimensional analysis method,

$$0.02 \text{ g} \times \frac{500 \text{ mL}}{1 \text{ g}} = 10 \text{ mL}$$

Determine the volume to be prepared for each ordered injectable solution using the labels provided. (Round to the hundredths place.)

Note: *Questions 1–10 have accompanying handouts that must be obtained from your instructor.*

1. How many milliliters of solution are needed to provide 50 mg of Xylocaine? On the handout that you obtained from your instructor, indicate the correct volume on the measuring device.

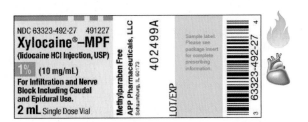

2. How many milliliters of solution are needed to provide 60 mg of furosemide? On the handout that you obtained from your instructor, indicate the correct volume on the measuring device.

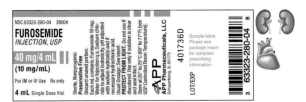

3. How many milliliters of solution are needed to provide 80 mg of furosemide? On the handout that you obtained from your instructor, indicate the correct volume on the measuring device.

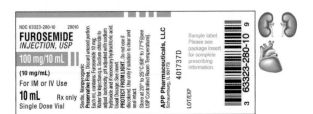

4. How many milliliters of solution are needed to provide 0.75 mg of indomethacin in this 1 mg/1 mL vial? On the handout that you obtained from your instructor, indicate the correct volume on the measuring device.

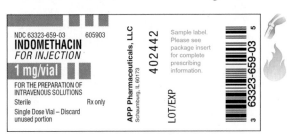

5. How many milliliters of solution are needed to provide 100 mg of diphenhydramine? On the handout that you obtained from your instructor, indicate the correct volume on the measuring device.

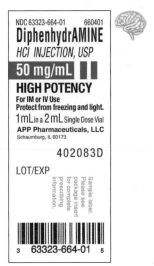

6. How many milliliters of solution are needed to provide 30 mg of famotidine? On the handout that you obtained from your instructor, indicate the correct volume on the measuring device.

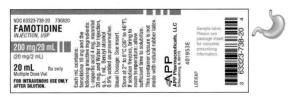

7. How many milliliters of solution are needed to provide 40 mg of famotidine? On the handout that you obtained from your instructor, indicate the correct volume on the measuring device.

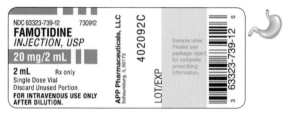

8. How many milliliters of solution are needed to provide 250 mg of azithromycin? On the handout that you obtained from your instructor, indicate the correct volume on the measuring device.

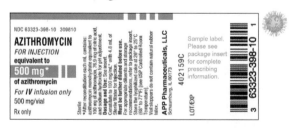

9. How many milliliters of solution are needed to provide 400 mg of azithromycin? On the handout that you obtained from your instructor, indicate the correct volume on the measuring device.

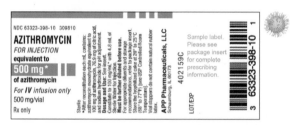

10. How many milliliters of solution are needed to provide 50 mg of cisplatin? On the handout that you obtained from your instructor, indicate the correct volume on the measuring device.

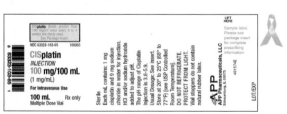

Calculate the quantity of drug in the injectable solution using the provided vial labels.

11. How many milligrams of ketorolac are contained in 0.5 mL?

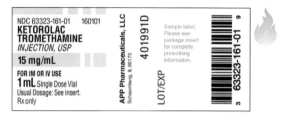

12. How many milligrams of ketorolac are contained in 1.75 mL?

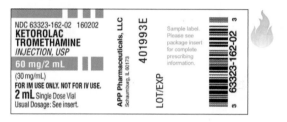

13. How many milligrams of lidocaine HCl are contained in 3.75 mL?

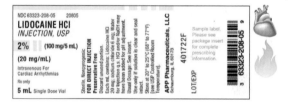

14. How many milligrams of midazolam HCl are contained in 1.3 mL?

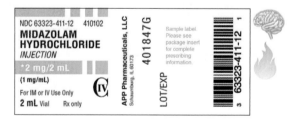

15. How many milligrams of midazolam HCl are contained in 5 mL?

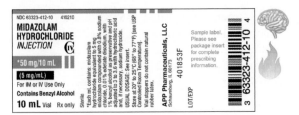

16. How many milligrams of midazolam HCl are contained in 5 mL?

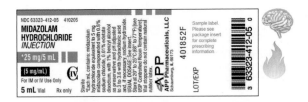

17. How many milligrams of midazolam HCl are contained in 5 mL?

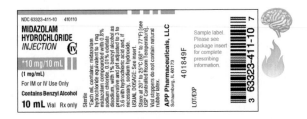

18. How many milligrams of dexamethasone are contained in 8 mL?

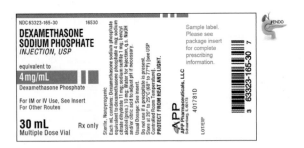

19. How many milligrams of ondansetron are contained in 1.5 mL?

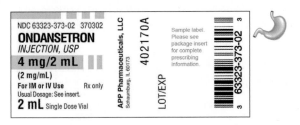

20. How many milligrams of progesterone are contained in 2.5 mL?

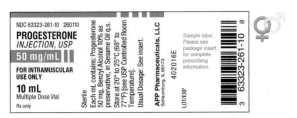

Calculate the amount of pure drug in a ratio solution.

21. How many milligrams are in 2 mL of a 1:1000 solution?

22. How many micrograms are in 1 mL of a 1:5000 solution?

23. How many micrograms are in 1.5 mL of a 1:10,000 solution?

24. How many micrograms are in 1.4 mL of a 1:2000 solution?

25. How many micrograms are in 2.5 mL of a 1:10,000 solution?

Calculate the volume of solution needed for each requested dose to be infused intravenously.

26. How many milliliters of 1:1000 solution are needed to provide a 500 mg dose?

27. How many milliliters of 1:10,000 solution are needed to provide a 50 mg dose?

28. How many milliliters of 1:300 solution are needed to provide a 600 mg dose?

29. How many milliliters of 1:500 solution are needed to provide a 250 mg dose?

30. How many milliliters of 1:750 solution are needed to provide a 0.01 g dose?

Self-check your work in Appendix A.

6.2 Other Units of Measure

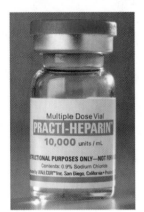

Heparin is a medication that is dosed in units.

Although most medications are dosed using the units of the metric system, such as milligrams or grams, doses of some medications are calculated using other units of measure. Some of these substances are as simple as salts, but others are complicated proteins or hormones such as insulin. Other examples include penicillin V, whose unit is based on the number of bacteria affected, and heparin, whose unit is based on the amount of anticoagulant property present. Although these substances do have weights, they will be dosed based on their activity, and the weight will often be disregarded.

Calculating Milliequivalents

Many fluids in pharmacy contain dissolved mineral salts known as **electrolytes**. They are so named because they conduct a charge through the solution when connected to electrodes.

Most electrolyte solutions are measured by milliequivalents, which are related to molecular weight. Molecular weights are based on the atomic weight of common elements. The **atomic weight** of an element is the weight of a single atom of that element compared with the weight of a single atom of hydrogen. The **molecular weight** of a compound is the sum of the atomic weights of all atoms in one molecule of the compound. A **millimole (mM)** is the molecular weight expressed as milligrams.

A **milliequivalent (mEq)** is the ratio of the weight of a molecule to its **valence**, or the likely charge or ability to bond with an equally charged molecule.

$$mEq = \frac{molecular\ weight}{valence}$$

Valence is most familiar as the plus or minus sign next to chemical abbreviations or symbols such as Na^+, Cl^-, or Ca^{++}. The valence of substances used in pharmacy preparations is most commonly plus or minus 1, 2, or 3. Milliequivalents represent both the amount of active substance and the likelihood that the substance, once in the body, will cause a change in the way two compounds are bonded.

Electrolyte solutions and certain drugs, besides being measured by weight at the manufacturer, are also measured in millimoles and milliequivalents. These types of measure are particularly important when working with IV solutions. For example, you may be asked to add 28 mEq of sodium chloride to an IV bag. You would then need to calculate the total volume in milliliters of sodium chloride solution to add to the IV bag, given an available solution of 4 mEq/mL.

Fortunately, medications commonly used today are standardized, and the calculations needed in the pharmacy will involve determining the volume of a substance that has an electrolyte as its primary ingredient. The two most common electrolytes that are supplemented or replaced due to loss are potassium and sodium. These electrolytes are required for normal body functions and are typically obtained through nutrition. When administered as medications, they are used to restore a natural balance and may affect many body systems.

You are requested to add 44 mEq of sodium chloride (NaCl) to an IV bag. Sodium chloride is available as a 4 mEq/mL solution. How many milliliters will you add to the bag?

Solution 1: Using the ratio-proportion method,

$$\frac{x \, \text{mL}}{44 \, \text{mEq}} = \frac{1 \, \text{mL}}{4 \, \text{mEq}}$$

$$x \, \text{mL} = \frac{(44 \, \text{mEq}) \times 1 \, \text{mL}}{4 \, \text{mEq}} = 11 \, \text{mL}$$

Solution 2: Using the dimensional analysis method,

$$44 \, \text{mEq} \times \frac{1 \, \text{mL}}{4 \, \text{mEq}} = 11 \, \text{mL}$$

Medications to replace potassium can be administered as an IV solution, or a patient may take potassium orally by tablet or oral solution. The calculations are performed using the same process as previously discussed.

A patient needs to take a solution of potassium chloride to replace potassium lost due to diuresis. The available solution is shown in the label below. The physician has indicated that the patient needs 15 mEq. How many milliliters will be prepared for the patient?

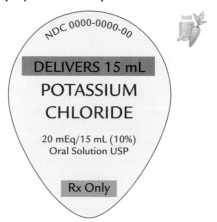

Solution 1: Using the ratio-proportion method,

$$\frac{x \, \text{mL}}{15 \, \text{mEq}} = \frac{15 \, \text{mL}}{20 \, \text{mEq}}$$

$$x \, \text{mL} = \frac{(15 \, \text{mEq}) \times 15 \, \text{mL}}{20 \, \text{mEq}} = 11.25 \, \text{mL, rounded to 11 mL}$$

Solution 2: Using the dimensional analysis method,

$$15 \text{ mEq} \times \frac{15 \text{ mL}}{20 \text{ mEq}} = 11.25 \text{ mL, rounded to 11 mL}$$

Example 6.2.3

You are instructed to add 20 mEq of potassium chloride to a patient's IV solution bag. Using the multiple-dose vial label provided, how many milliliters should be drawn up?

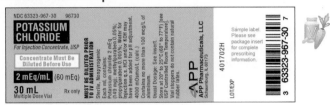

Solution 1: Using the ratio-proportion method,

$$\frac{x \text{ mL}}{20 \text{ mEq}} = \frac{1 \text{ mL}}{2 \text{ mEq}}$$

$$x \text{ mL} = \frac{(20 \text{ mEq}) \times 1 \text{ mL}}{2 \text{ mEq}} = 10 \text{ mL}$$

Solution 2: Using the dimensional analysis method,

$$20 \text{ mEq} \times \frac{1 \text{ mL}}{2 \text{ mEq}} = 10 \text{ mL}$$

Example 6.2.4

You are instructed to add 16 mEq of potassium chloride to a patient's IV bag. Using the single-dose vial labels, select the correct vial and then calculate how many milliliters you will prepare.

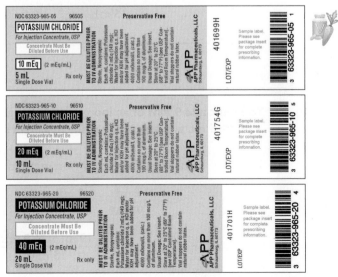

Part I. Analyze the total milliequivalents in each vial to choose the correct vial. In the labels shown, the manufacturer has highlighted the milliequivalents in each vial. Because your order calls for 16 mEq, you will select the potassium chloride vial labeled "20 mEq." The total volume is 10 mL.

Part II. Determine the number of milliliters needed to fill the order.

Solution 1: Using the ratio-proportion method,

$$\frac{x \text{ mL}}{16 \text{ mEq}} = \frac{10 \text{ mL}}{20 \text{ mEq}}$$

$$x \text{ mL} = \frac{(16 \text{ mEq}) \times 10 \text{ mL}}{20 \text{ mEq}} = 8 \text{ mL}$$

Solution 2: Using the dimensional analysis method,

$$16 \text{ mEq} \times \frac{10 \text{ mL}}{20 \text{ mEq}} = 8 \text{ mL}$$

Example 6.2.5

You have been instructed to add 15 mL of sodium chloride to a patient's IV bag for dilution. The medication label states that the concentration of sodium chloride is 4 mEq/mL. Calculate how many milliequivalents of sodium chloride will be in 15 mL of solution.

Solution 1: Using the ratio-proportion method,

$$\frac{x \text{ mEq}}{15 \text{ mL}} = \frac{4 \text{ mEq}}{1 \text{ mL}}$$

$$x \text{ mEq} = \frac{(15 \text{ mL}) \times 4 \text{ mEq}}{1 \text{ mL}} = 60 \text{ mEq}$$

Solution 2: Using the dimensional analysis method,

$$15 \text{ mL} \times \frac{4 \text{ mEq}}{1 \text{ mL}} = 60 \text{ mEq}$$

Example 6.2.6

You must add 9 mM of an inorganic phosphate to an IV solution. You have 15 mM/5 mL available. How many milliliters should you add?

Solution 1: Using the ratio-proportion method,

$$\frac{x \text{ mL}}{9 \text{ mM}} = \frac{5 \text{ mL}}{15 \text{ mM}}$$

$$x \text{ mL} = \frac{(9 \text{ mM}) \times 5 \text{ mL}}{15 \text{ mM}} = 3 \text{ mL}$$

Solution 2: Using the dimensional analysis method,

$$9 \text{ mM} \times \frac{5 \text{ mL}}{15 \text{ mM}} = 3 \text{ mL}$$

Calculating Units

Safety in Numbers

Pharmacy technicians should not abbreviate international units as IU or U but should write out "units."

For Good Measure

The number of units used should correspond to the size of insulin syringe that the patient uses.

Safety in Numbers

Only insulin syringes should be used to administer or dispense insulin.

A number of drugs—including insulin, heparin, corticotropin (ACTH), Factor VIII, penicillin, and some vitamins—are measured in units. A **unit** describes the amount of activity within a unique test system. Drugs that are derived mainly from biological products are expressed in international units or United States Pharmacopeia (USP) units. Both are expressed as "units."

Each drug has a unique biological assay to define its unit of activity. For example, insulin is dosed in units, and the units are based on the amount of glucose that a specific amount of insulin can make available to the cells in a living human being. The degree of activity in this case refers to the insulin's activity. When insulin is prescribed and administered, the dose is based on how much assistance the patient's body will need. Different types and brands of insulin have different weights, but all insulins use a common "unit" of activity. Thus, the weight can be disregarded, and the unit becomes a universal dose for insulin. Insulin syringes are prepared and marked according to these standard units. Manufacturers maintain the same concentration of insulin from brand to brand so that the standard insulin syringe will measure out a uniform unit of insulin with a known activity level in the body.

Insulin doses are always calculated in units. Although it is important to know the approximate volume in milliliters, the preparation will most likely involve the use of syringes that are specially marked with units instead of milliliters. Insulin is concentrated as "U-100" insulin, which means that there are 100 units in 1 mL (or 100 units/mL). Insulin syringes are available in standard unit sizes as illustrated in Figure 6.1.

FIGURE 6.1
Standard Insulin Syringe Sizes

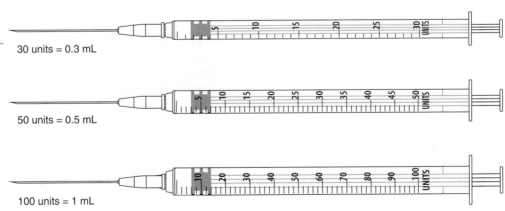

30 units = 0.3 mL

50 units = 0.5 mL

100 units = 1 mL

Example 6.2.7

A patient is to receive a bolus (concentrated) dose of heparin. If the dose is 7500 units and you have a vial with the label shown below, how many milliliters will you prepare?

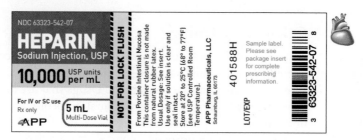

Solution 1: Using the ratio-proportion method,

$$\frac{x \text{ mL}}{7500 \text{ units}} = \frac{1 \text{ mL}}{10,000 \text{ units}}$$

$$x \text{ mL} = \frac{(7500 \text{ units}) \times 1 \text{ mL}}{10,000 \text{ units}} = 0.75 \text{ mL}$$

Solution 2: Using the dimensional analysis method,

$$7500 \text{ units} \times \frac{1 \text{ mL}}{10,000 \text{ units}} = 0.75 \text{ mL}$$

Example 6.2.8

A patient is to receive 1000 units/kg of bacitracin IM indicated on the label below. The patient weighs 15 kg. How many milliliters of bacitracin are needed?

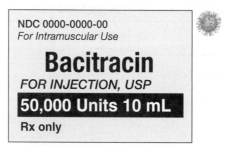

Begin by determining the number of units in a dose, based on the patient's weight of 15 kg.

$$15 \text{ kg} \times \frac{1000 \text{ units}}{1 \text{ kg}} = 15,000 \text{ units}$$

Then, calculate the amount of milliliters needed, using either the ratio-proportion method or the dimensional analysis method.

Solution 1: Using the ratio-proportion method,

$$\frac{x \text{ mL}}{15{,}000 \text{ units}} = \frac{10 \text{ mL}}{50{,}000 \text{ units}}$$

$$x \text{ mL} = \frac{(15{,}000 \text{ units}) \times 10 \text{ mL}}{50{,}000 \text{ units}} = 3 \text{ mL}$$

Solution 2: Using the dimensional analysis method,

$$15{,}000 \text{ units} \times \frac{10 \text{ mL}}{50{,}000 \text{ units}} = 3 \text{ mL}$$

Safety in Numbers

Pharmacy technicians should check insulin labels three times to ensure that they have selected the correct product.

As discussed earlier in this section, insulin is dosed with the concentration of 100 units/mL, and all insulin is dosed and calibrated to the standard U-100 or "unit." Despite this consistency, many types of insulin products are available. Some insulin products require the patient to withdraw medication from a vial. Other insulin products come in a prefilled syringe or "pen" with a disposable needle on the tip. Only insulin syringes should be used to administer or dispense insulin.

Reading insulin labels can be challenging because labels may have only slight differentiations from one product to another (see Figure 6.2). Even though insulins dispensed to patients have a standard U-100 concentration, they are not interchangeable. They differ by onset and duration of action and have the potential to harm a patient who uses the wrong brand or type. When preparing an insulin dose or prescription, triple-check the medication's label against the printed label and the ordered medication. Confirm that the NDC numbers match. If the pharmacy is equipped with a bar-code scanner, such a device will be helpful in confirming that the correct medication is being used. Insulins with a higher concentration of U-500 are administered only in hospital settings under specific circumstances.

FIGURE 6.2   Insulin Labels

Although it is true for all drug labels, it is especially important to read insulin labels carefully.

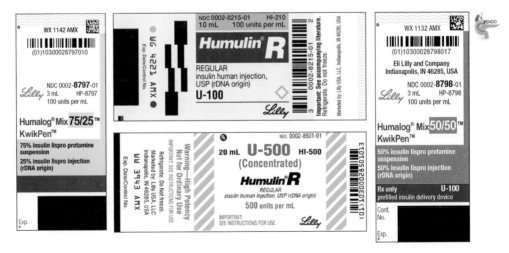

The following examples demonstrate the calculation of a volume of insulin in milliliters (vs. standard units). Calculating the volume of insulin in milliliters is helpful when determining how long an insulin vial or pen will last a patient.

Example 6.2.9

A patient is to receive 32 units of regular insulin each morning before breakfast. Insulin comes in a concentration of 100 units/mL. How many milliliters will the patient receive with each dose? How many days will the vial last?

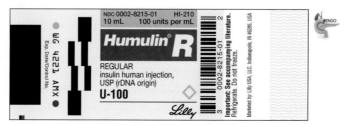

Part I. Calculate the volume the patient will receive with each dose by using either the ratio-proportion method or the dimensional analysis method.

Solution 1: Using the ratio-proportion method,

$$\frac{x \text{ mL}}{32 \text{ units}} = \frac{1 \text{ mL}}{100 \text{ units}}$$

$$x \text{ mL} = \frac{(32 \text{ units}) \times 1 \text{ mL}}{100 \text{ units}} = 0.32 \text{ mL}$$

Solution 2: Using the dimensional analysis method,

$$32 \text{ units} \times \frac{1 \text{ mL}}{100 \text{ units}} = 0.32 \text{ mL}$$

Part II. Using the volume per dose just calculated, determine the number of days a single vial will last. In this example, the patient takes a single dose a day.

Solution 1: Using the ratio-proportion method,

$$\frac{x \text{ days}}{10 \text{ mL}} = \frac{1 \text{ day}}{0.32 \text{ mL}}$$

$$x \text{ days} = \frac{(10 \text{ mL}) \times 1 \text{ day}}{0.32 \text{ mL}} = 31.25 \text{ days, or 31 days}$$

Solution 2: Using the dimensional analysis method,

$$10 \text{ mL} \times \frac{1 \text{ day}}{0.32 \text{ mL}} = 31.25 \text{ days, or 31 days}$$

Example 6.2.10

A patient is to receive 49 units of Humulin 70/30 insulin. Insulin comes in a concentration of 100 units/mL. How many milliliters will the patient receive in each dose? How many vials will the patient need to last 30 days (1 month)?

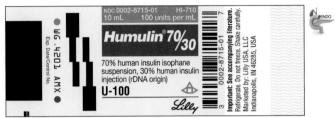

Part I. Calculate the volume the patient will receive with each dose by using either the ratio-proportion method or the dimensional analysis method.

Solution 1: Using the ratio-proportion method,

$$\frac{x \text{ mL}}{49 \text{ units}} = \frac{1 \text{ mL}}{100 \text{ units}}$$

$$x \text{ mL} = \frac{(49 \text{ units}) \times 1 \text{ mL}}{100 \text{ units}} = 0.49 \text{ mL}$$

Solution 2: Using the dimensional analysis method,

$$49 \text{ units} \times \frac{1 \text{ mL}}{100 \text{ units}} = 0.49 \text{ mL}$$

Part II. Using the volume per dose just calculated, determine the number of milliliters needed for 30 days.

Solution 1: Using the ratio-proportion method,

$$\frac{x \text{ mL}}{30 \text{ days}} = \frac{0.49 \text{ mL}}{1 \text{ day}}$$

$$x \text{ mL} = \frac{(30 \text{ days}) \times 0.49 \text{ mL}}{1 \text{ day}} = 14.7 \text{ mL}$$

Solution 2: Using the dimensional analysis method,

$$30 \text{ days} \times \frac{0.49 \text{ mL}}{1 \text{ day}} = 14.7 \text{ mL}$$

Since 1 vial = 10 mL, 2 vials will be needed to last 30 days.

Example 6.2.11

Humalog Mix 75/25 KwikPen is useful for patients with busy lifestyles or those "trying out" a new formula of insulin. How many units are in the KwikPen with the following label? If a patient uses 23 units daily, how many days will this KwikPen last?

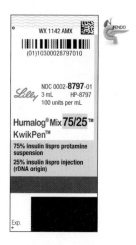

Part I.   Calculate the total number of units in a single pen.

Solution 1: Using the ratio-proportion method,

$$\frac{x \text{ units}}{3 \text{ mL}} = \frac{100 \text{ units}}{1 \text{ mL}}$$

$$x \text{ units} = \frac{(3 \text{ mL}) \times 100 \text{ units}}{1 \text{ mL}} = 300 \text{ units}$$

Solution 2: Using the dimensional analysis method,

$$3 \text{ mL} \times \frac{100 \text{ units}}{1 \text{ mL}} = 300 \text{ units}$$

Part II.   Calculate the number of days a single pen will last using the patient's daily units. Again, you can use either the ratio-proportion method or the dimensional analysis method.

Solution 1: Using the ratio-proportion method,

$$\frac{x \text{ days}}{300 \text{ units}} = \frac{1 \text{ day}}{23 \text{ units}}$$

$$x \text{ days} = \frac{(300 \text{ units}) \times 1 \text{ day}}{23 \text{ units}} = 13.04 \text{ days, or } 13 \text{ days}$$

Solution 2: Using the dimensional analysis method,

$$300 \text{ units} \times \frac{1 \text{ day}}{23 \text{ units}} = 13.04 \text{ days, or } 13 \text{ days}$$

Perform the necessary calculations to answer each of the following. (Round to the hundredths place.)

Note: Questions 1, 2, 4, 6, 7, 8, 13, 14, and 16 have accompanying handouts that must be obtained from your instructor.

1. An order requires 30 mEq of potassium phosphate. You have a 4.4 mEq/mL solution available. How many milliliters should you put in the IV bag? On the handout that you obtained from your instructor, indicate the correct volume on the measuring devices.

2. An order requires 45 mEq of potassium phosphate. You have a 4.4 mEq/mL solution available. How many milliliters should you put in the IV solution? On the handout that you obtained from your instructor, indicate the correct volume on the measuring devices.

3. A prescription states that a patient must take 32 mEq of potassium. The potassium replacement selected has 8 mEq per tablet. How many tablets would the patient need to take?

4. A patient is to use a sugar- and alcohol-free solution of potassium that contains 40 mEq/15 mL. He is to take 30 mEq daily in two equally divided doses. How many milliliters will each dose be? On the handout that you obtained from your instructor, indicate the correct volume on the measuring devices.

5. A prescription has been filled for 15 mL Rum-K with breakfast. Rum-K contains 20 mEq/10 mL. How many milliequivalents is the patient taking with each dose?

6. A patient needs to take 30 mEq of potassium orally. The solution on hand has 20 mEq/15 mL. How much should be prepared for the patient? On the handout that you obtained from your instructor, indicate the correct volume on the measuring device.

For questions 7–10, select the vial that is needed to fill each order with the required number of milliequivalents of potassium chloride, and then calculate the volume to be withdrawn from the selected vial for the order.

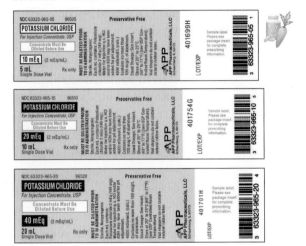

7. Add 14 mEq potassium chloride to the patient's IV solution. On the handout that you obtained from your instructor, indicate the correct volume on the measuring devices.

8. Add 19 mEq potassium chloride to the patient's IV solution. On the handout that you obtained from your instructor, indicate the correct volume on the measuring device.

9. Add 27 mEq potassium chloride to the patient's IV solution.

10. Add 50 mEq potassium chloride to the patient's IV solution.

For each of the following questions, use the label provided to calculate the volume or amount requested.

11. How many milliequivalents of potassium chloride are in 8 mL of the solution?

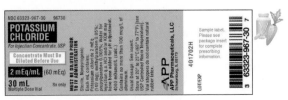

12. How many milliequivalents of potassium chloride are in 15 mL of the solution?

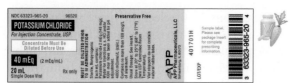

13. The following order is received by the pharmacy. Sodium chloride is available as a 4 mEq/mL solution. How many milliliters should you add to the bag? On the handout that you obtained from your instructor, indicate the correct volume on the measuring device.

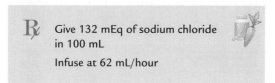

Give 132 mEq of sodium chloride in 100 mL

Infuse at 62 mL/hour

14. An order is received indicating that you should add 120 mEq sodium chloride to an IV bag of dextrose 5% in water (D_5W). Using a vial that is labeled 4 mEq/mL, how many milliliters should you add to the bag? On the handout that you obtained from your instructor, indicate the correct volume on the measuring device.

Use the following label to answer questions 15 and 16.

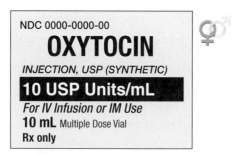

NDC 0000-0000-00

OXYTOCIN

INJECTION, USP (SYNTHETIC)

10 USP Units/mL

For IV Infusion or IM Use

10 mL Multiple Dose Vial

Rx only

15. A patient is to receive 4 units of oxytocin. Using the vial with the label shown above, how many milliliters will be needed?

16. A patient has received 2.8 mL of the oxytocin solution shown in the label above. How many units is this? On the handout that you obtained from your instructor, indicate the correct volume on the measuring device.

17. A patient is to receive 3500 units heparin, and the following label shows the drug you are to dispense. How many milliliters is this?

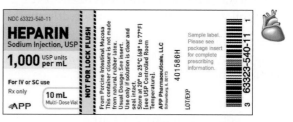

18. A patient needs an injection of heparin. An order for 0.43 mL has been prepared. How many units of heparin are in the dose if it contains 20,000 units/0.8 mL?

19. Prepare 7,000 units of heparin from the vial with the label shown below. How many milliliters is this?

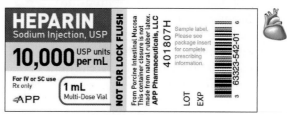

20. Prepare 24,000 units of heparin from the vial with the label shown below. How many milliliters is this?

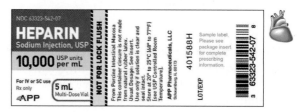

21. Prepare two syringes for a patient on the orthopedic floor. Each syringe should contain 30 mg of Lovenox. How many milliliters will be in each syringe?

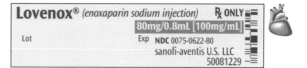

Calculate the following volumes or amount of units.

22. Pen VK (penicillin V–potassium) can be reconstituted to many different concentrations. You are filling an order for 175,000 units and have available a concentration that has already been concentrated to 500,000 units/mL. How many milliliters is the dose?

23. Bicillin CR is given as an IM injection preparation. It comes as 600,000 units/mL, and the dose is 1.5 million units. What is the volume to be administered?

24. A physician has ordered 385,000 units of Pen VK (penicillin V–potassium) for a patient. Your stock preparation has 50,000 units/mL. How many milliliters should the dose be?

25. A patient is to receive Humulin 70/30 insulin at a dose of 45 units at 8:00 every morning. Using the vial with the following label, how many milliliters should be drawn into the syringe?

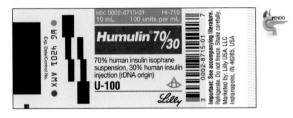

26. A patient uses 18 units of insulin each morning and 10 units at 7:00 p.m. How long will the vial shown in the following label last?

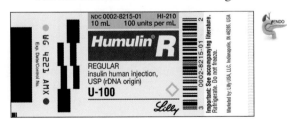

27. A patient uses 20 units of insulin every morning and 18 units of insulin every evening. Using the label below, answer the following questions.

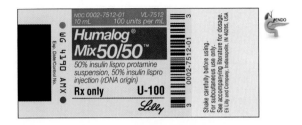

a. How many total units does the patient use daily?

b. How many vials are needed for 30 days?

28. A patient uses 10 units of Humulin R each morning and 15 units of Humulin 70/30 at lunch and supper. Using the labels below, how many vials of each will the patient need for 30 days?

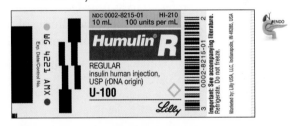

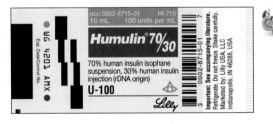

29. A patient uses 0.5 mL daily of Lantus shown in the following label. How many units is this?

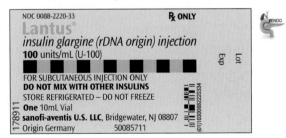

30. Using the label shown below, how long will
    two vials of Apidra last a patient who uses
    20 units twice daily?

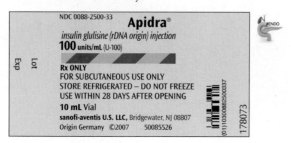

Self-check your work in Appendix A.

6.3 Solutions Using Powders

In the preparation of solutions, the active ingredient is discussed in terms of weight, but it also occupies a certain amount of space. For lyophilized (freeze-dried) pharmaceuticals that are packaged in a sterile vial and used for reconstitution, this space is referred to as **powder volume (pv)**. It is equal to the difference between the final volume (fv) and the volume of the diluting ingredient, or the diluent volume, (dv), as expressed in the following equation:

$$\text{powder volume (pv)} = \text{final volume (fv)} - \text{diluent volume (dv)}$$

or

$$pv = fv - dv$$

Example 6.3.1

A powdered antibiotic must be reconstituted for use. The label states that the dry powder occupies 0.5 mL. Using the formula for solving for powder volume, determine the diluent volume (the amount of solvent added). You are given the final volume for three different examples below with the same powder volume.

Final Volume	Powder Volume
2 mL	0.5 mL
5 mL	0.5 mL
10 mL	0.5 mL

$dv = fv - pv$
$dv = 2 \text{ mL} - 0.5 \text{ mL} = 1.5 \text{ mL}$
$dv = 5 \text{ mL} - 0.5 \text{ mL} = 4.5 \text{ mL}$
$dv = 10 \text{ mL} - 0.5 \text{ mL} = 9.5 \text{ mL}$

Example 6.3.2

You are to reconstitute 1 g of dry powder. The label states that you are to add 9.3 mL of diluent to make a final solution of 100 mg/mL. What is the powder volume?

Begin by calculating the final volume. The strength of the final solution will be 100 mg/mL. Since you start with 1 g = 1000 mg of powder, for a final volume x of the solution, it will have strength 1000 mg/x mL.

Solution 1: Using the ratio-proportion method,

$$\frac{x \text{ mL}}{1000 \text{ mg}} = \frac{1 \text{ mL}}{100 \text{ mg}}$$

$$x \text{ mL} = \frac{(1000 \text{ mg}) \times 1 \text{ mL}}{100 \text{ mg}} = 10 \text{ mL}$$

Solution 2: Using the dimensional analysis method,

$$1000 \text{ mg} \times \frac{1 \text{ mL}}{100 \text{ mg}} = 10 \text{ mL}$$

Then, using the calculated final volume and the given diluent volume, determine the powder volume.

$$\text{pv} = \text{fv} - \text{dv}$$

$$\text{pv} = 10 \text{ mL} - 9.3 \text{ mL} = 0.7 \text{ mL}$$

Example 6.3.3

A label states that a 5 g quantity of an antibiotic in a bottle should be reconstituted with 8.7 mL saline for injection. The resulting concentration will be 500 mg/mL. What is the powder volume contained in the vial?

First, convert 500 mg to grams.

$$500 \text{ mg} \times \frac{1 \text{ g}}{1000 \text{ mg}} = 0.5 \text{ g}$$

Second, determine the total number of milliliters that will contain the resultant concentration of 0.5 g/mL.

$$\frac{x \text{ mL}}{5 \text{ g}} = \frac{1 \text{ mL}}{0.5 \text{ g}}$$

$$x \text{ mL} = 10 \text{ mL}$$

Third, subtract the diluent volume from the final volume.

$$10 \text{ mL (fv)} - 8.7 \text{ mL (dv)} = 1.3 \text{ mL (pv)}$$

6.3 Problem Set

Solve the following.

1. You need to make an injectable solution with a final concentration of 375 mg/mL. After checking your supply, you have a vial that contains 1.5 g with the instructions to add 3.3 mL. What is the powder volume?

2. You must add water to an oral suspension before it can be dispensed to the patient. The dose is to be 250 mg/tsp, and the dry powder is 5 g with a powder volume of 8.6 mL. How much water must you add?

3. An injectable preparation comes packaged as a 1 g vial, and you want a final concentration of 125 mg/2 mL. The vial states that you are to add 14.4 mL diluent. What is the powder volume?

4. The label of a 2 g vial states that you are to add 6.8 mL to get a concentration of 250 mg/mL. What is the powder volume?

5. In question 4, to make a final concentration of 125 mg/mL, how much diluent must you add?

6. The label of a 4 g vial states that you are to add 11.7 mL to get a concentration of 250 mg/mL. What is the powder volume?

7. The label of a 6 g vial says that if you add 12.5 mL of diluent to the vial's contents you will get a concentration of 1 g/2.5 mL. What concentration do you get if you add 2.5 mL?

8. You have added 3.3 mL of diluent to a 1 g vial and now have a final volume of 4 mL. What is the powder volume?

9. How many milliliters of the medication in question 8 do you need for a 100 mg dose?

10. If you add 8.8 mL of diluent to a 2 g vial and get a final concentration of 200 mg/mL, what is the powder volume?

11. A 10 g vial must have 45 mL of diluent added to it. It has a powder volume of 5 mL. How many milligrams will be in each milliliter of the final solution?

12. For an oral suspension, you add 170 mL of fluid and get a final volume of 200 mL. If it contains 8 g of medication, how many milligrams will be in 1 tsp?

13. A 20 g bulk vial label states that if you add 106 mL of diluent, the concentration will be 1 g/6 mL. How much diluent would you add to get a concentration of 1 g/3 mL?

14. You need a concentration of 375 mg/mL. Your vial contains 2 g with instructions to add 3.5 mL of diluent. What is the powder volume?

15. An oral medication requires reconstitution. The dose is 300 mg/tsp. The dry powder is 2.5 g with a volume of 9.6 mL. How much water do you add?

16. A 5 g vial requires that 8.6 mL diluent be added to get a concentration of 250 mg/mL. What is the powder volume?

17. A 10 g vial label says to add 20 mL of diluent to get 1 g per 2.5 mL. What concentration would you get if you added 35 mL?

18. You add 4.3 mL of diluent to a 1 g vial and have a final volume of 5 mL. What is the powder volume?

19. A 5 g vial requires 25 mL to be added. It has a powder volume of 5 mL. How many milligrams are in each milliliter of the final solution?

20. A 20 g vial must have 90 mL of diluent added. It has a powder volume of 10 mL. How many milligrams will be in each milliliter of the final solution?

21. A 3 g vial requires 20 mL of diluent to be added. It has a powder volume of 5 mL. How many milligrams are in each milliliter of the final solution?

22. A pediatric antibiotic requires 67 mL to be added to the bottle for reconstitution. The final volume will be 100 mL. What is the powder volume?

23. If the bottle in question 22 is reconstituted and there are 35 g of active ingredient in the bottle, what will the resulting strength be in milligrams per milliliters?

Solve the following compounding problems.

24. The pharmacy receives the following compound. What is the final concentration in milligrams per milliliters?

25. The pharmacy receives the following compound.

a. What concentration is the vial of cephalosporin when you reconstitute it in milligrams per milliliters?

b. What milligram dose is the patient receiving?

Self-check your work in Appendix A.

Chapter Summary

- The three common types of injections are subcutaneous (SC), intramuscular (IM), and intravenous (IV).
- SC and IM injections are small-volume injections given over a short period.
- IV infusions range from 50–1000 mL and are administered in a vein over a period of minutes to hours, depending on the volume.
- Syringe barrel size is selected by choosing the smallest volume barrel that will accurately measure the desired amount.
- Small volumes may be rounded off to the nearest tenth or hundredth, depending on the accuracy of the measuring device available.
- Larger volumes may be rounded off to the nearest tenth or whole milliliter, depending on the accuracy of the measuring device available.
- Ratio strength (example 1:1000) is used to represent the concentration when the amount of drug in the vehicle is very small.
- The units of measure for a 1:100 ratio solution are 1 g:100 mL when a solid medication has been dissolved in a liquid.

- Electrolytes are measured in milliequivalents.
- Milliequivalents represent the amount of active charged electrolytes, not the amount of drug by weight.
- The two most common electrolytes administered intravenously are potassium and sodium.
- Drugs derived from biological sources are sometimes dosed in "units."
- Units represent a certain amount of anticipated biological activity in a specific manner or body system.
- Insulin and heparin are the two most common medications dosed in units.
- Insulin is concentrated as standard "U-100," which means that there are 100 units in 1 mL.
- Even though there are many brands and types of insulin that use the standard U-100 concentration, they are not interchangeable.
- Powder volume is the amount of space taken up by the freeze-dried drug in a sterile vial; this type of medication is used for reconstitution.

Formulas for Success

$$\text{mEq} = \frac{\text{molecular weight}}{\text{valence}}$$

Key Terms

atomic weight the weight of a single atom of an element compared with the weight of a single atom of hydrogen

electrolytes substances such as mineral salts that carry an electrical charge when dissolved in a solution

infusion the administration of a large volume of liquid medication given parenterally over a long period

injection a method of administering medications in which a syringe with a needle or cannula is used to penetrate through the skin or membrane into the tissue below

intramuscular (IM) injection an injection given into the aqueous muscle tissue

intravenous (IV) infusion the injection of fluid into the veins

milliequivalent (mEq) the ratio of the weight of a molecule to its valence, used to measure the concentration of electrolytes in a volume of solution; also an amount of medication that will provide the patient with a specific amount (equivalent amount) of an electrolyte

millimole (mM) molecular weight expressed in milligrams

molecular weight the sum of the atomic weights of all atoms in one molecule of a compound

parenteral administered by injection or infusion and not by way of the GI system

powder volume (pv) the space occupied by dry pharmaceuticals, calculated as the difference between the final volume and the volume of the diluting ingredient, or the diluent volume; the amount of space occupied by lyophilized (freeze-dried) medication in a sterile vial, used for reconstitution

ratio strength a means of describing the concentration of a liquid medication based on a ratio such as *a* grams:*b* milliliters

subcutaneous (SC) injection an injection given into the vascular, fatty layer of tissue under the skin

unit the amount of activity associated with a medication that has a biological impact on a patient

valence the ability of a molecule to bond, as indicated by its positive or negative charge; represented by a superscript plus or minus sign next to an element's chemical symbol

Chapter Review

Assessing Comprehension

To check your comprehension of this chapter's key concepts, read the following multiple-choice questions and then record your answers on a separate sheet of paper. Write your answers as modeled in these examples: 1d; 2c; 3b; etc.

1. Which of the following is associated with administering a large volume of fluid?
   a. IM
   b. SC
   c. IV infusion
   d. U-100

2. Injectable solutions are typically measured in the pharmacy using
   a. IV bags.
   b. syringes.
   c. graduated cylinders.
   d. ampules.

3. What unit should pharmacy personnel use with the variable *x* when calculating the volume needed for an injection?
   a. liters
   b. milliliters
   c. teaspoons
   d. milligrams

4. What unit should pharmacy personnel use with the variable *x* when calculating the amount of drug in an injection?
   a. liters
   b. milliliters
   c. teaspoons
   d. milligrams

5. What two units are used when describing the ratio strength of a solution?
   a. g/mL
   b. mg/mL
   c. g/L
   d. mg/L

6. Milliequivalents are associated with
   a. ratio strength.
   b. charged electrolytes.
   c. insulin.
   d. freeze-dried drugs.

7. Insulin is dosed in
   a. units.
   b. milliequivalents.
   c. milliliters.
   d. grams.

8. Insulin and insulin syringes use a standard called
   a. milliequivalents.
   b. U-100.
   c. milliliters.
   d. millimoles.

9. Powdered or freeze-dried medications must be _____ before use.
   a. reconstituted
   b. lyophilized
   c. concentrated
   d. sterilized

10. The diluent added to the lyophilized dry powder is the
    a. concentration.
    b. final volume.
    c. powder volume.
    d. solvent.

Finding Solutions

To gain practice in handling challenging situations in the workplace, consider the following real-world scenarios and then use the guiding questions to help you formulate your responses.

Note: *To indicate your answer for Scenario A, Question 2, ask your instructor for the handout depicting 1 mL, 3 mL, and 5 mL syringes. For Scenario B, use the handout to select the correct insulin syringe.*

Scenario A: Lin Nguyen, a 23-year-old patient in the postsurgical unit, weighs 120 pounds. You have an order to prepare 100 mg of progesterone injection in a syringe for IM administration. You have on hand a 50 mL multi-dose vial of progesterone 50 mg/mL as well as 1 mL, 3 mL, and 5 mL syringes.

1. How many milliliters will be given at each dose?

2. On the handout that you obtained from your instructor, select the correct syringe size and indicate the amount of medication that should be administered to the patient.

3. How many milligrams are in the 50 mL multi-dose vial?

4. How many 100 mg doses can be obtained from this vial?

Scenario B: MaryEllen Wainwright is a patient who uses insulin to control her diabetes. She normally gets two vials of insulin each month, but the doctor has just reduced her dose of insulin from 55 units daily to 30 units daily. She also needs new insulin syringes that are smaller and easier to read.

5. How many 10 mL vials will be needed to administer the lowered dose for one month?

6. What size insulin syringe will the patient need? Select which insulin syringes will be used from the handout.

7. If the doctor has the patient reduce her dose by 2 units after 10 days, and 2 units on day 20, and 2 units on day 30, how many units will she be using daily after 30 days? Fill in the correct amount that the patient will be using after 30 days.

Sampling the Certification Exam

To provide you with practice for the Certification Exam, read the following questions that have been patterned after the test format and then record your answers on a separate sheet of paper. Write your answers as modeled in these examples: 1d; 2c; 3b; etc.

1. How many 25 mg doses can be obtained from a 10 mL multi-dose vial of medication whose concentration is 10 mg/mL?
   a. 1 dose
   b. 4 doses
   c. 8 doses
   d. 12 doses

2. You have an order for 10,000 units of heparin to be administered to a patient. The vial you have on hand contains 5,000 units/mL and contains 10 mL. How many milliliters will you need to fill the order?
   a. 1 mL
   b. 1.5 mL
   c. 2 mL
   d. 2.5 mL

3. A patient who is self-administering Humulin R uses 20 units in the morning and 15 units in the afternoon. How many days will a 10 mL vial of U-100 insulin last?
   a. 10 days
   b. 15 days
   c. 21 days
   d. 28 days

4. How many milligrams of lidocaine are contained in 1.5 mL of a 2% solution (20 mg/mL)?
   a. 13 mg
   b. 20 mg
   c. 25 mg
   d. 30 mg

5. You need to prepare a 50 mg dose of Lovenox. The medication is in a vial containing 80 mg/0.8 mL. How much will you need?
   a. 0.5 mL
   b. 0.8 mL
   c. 1.5 mL
   d. 5 mL

To put your pharmacy calculation skills to the test, read the following questions and then record your answers on a separate sheet of paper.

Determine the volume to prepare for each ordered injectable solution using the labels provided. (Round to the hundredths place.)

Note: *Questions 1–4 have accompanying handouts that must be obtained from your instructor.*

1. How many milliliters of solution are needed to provide 2 g of cefazolin? On the handout that you obtained from your instructor, indicate the correct volume on the measuring device.

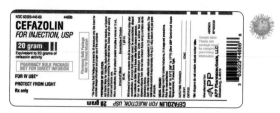

2. How many milliliters of solution are needed to provide 60 mg of furosemide? On the handout that you obtained from your instructor, indicate the correct volume on the measuring device.

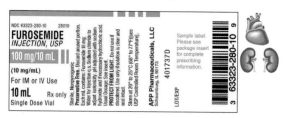

3. How many milliliters of solution are needed to provide 25 mg of diphenhydramine HCl? On the handout that you obtained from your instructor, indicate the correct volume on the measuring device.

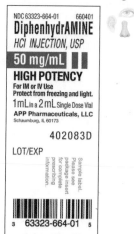

4. How many milliliters of solution are needed to provide 10 mg of famotidine? On the handout that you obtained from your instructor, indicate the correct volume on the measuring device.

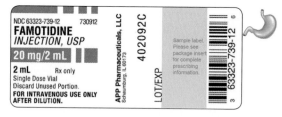

Calculate the quantity of drug in an injectable solution using the provided vial labels.

5. How many milligrams of ketorolac are contained in 1.4 mL?

6. How many milligrams of lidocaine HCl are contained in 3.1 mL?

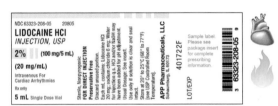

7. How many milligrams of midazolam are contained in 0.8 mL?

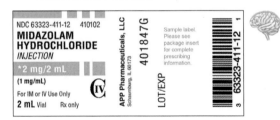

8. How many milligrams of progesterone are contained in 1.8 mL?

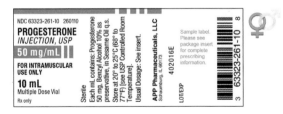

Calculate the quantity of a drug using ratio strength.

9. How many grams are in 600 mL of a 1:200 solution of drug product?

10. How many milligrams are in 5 mL of a 1:5000 solution?

11. How many milligrams are in 0.5 mL of a 1:1000 solution?

12. How many micrograms are in 0.5 mL of a 1:1000 solution?

Perform the necessary calculations to determine the amount of medication needed to prepare the following orders.

13. Using the following order and the stock solutions of lidocaine and furosemide, determine how many milliliters of each solution should be added to the IV bag.

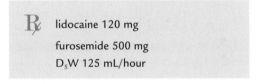

℞ lidocaine 120 mg

furosemide 500 mg

D₅W 125 mL/hour

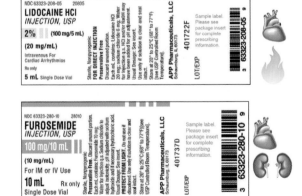

14. Using the following order and the stock solution of potassium chloride with the label shown below, how many milliliters of potassium chloride will be added to the IV bag?

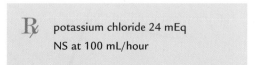

R̸ potassium chloride 24 mEq
NS at 100 mL/hour

NDC 63323-967-30   96730
POTASSIUM CHLORIDE
For Injection Concentrate, USP
Concentrate Must Be Diluted Before Use
2 mEq/mL (60 mEq)
30 mL   Rx only
Multiple Dose Vial

15. Fill the order below given the following preparations. How much of each medication is needed?

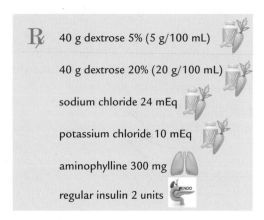

R̸ 40 g dextrose 5% (5 g/100 mL)

40 g dextrose 20% (20 g/100 mL)

sodium chloride 24 mEq

potassium chloride 10 mEq

aminophylline 300 mg

regular insulin 2 units

a. 40 g dextrose using dextrose 5% (5 g/100 mL)

b. 40 g dextrose using dextrose 20% (20 g/100 mL)

c. sodium chloride, 4 mEq/mL

d. potassium chloride, 2 mEq/mL

e. aminophylline, 25 mg/mL

f. insulin, 100 units/mL

16. Fill the given order with the stock solutions that have the following labels. How much of each medication is needed?

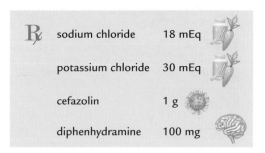

R̸ sodium chloride   18 mEq

potassium chloride   30 mEq

cefazolin   1 g

diphenhydramine   100 mg

a. sodium chloride, 4 mEq/mL

b. potassium chloride, 40 mEq/20 mL

c. cefazolin, 500 mg/mL

d. diphenhydramine, 50 mg/mL

Calculate the milliliters needed to provide the following quantities of drug. (Round to the nearest hundredths place.)

17. Pen VK (penicillin V–potassium) can be reconstituted to many different concentrations. You are filling an order for 230,000 units and have available a concentration that has already been reconstituted to 500,000 units/mL. How many milliliters is the dose?

18. Prepare 15,000 units of heparin from the vial with the label shown below. How many milliliters is this?

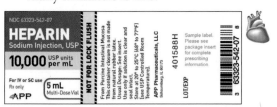

NDC 63323-542-07
HEPARIN
Sodium Injection, USP
10,000 USP units per mL
For IV or SC use
Rx only
APP
5 mL
Multi-Dose Vial
NOT FOR LOCK FLUSH
From Porcine Intestinal Mucosa
This container closure is not made from natural rubber latex.
Usual Dosage: See insert.
Use only if solution is clear and seal intact.
Store at 20° to 25°C (68° to 77°F)
[see USP Controlled Room Temperature].
APP Pharmaceuticals, LLC
Schaumburg, IL 60173
401588H
LOT/EXP
Sample label.
Please see package insert for complete prescribing information.
3 63323-542-07 8

19. How many milliequivalents of sodium chloride are in 3.5 mL of a solution that contains 4 mEq/mL?

20. Prepare two syringes for a patient on the orthopedic floor. Each syringe should contain 35 mg of Lovenox. How many milliliters will be in each syringe?

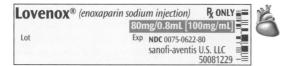

21. A patient is to receive 0.42 mL of Lantus daily. Using the label shown below, how many units is this?

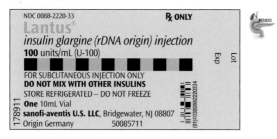

22. A patient uses 18 units of insulin twice daily. How long will the two vials shown in the following label last?

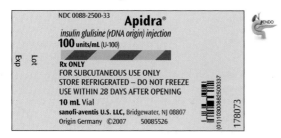

For questions 23 and 24, select the vial that is needed to fill each order with the required number of milliequivalents of potassium chloride, and then calculate the volume to be withdrawn from the selected vial for the order.

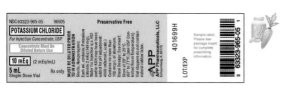

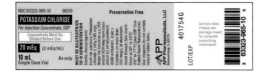

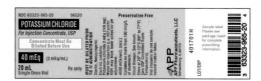

23. Add 16 mEq of potassium chloride to the patient's IV solution.

24. Add 38 mEq of potassium chloride to the patient's IV solution.

Solve the following problems involving powders that are reconstituted.

25. The label of a vial states that it contains 1 g in 10 mL. You know that 9.6 mL were added. What is the powder volume?

26. Your bottle of Amoxil (amoxicillin) says to add 39 mL to the bottle to get a solution of 150 mg/tsp. The total amount in the bottle is 2 g. What is the powder volume?

27. A 10 g vial label states that the concentration is 100 mg/mL if you add 87 mL. How much would you need to add to get a concentration of 50 mg/mL?

28. An oral suspension once reconstituted is to have a dose of 250 mg/tsp, and the dry powder is 4 g with a powder volume of 11.3 mL. How much water must you add?

29. A 30 g vial must have 76 mL added and has a powder volume of 12.6 mL. How many milligrams per milliliter will be in the final solution?

30. A 1 g vial requires 8.9 mL to be added to have a concentration of 100 mg/mL. What is the powder volume?

Preparing Parenteral Solutions

Lisa McCartney, BAAS, CPhT, PhTR

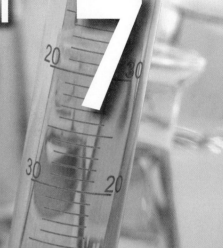

Learning Objectives

- Calculate the amount of medication in a solution based on a given percentage strength.

- Calculate the percentage strength of medication in a given solution.

- Describe the types of intravenous sets by drop factor.

- Calculate intravenous drip rates and flow rates using various intravenous sets.

- Estimate and calculate time for intravenous administration.

- Calculate rates of intravenous infusion and intravenous piggyback infusion.

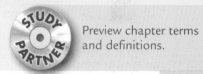

Preview chapter terms and definitions.

7.1 Percentage and Ratio Strength Dilutions

A **solution** is a mixture of two or more substances. Solutions may be comprised of any of the three states of matter: gas, liquid, or solid. Solutions can also exist in the following combinations of components:

- solid in a liquid (e.g., salt water)
- two liquids (e.g., a mixed drink)
- solid in a solid (e.g., fruit in gelatin)
- gas in a liquid (e.g., soda water)

In a solution, the substance dissolved in the liquid is called the **solute**, and the liquid is the **solvent**. If both substances are liquids, usually the component representing the greater amount is considered the solvent, and the component representing the smaller amount is the solute. The goal in preparing pharmaceutical solutions is to mix concentrations that result in accurately measured doses.

In general, in comparing two solutions containing the same components, the solution containing the smaller amount of solute is considered dilute. The solution containing the larger amount of solute is considered concentrated. As discussed in Chapter 6, the concentration of one substance dissolved in another substance may be expressed as either a percentage strength (e.g., 25%) or a ratio strength (e.g., $^{25}/_{100}$ or ¼). The ratio strength or percentage strength of a solution refers to the number of grams/100 mL. How the concentration of the solute in the solvent is expressed as a percentage strength depends on which is a solid and/or which is a liquid. The concentrations can also be expressed as fractions.

Within the context of preparing sterile, parenteral solutions, the percentage strength or ratio strength may be further classified as a solid in a liquid, sometimes referred to as weight in volume (w/v) or a liquid in a liquid, sometimes referred to as volume in volume (v/v). There are two common scenarios that require calculations based on percentage strength or ratio strength. These scenarios include the preparation of a solid-in-a-liquid solution and the preparation of a two-liquid solution.

Solid in a Liquid

weight in volume (w/v) = number of grams of drug in = $\dfrac{x \text{ g of drug}}{100 \text{ mL of final solution}}$
100 mL of final solution

Two Liquids

volume in volume (v/v) = number of milliliters of drug = $\dfrac{x \text{ mL drug}}{100 \text{ mL of final solution}}$
in 100 mL of final solution

Example 7.1.1

A 9% solution means there are 9 parts of the drug (or active ingredient) in 100 parts of the solution. Express this percentage strength as w/v and v/v.

w/v = 9 g of drug in 100 mL of final solution (or 9 g/100 mL)

v/v = 9 mL of drug in 100 mL of final solution (or 9 mL/100 mL)

Example 7.1.2

Express the components of a 4% solution of sodium chloride (NaCl) in the form of a w/v solution.

A 4% NaCl solution contains 4 g of NaCl in each 100 mL of fluid. Another way of saying this is that an IV solution with a concentration of 4% NaCl will provide 4 g of NaCl for every 100 mL of fluid that is administered to the patient.

$$\dfrac{4 \text{ g of NaCl}}{100 \text{ mL of fluid}}$$

For ease of understanding and computation, this type of ratio is usually expressed as:

$$\dfrac{4 \text{ g}}{100 \text{ mL}}$$

Example 7.1.3

Express the components of a 3% solution of acetic acid in the form of a v/v solution.

A 3% acetic acid solution contains 3 mL of pure acetic acid in each 100 mL of fluid. Another way of saying this is that an irrigation solution with a concentration of 3% acetic acid will provide 3 mL of pure acetic acid for every 100 mL of fluid that is administered to the patient.

$$\frac{3 \text{ mL of 3\% acetic acid}}{100 \text{ mL of fluid}}$$

For ease of understanding and computation, this type of ratio is usually expressed as:

$$\frac{3 \text{ mL}}{100 \text{ mL}}$$

The following ratios are important to remember when setting up problems involving solutions. Weight-in-volume (w/v) problems involve adding a solid drug (e.g., an active ingredient) to a liquid, such as sodium chloride dissolved in water.

$$\text{percentage strength of w/v solution} = \frac{\text{g of active ingredient}}{100 \text{ mL of solution}} \times 100$$

Volume-in-volume (v/v) problems involve mixing a pure liquid and another liquid, such as pure acetic acid and water.

$$\text{percentage strength of v/v solution} = \frac{\text{mL of active ingredient}}{100 \text{ mL of solution}} \times 100$$

Intravenous (IV) solutions that are given in large quantities are labeled as a percentage strength, such as dextrose 5%, which is also written as D_5W or D5W. Normal saline (NS) is a solution of water and sodium chloride at 0.9% concentration. Water that is germ-free but has no dextrose or sodium chloride added to it is referred to as *sterile water*. The labels below show examples of how IV and injectable products are labeled. The striking difference between these labels and the previous label examples is that there is no milligrams-per-milliliter designation.

When the percentage concentration of a solution is known, that percentage can be used to determine the amount of active ingredient, as demonstrated in the following example.

For Good Measure

Pharmacy technicians should be familiar with the frequently used abbreviation NS, which refers to normal saline.

Example 7.1.4

How many grams of dextrose are in 1 L of D₅W?

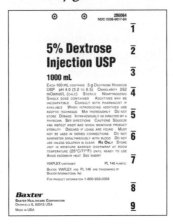

Note that D_5W means 5% dextrose in water, or a concentration of 5 g/100 mL. Solve this problem by using the ratio-proportion method, but first note that 1 L equals 1000 mL.

$$\frac{5 \text{ g}}{100 \text{ mL}} = \frac{x \text{ g}}{1000 \text{ mL}}$$

Cross multiply: $5 \times 1000 = 5000$; then divide $5000/100 = 50$

$$x \text{ g} = 50 \text{ g}$$

There are 50 g of dextrose in 1 L of D_5W.

For Good Measure

In practice, you will not typically be required to calculate the number of grams of dextrose or sodium chloride, but knowing how to solve these types of pharmacy calculations is important to your overall understanding of pharmacy math applications.

Example 7.1.5

How many grams of sodium chloride (NaCl) are in 1 L of NS?

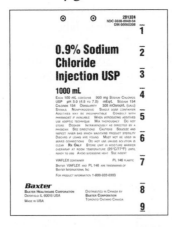

Remember that NS is 0.9% NaCl or a concentration of 0.9 g/100 mL. Solve this problem by using the ratio-proportion method, but first note the following: 1 L equals 1000 mL; 1000 mg equals 1 g.

$$\frac{0.9 \text{ g}}{100 \text{ mL}} = \frac{x \text{ g}}{1000 \text{ mL}}$$

Cross multiply: $0.9 \times 1000 = 900$; then divide $900/100 = 9$

$$x \text{ g} = 9 \text{ g}$$

There are 9 g of NaCl in 1 L of NS.

When the amount of active ingredient and the total volume of the final solution are known, the percentage strength of the concentration can be calculated as shown in the following example.

Example 7.1.6

If there are 30 g of dextrose in a 500 mL IV bag, what is the percentage strength of the solution?

Insert the values into the w/v equation.

$$x\% \text{ w/v} = \frac{30 \text{ g}}{500 \text{ mL}} \times 100 = 0.06 \text{ g/mL} \times 100$$

$$x\% \text{ w/v} = 6\% \text{ w/v}$$

This problem could also be solved using the ratio-proportion method:

$$\frac{x\%}{100 \text{ mL}} = \frac{30 \text{ g}}{500 \text{ mL}}$$

Cross multiply: $100 \times 30 = 3000$; then divide $3000/500 = 6$

$$x = 6 \text{ g}; 6 \text{ g}/100 \text{ mL} = 6\% \text{ w/v}$$

The percentage strength of a solution that contains 30 g of dextrose and has a total volume of 500 mL is 6%.

Example 7.1.7

If there are 5 g of lipids in a 250 mL IV fat emulsion, what is the percentage strength of the solution?

Insert the values into the w/v equation.

$$x\% \text{ w/v} = \frac{5 \text{ g}}{250 \text{ mL}} \times 100 = 0.02 \text{ g/mL} \times 100$$

$$x\% \text{ w/v} = 2\% \text{ w/v}$$

This problem could also be solved using the ratio-proportion method:

$$\frac{x\%}{100 \text{ mL}} = \frac{5 \text{ g}}{250 \text{ mL}}$$

Cross multiply: $100 \times 5 = 500$; then divide $500/250 = 2$

$$x = 2 \text{ g}; \ 2 \text{ g}/100 \text{ mL} = 2\% \text{ w/v}$$

The percentage strength of a solution that contains 5 g of lipids and has a total volume of 250 mL is 2%.

Example 7.1.8

Name Exchange

The generic drug furosemide is commonly known among pharmacy personnel by the brand name Lasix.

Use the label provided to determine the percentage strength of the solution.

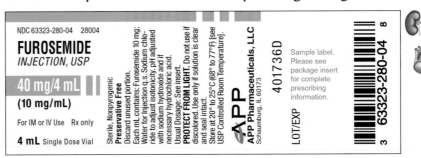

Insert the values into the w/v equation.

$$x\% \text{ w/v} = \frac{0.04 \text{ g}}{4 \text{ mL}} \times 100 = 0.01 \text{ g/mL} \times 100$$

$$x\% \text{ w/v} = 1\% \text{ w/v}$$

This problem could also be solved using the ratio-proportion method:

$$\frac{x\%}{100 \text{ mL}} = \frac{0.04 \text{ g}}{4 \text{ mL}}$$

Cross multiply: $100 \times 0.04 = 4$; then divide $\frac{4}{4} = 1$

$$x = 1 \text{ g}; \ 1 \text{ g}/100 \text{ mL} = 1\% \text{ w/v}$$

The percentage strength of a furosemide solution that has a concentration of 40 mg/4 mL is 1%.

Express the following items as weight-in-volume (w/v) or volume-in-volume (v/v) solutions.

1. the components of 10% dextrose as a w/v solution

2. the components of 0.45% NaCl as a w/v solution

3. the components of acetic acid 0.25% as a v/v solution

4. the components of Aminosyn 7% as a v/v solution

Perform calculations to answer the following questions.

5. If a patient receives an IV solution containing 500 mL of a 10% IV fat emulsion, how many grams of fat did he or she receive?

6. An injection of 1.3 mL lidocaine 2% was given. How many milligrams of lidocaine are in this solution?

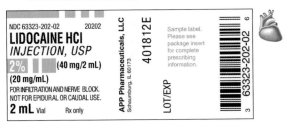

7. A total parenteral nutrition (TPN) order calls for 15 g of dextrose per 100 mL of solution. The total volume of the TPN solution is 2 L. What is the percentage strength of dextrose?

8. What is the percentage strength of the following solution: NaCl 20 g in a 500 mL solution?

Based on the labels provided below, determine the percentage strength of each drug in the following solutions.

9.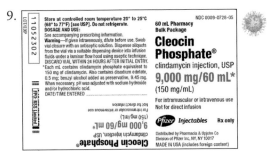

10.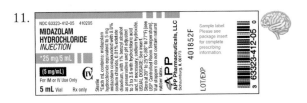

11.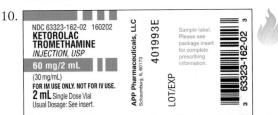

12.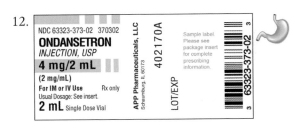

13.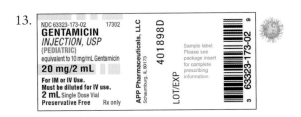

14.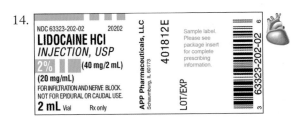

Calculate the amount of drug or active ingredient (in grams) for each of the following solutions.

15. amino acid 3.5%, 2.5 L

16. dextrose 10%, 1000 mL

17. acetic acid 0.25%, 1000 mL

18. sodium chloride 0.9%, 100 mL

19. NaCl 4%, 500 mL

20. NaCl 0.45%, 1 L

21. D$_5$W, 1000 mL

22. aminophylline 0.4%, 500 mL

23. lidocaine 4%, 0.5 L

24. dopamine 2%, 250 mL

Calculate the amount of drug or active ingredient (in milligrams) in the following doses.

25. You have 7.5% solution of dextrose on hand. If the dose is 5 mL, how many milligrams are in one dose?

26. How many milligrams are in 50 mL of a 0.5% drug product?

27. How many milligrams are in 0.5 mL of a 1% solution?

28. How many milligrams of epinephrine are in 1 mL of a 1:1000 solution?

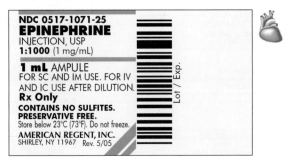

29. You have a 1:5000 solution on hand. If the dose is 5 mL, how many milligrams are in one dose?

Using the medication order below, perform calculations to answer questions 30 and 31.

ID#: L0382201			Memorial Hospital
Name: Luke, Tamika			
DOB: 03/04/67			
Room: 299			
Dr: Dr. Ahmed Vincelette			Physician's Medication Order
ALLERGY OR SENSITIVITY		DIAGNOSIS	
NKA		diverticulitis	
DATE	TIME	ORDERS	PHYSICIAN'S SIG.
10/21/2018	3:16 PM	Change TPN base solution to	
		deliver 100 grams of	
		dextrose per liter of TPN fluid	
			Dr. Ahmed Vincelette

30. What is the final percentage strength of dextrose?

31. If the patient receives 3000 mL/24 hours of the TPN solution described above, how many grams of dextrose will she receive in one day?

Using the medication order below, perform calculations to answer questions 32 and 33.

ID#: L0382201			Memorial Hospital
Name: Ransom, Harold G.			
DOB: 12/01/39			
Room: 454			
Dr: Bettina Kelly, M.D.			Physician's Medication Order
ALLERGY OR SENSITIVITY		DIAGNOSIS	
PCN		dehydration	
DATE	TIME	ORDERS	PHYSICIAN'S SIG.
04/26/2017	0220	IVF: D5NS w/20 mEq	
		potassium chloride @ 150 mL/hour	
			Bettina Kelly, M.D.

32. What is the percentage strength of NaCl?

33. How many grams of NaCl will the patient receive in a 24-hour period?

How many grams of NaCl are in the following volumes of NS (0.9% NaCl)?

How many grams of dextrose are in the following volumes of D$_5$W (5%)?

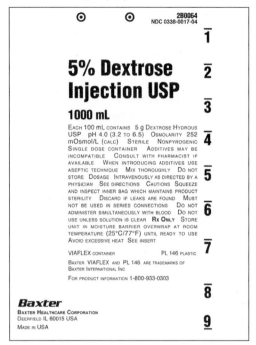

34. 250 mL

35. 500 mL

36. 1000 mL

37. 2225 mL

How many grams of NaCl are in the following volumes of ½ NS (0.45% NaCl)?

38. 125 mL

39. 250 mL

40. 750 mL

41. 1800 mL

42. 2600 mL

43. 75 mL

44. 385 mL

45. 525 mL

46. 1350 mL

How many grams of dextrose are in the following volumes of D$_{10}$W (10%)?

47. 100 mL

48. 325 mL

49. 450 mL

50. 875 mL

Self-check your work in Appendix A.

7.2 IV Flow Rates

Pharmacy staff members use the **flow rate** of an IV solution to determine the answers to various questions encountered in daily practice. These questions may address the days' supply of a patient's IV solution or the administration of a particular parenteral dose. The IV flow rate typically refers to the number of milliliters of medication a patient should receive in an hour. Depending on the particular medication, the physician may order the IV flow rate in units per hour (units/hr), or by the drops per minute (gtts/min) a patient should receive. The flow rate may also be expressed in terms of how much IV fluid should be administered per dose, or per day. The IV flow rate is often referred to as the *infusion rate* or *rate of infusion*.

The physician typically orders the type of IV fluid to be given (referred to as the IV's base solution) and any additives (such as a medication or an electrolyte) that are required. The physician also indicates the rate at which the IV solution should be administered in milliliters per hour (mL/hr). The nursing staff closely monitors IV fluid administration to ensure that an appropriate volume of fluid—and the corresponding amount or dosage of any additive—is given over the specified period to achieve the intended therapeutic response.

The days' supply of an IV preparation may be calculated using the following formula:

$$\frac{\text{volume}}{\text{flow rate}} = \text{number of hours a single IV bag will last}$$

When calculating the duration of therapy, always round down your answer to the whole hour.

For the examples below, note the following conversion: 1 L = 1000 mL.

Example 7.2.1

A 1 L IV is administered at a flow rate of 125 mL/hr. How long will the IV bag last?

$$\frac{\text{volume}}{\text{flow rate}} = x \text{ number of hours a single IV bag will last}$$

$$\text{volume} = 1000 \text{ mL}$$

$$\text{flow rate} = 125 \text{ mL/hr}$$

$$\frac{1000 \text{ mL}}{125 \text{ mL/hr}} = x \text{ hr}$$

$$x \text{ hr} = 8 \text{ hr}$$

A 1 L IV bag administered at 125 mL/hr will last 8 hours.

This problem can also be solved using the ratio-proportion method:

$$\frac{125 \text{ mL}}{1 \text{ hr}} = \frac{1000 \text{ mL}}{x \text{ hr}}$$

Cross multiply 1 × 1000 = 1000; then divide 1000/125 = 8.

$$x \text{ hr} = 8 \text{ hr}$$

This problem can also be solved using the dimensional analysis method:

$$x \text{ hr} = \frac{1\cancel{L} \times 1000 \cancel{mL}}{1 \cancel{L}} \times \frac{1 \text{ hr}}{125 \cancel{mL}} = 8 \text{ hr}$$

Example 7.2.2

The prescriber has ordered D$_5$NS to run at 150 mL/hr. How many bags will be needed in a 24-hour period?

First, determine how long a single bag will last:

$$\frac{\text{volume}}{\text{flow rate}} = x$$

$$\text{volume} = 1000 \text{ mL } (1 \text{ L} = 1000 \text{ mL})$$

$$\text{flow rate} = 150 \text{ mL/hr}$$

$$\frac{1000 \text{ mL}}{150 \text{ mL/hr}} = x$$

$$x = 6.67 \text{ hr}$$

Then determine how many bags will be needed for 24 hours:

$$24/6.67 = 3.6 \text{ (rounded up to 4)}$$

Four bags will be needed for a 24-hour period.

This problem can also be solved using the ratio-proportion method. *Note:* When determining days' supply for an IV bag, always round up to the nearest 1 L.

$$\frac{150 \text{ mL}}{1 \text{ hr}} \times \frac{x \text{ mL}}{24 \text{ hr}}$$

Cross multiply $150 \times 24 = 3600$; then divide $3600/1 = 3600$ mL, rounded up to 4000 mL or 4 bags per day.

This problem can also be solved using the dimensional analysis method:

$$x \text{ bags} = \frac{1 \text{ bag}}{1000 \cancel{mL}} \times \frac{24 \cancel{hr}}{1 \text{ day}} \times \frac{150 \cancel{mL}}{1 \cancel{hr}} = \frac{3600}{1000}$$

$$\frac{3600}{1000} = 3.6 \text{ (rounded up to 4 bags per day)}$$

Safety in Numbers

When determining days' supply for an IV bag, technicians should always round up to the nearest 1 L.

When an order specifies a certain volume to be infused over a specific period (also known as the *duration of therapy*), the IV flow rate can be calculated using the following formula:

$$\text{IV flow rate} = \frac{\text{volume of fluid or amount to be infused}}{\text{duration of therapy}}$$

Example 7.2.3

The physician has ordered a 1 L IV bag to be infused over 10 hours. What is the IV flow rate in milliliters per hour (mL/hr)?

$$\text{IV flow rate} = \frac{\text{volume of fluid or amount to be infused}}{\text{duration of therapy}}$$

$$\text{volume} = 1000 \text{ mL } (1 \text{ L} = 1000 \text{ mL})$$

$$\text{duration of therapy} = 10 \text{ hr}$$

$$\frac{1000 \text{ mL}}{10 \text{ hr}} = 100 \text{ mL/hr}$$

A 1 L IV bag infused over 10 hours has an IV flow rate of 100 mL/hr.

When a medication order specifies an amount or a dosage of a drug that is to be administered over a specific period, the amount of drug administered per hour (expressed as milligrams/hour, or mg/hr) can be calculated using the following formula:

$$\text{amount of drug in milligrams/hour} = \frac{\text{total amount of drug}}{\text{duration of therapy}}$$

Example 7.2.4

The physician has ordered a 250 mL intravenous piggyback (IVPB) with 500 mg of Solu-Cortef to be infused over 4 hours. What is the dose of drug being administered per hour?

$$\text{amount of drug in milligrams/hour} = \frac{\text{total amount of drug}}{\text{duration of therapy}}$$

$$\text{total amount of drug} = 500 \text{ mg}$$

$$\text{duration of therapy} = 4 \text{ hr}$$

$$\frac{500 \text{ mg}}{4 \text{ hr}} = 125 \text{ mg/hr}$$

The patient is receiving 125 mg of Solu-Cortef per hour.

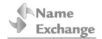

Example 7.2.5

The following order is received in the IV room.

> **Medication: cefazolin, 1 g**
>
> Fluid volume: D₅W, 150 mL
> Administration rate: over 120 minutes

What volume of fluid is administered per hour, and what amount of drug is given per hour?

Step 1. Determine the volume of fluid given per hour (in mL/hr).
   Note that 120 minutes = 2 hours.

$$\text{IV flow rate} = \frac{\text{volume of fluid or amount to be infused}}{\text{duration of therapy}}$$

$$\frac{150 \text{ mL}}{2 \text{ hr}} = 75 \text{ mL/hr}$$

Step 2. Calculate the amount of drug given per hour (in mg/hr).
   Note that 1 g = 1000 mg.

$$\text{amount of drug in milligrams/hour} = \frac{\text{total amount of drug}}{\text{duration of therapy}}$$

$$\frac{1000 \text{ mg}}{2 \text{ hr}} = 500 \text{ mg/hr}$$

7.2 Problem Set

Perform calculations to answer the following questions.

1. A 1 L IV bag is running at 50 mL/hour. How long will it last?

2. A 1 L bag of IV fluid is hung at 7 PM and runs at 100 mL/hr. What time will the next bag be needed?

3. A 500 mL bag of IV fluid is running at 30 mL/hr. How long will it last?

4. If a patient is given 60 mg of medication in 75 mL over 45 minutes, what is the flow rate in milliliters per hour?

5. A patient receives 20,000 units of heparin in an IV of 100 mL over 45 minutes. What is the flow rate in milliliters per hour?

> *****IV Piggyback*****
> Memorial Hospital
>
> **Name:** Washington, Deandra   **Room:** ICU-4
> **Pt. ID#:** 776263663   **Rx#:** 77283993
>
> ---
>
> **Vancomycin 1500 mg**
> **Dextrose 5% in water (D₅W) 250 mL**
> **Rate: over 5 hr**
>
> Expires _____
> RPh _____
> Tech _____
>
> Keep refrigerated – warm to room temperature
> before use.

Based on the IVPB label above, answer questions 6 and 7.

6. What is the flow rate in milliliters per hour?

7. What is the vancomycin dosage in milligrams per hour?

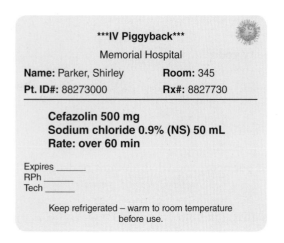

IV Piggyback

Memorial Hospital

Name: Parker, Shirley   **Room:** 345

Pt. ID#: 88273000   **Rx#:** 8827730

Cefazolin 500 mg
Sodium chloride 0.9% (NS) 50 mL
Rate: over 60 min

Expires _____
RPh _____
Tech _____

Keep refrigerated – warm to room temperature
before use.

Based on the IVPB label above, answer questions 8 and 9.

8. What is the flow rate in milliliters per hour?

9. What is the cefazolin dosage in milligrams per hour?

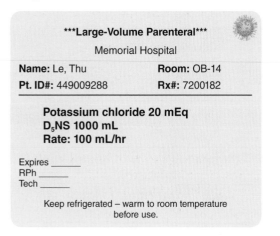

Large-Volume Parenteral

Memorial Hospital

Name: Le, Thu   **Room:** OB-14

Pt. ID#: 449009288   **Rx#:** 7200182

Potassium chloride 20 mEq
D$_5$NS 1000 mL
Rate: 100 mL/hr

Expires _____
RPh _____
Tech _____

Keep refrigerated – warm to room temperature
before use.

Based on the IV label above, answer questions 10–15.

10. What is the flow rate in milliliters per hour?

11. How many hours will this IV bag last?

12. How many IV bags will be needed in a 24-hour period? (Round up to the nearest 1 L bag.)

13. What is the potassium dosage in milliequivalents per hour?

14. How many grams of dextrose are in this IV bag?

15. How many grams of NaCl are in this IV bag?

For each rate, determine the quantity of 1 L bags needed for 24 hours. (Round up to the nearest 1 L bag.)

16. 50 mL/hr

17. 75 mL/hr

18. 100 mL/hr

19. 120 mL/hr

20. 125 mL/hr

21. 130 mL/hr

22. 150 mL/hr

23. 175 mL/hr

24. 200 mL/hr

25. 225 mL/hr

Use what you have learned to interpret the prescriptions and perform the necessary calculations to answer each of the questions below.

26. Medication: Solu-Cortef (hydrocortisone) 250 mg
Fluid volume: 250 mL
Time of infusion: 4 hr

a. How many milliliters per hour?

b. How many milligrams per hour?

27. Medication: penicillin G 12 million units
Fluid volume: 500 mL
Time of infusion: 12 hr

a. How many milliliters per hour?

b. How many units per hour?

28. Medication: lidocaine 4%
    Fluid volume: 500 mL
    Rate: 800 mg/hr

    a. How many milliliters per hour?

    b. How many hours will it take until the entire IV bag has been administered?

29. Medication: Solu-Medrol (methylprednisolone) 250 mg
    Fluid volume: 500 mL
    Rate: 20 mg/hr

    a. How many milliliters per hour?

    b. How many hours will it take until the entire dose has been administered?

30. Medication: dopamine 1600 mcg in D_5W
    Fluid volume: 500 mL
    Dose: 4 mcg/min

    a. How many milliliters per hour?

    b. How many micrograms per hour?

31. A physician has ordered an IV infusion of dopamine hydrochloride (Intropin) 800 mg in 250 mL of D5W to run at 5 mg/hr. Dopamine is available in a 20 mL vial at a concentration of 200 mg/5 mL.

    a. How many milliliters of dopamine must be drawn up to prepare this dose?

    b. What is the IV flow rate in milliliters per hour?

32. A physician has ordered an IVPB of gentamicin 2 mg/kg q8h for a patient who weighs 176 lb. The IVPB will be prepared in a base solution of of D5W 100 mL and will be administered over 60 min. Gentamicin is available in a 20 mL vial at a concentration of 40 mg/mL.

    a. How many milliliters of gentamicin must be drawn up to prepare a single dose?

    b. What is the administration rate in milliliters per hour?

    Self-check your work in Appendix A.

7.3 Drop Factor and Infusion Rates

For Good Measure

When performing drop factor equations, pharmacy technicians must examine the IV set or tubing package to determine the drop size in gtts/mL.

Nursing staff—and, occasionally, pharmacy staff—are required to calculate the rate of administration for an IV fluid in *drops per minute* (expressed as gtts/min). Most inpatient facilities now use electronic infusion pumps to regulate both the volume and the rate of a patient's IV medication. Nursing personnel program the prescribed rate into the electronic infusion pump at the patient's bedside to administer the prescribed number of drops per minute. The rate can be digitally adjusted, which causes the pump's internal clamp to slow or quicken the rate at which the fluid flows through tubing routed through a chamber in the pump. Pumps can be set to give IV fluids in milliliters per hour or drops per minute.

Occasionally, nursing staff will be required to manually adjust the IV flow rate using the tubing's roll clamp, which controls the rate of the fluid volume being administered to the patient. The rate in drops per minute can be calculated manually by counting the number of drops of fluid that fall into the drip chamber over a minute. The nurse can then manually adjust the rate up or down by using the roll clamp.

Calculating the flow rate in drops per minute is complicated by the variety of IV tubing—sometimes called IV tubing sets, or simply IV sets—that is available. Manufacturers produce calibrated IV sets that have different size drops. An IV set is identified by the number of drops it takes to make 1 mL. This calibration may be referred to as a drop set or a drip set but is most commonly called the IV set's **drop factor**. The most common IV sets are 10, 15, 20, and 60, meaning 10 gtts/mL, 15 gtts/mL, 20 gtts/mL, and 60 gtts/mL, respectively. The drop sizes for the 10, 15, and 20 calibrations produce macrodrops; this type of tubing is referred to as *macrodrip IV tubing*. The 60 calibration produces microdrops and is referred to as microdrip tubing, or a **minidrip set**. Figure 7.1 on the following page illustrates these different drop sizes.

When an IV tubing set is used to administer fluids, the drop factor for the IV set will be prominently displayed on the outside of the package. The 10 drop and 15 drop sets are commonly used for adult patients, whereas the 60 drop set is used for pediatric patients or patients who are critically ill and are being given medications that have a narrow therapeutic window.

To determine the rate in drops per minute, when the total volume and infusion time are known, the following formula is used:

$$\frac{\text{total volume (TV)}}{\text{infusion time (IT) in minutes}} \times \text{drop factor (DF)} = \text{drops/minute}$$

$$\frac{\text{TV}}{\text{IT}} \times \text{DF} = \text{gtts/min}$$

The following examples will demonstrate the use of this formula in various scenarios. It should be noted that dimensional analysis may also be used to solve this type of equation. It is common practice to round down in the event a partial drop or minute is calculated. For example, 20.6 gtts/min would be rounded down to 20 gtts/min.

FIGURE 7.1
IV Drop Sets

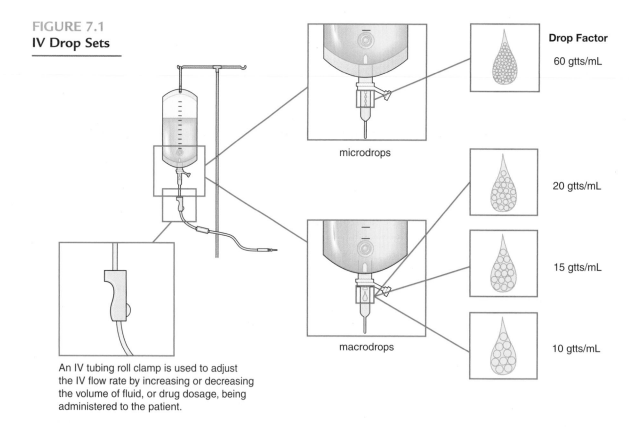

Drop Factor

60 gtts/mL

microdrops

20 gtts/mL

15 gtts/mL

macrodrops

10 gtts/mL

An IV tubing roll clamp is used to adjust the IV flow rate by increasing or decreasing the volume of fluid, or drug dosage, being administered to the patient.

Example 7.3.1

An IV has a total volume of 250 mL and is being administered over 60 minutes using macrodrip tubing with a drop factor of 15 gtts/mL. What is the rate in drops per minute?

$$\frac{TV}{IT} \times DF = drops/minute$$

$$\frac{250 \text{ mL}}{60 \text{ min}} \times 15 \text{ gtts/mL}$$

$250/60 = 4.17 \times 15 = 62.5 = 62$ gtts (rounded down to the nearest whole drop)

The IV rate in drops per minute is 62 gtts/min.

To determine the rate in drops per minute, when the IV flow rate (in milliliters per hour) and the drop factor are known, the following formula is used:

$$\frac{IV \text{ flow rate (IVFR)}}{60 \text{ min/hr}} \times drop \text{ factor (DF)} = drops/minute$$

$$\frac{IVFR}{60 \text{ min/hr}} \times DF = gtts/min$$

Example 7.3.2

An IV of D₅W with 20,000 units of heparin is being administered at a rate of 40 mL/hr using macrodrip tubing with a drop factor of 20 gtts/mL. How many drops per minute is that?

Solution 1: Begin by identifying the amounts to insert into the formula:

$$\frac{IV \text{ flow rate (IVFR)}}{60 \text{ min/hr}} \times drop \text{ factor (DF)}$$

$$IVFR = 40 \text{ mL/hr}$$

$$drop \text{ factor} = 20 \text{ gtts/mL}$$

Insert the values from the problem statement into the formula to determine the drops per minute rate.

$$\frac{40}{60 \text{ min/hr}} \times 20 \text{ gtts/mL}$$

$$\frac{40}{60} = 0.66 \times 20 = 13.33 \text{ gtts/min}$$

The number of drops per minute is 13 gtts/min (rounded down to the nearest whole number).

Solution 2: This problem can also be solved using the dimensional analysis method:

$$x \text{ gtts/min} = 40 \text{ mL/hr} \times 20 \text{ gtts/mL} \times 1 \text{ hr/60 min} = 13.33 \text{ gtts/min}$$

13 gtts/min (rounded down to the nearest whole number)

Occasionally, pharmacy personnel use drop factor calculations to determine the amount of a drug that will be infused over a specific period. These types of problems are sometimes referred to as *IV drip rate calculations* and can be solved by using the following formula:

Step 1: Determine the concentration of the solution in milligrams/milliliter by dividing the total milligrams in the solution by the total volume in the solution.

$$\frac{\text{total milligrams}}{\text{total volume}} \text{ (TV)} = \frac{\text{concentration in milligrams}}{\text{milliliter}}$$

Step 2: Determine the number of milligrams in each drop, using the given drop factor.

$$\frac{\text{milligrams}}{\text{milliliters}} \div \text{drop factor (DF)} = \frac{\text{milligrams}}{\text{drop (mg/gtt)}}$$

The following example demonstrates this type of important calculation.

Example 7.3.3

The prescriber has ordered a dopamine drip of 800 mg in 250 mL D$_5$W. The IV will be administered at 10 mL/hr through tubing that has a drop factor of 10 gtts/mL. How many milligrams of dopamine are in each drop?

Step 1: Determine the concentration of the solution in milligrams/milliliter.

total milligrams = 800 mg
total volume (TV) = 250 mL
800/250 = 3.2 mg/mL

Step 2: Determine the number of milligrams of dopamine per drop (mg/gtt).

milligrams/milliliter = 3.2 mg (determined in Step 1 above)
DF = 10
3.2/10 = 0.32 mg/gtt

There are 0.32 mg of dopamine in each drop.

Perform calculations to answer the following questions.

1. An IV rate is 10 mL/hr. If an IV tubing set with a drop factor of 10 gtts/mL is used, what will the rate be in drops per minute?

2. What is the IV flow rate in drops per minute for an IV that is being administered at 35 mL/hr using a 60 drop set?

3. A patient is to receive 1 g of cefazolin in 100 mL of ½ NS over one hour using a 10 drop set. What is the rate in drops per minute?

4. A nurse will be administering 500 mg of medication in 50 mL over 30 minutes, using microdrip tubing. What is the flow rate in drops per minute?

5. A physician orders 20,000 units of heparin in an IV of D_5NS 500 mL to be administered continuously over 24 hours. Using a 15 drop set, what is the rate in drops per minute?

6. A physician orders 750 mg of vancomycin in 250 mL IVPB over one hour, using a 15 drop set. How many drops per minute will that be?

7. A patient is to be given 1000 mL of lactated Ringer's (LR) solution at 50 mL/hr. What will the rate in drops per minute be if tubing with a drop factor of 15 is used?

8. A patient is to be given TPN at 95 mL/hr. What will the drip rate be if a 20 drop set is used?

9. A physician orders 40 mEq of potassium chloride in 100 mL of D_5W to be administered over 4 hours. If a 10 drop set is used, how many milliequivalents of potassium will be in each drop?

10. A patient is to receive 20,000 units of heparin in 500 mL of D_5 ½ NS at a flow rate of 25 mL/hr. If tubing with a drop factor of 15 is used, what will the rate be in drops per minute?

11. The order below is received in the pharmacy. What is the rate in drops per minute if microdrip tubing is used?

ID#: Y7HH7992			Memorial Hospital
Name: Baldwin, Flora			
DOB: 11/22/90			
Room: 514			
Dr: Dr. Ahmed Vincelette			Physician's Medication Order
ALLERGY OR SENSITIVITY		DIAGNOSIS	
ASA, latex		pancreatitis	
DATE	TIME	ORDERS	PHYSICIAN'S SIG.
10/28/2019	2316	IVF — D5NS 1L w/20 mEq	
		potassium chloride, 1 mg folic acid,	
		and 1 amp MVI @ 50 mL/hr	
			Ahmed Vincelette, M.D.

12. The order below is received in the pharmacy. What is the rate in drops per minute if tubing with a drop factor of 20 is used?

ID#: MBYUU97II			Memorial Hospital
Name: Mosier, Bud			
DOB: 02/22/59			
Room: 716			
Dr: Jeremiah King, M.D.			Physician's Medication Order
ALLERGY OR SENSITIVITY		DIAGNOSIS	
PCN, Sulfa, shellfish, tape		asthmatic bronchitis	
DATE	TIME	ORDERS	PHYSICIAN'S SIG.
5/15/2017	3:27 PM	Aminophylline 1 g in 250 mL D5W	
		@ 10 mL/hr	
			Jeremiah King, M.D.

13. The order below is received in the pharmacy. If microdrip tubing is used, how many milligrams of amiodarone will be in each drop?

ID#: 9927739992			Memorial Hospital
Name: Brzyznski, Martha			
DOB: 01/09/48			
Room: ICU-24			
Dr: Amarite Gaya, M.D.			Physician's
			Medication Order
ALLERGY OR SENSITIVITY		DIAGNOSIS	
NKDA		myocardial infarction	
DATE	TIME	ORDERS	PHYSICIAN'S SIG.
8/8/2020		Administer amiodarone drip	
		450 mg in 250 mL NS at 8 mL/hr	
			Amarite Gaya, M.D.

14. The order below is received in the pharmacy. If tubing with a drop factor of 10 is used, how many milligrams per drop will be administered?

ID#: UHy08IIieX			Memorial Hospital
Name: Lazaar, Howard			
DOB: 07/20/50			
Room: CCU -03			
Dr: Thu Singh, M.D.			Physician's
			Medication Order
ALLERGY OR SENSITIVITY		DIAGNOSIS	
NSAIDs, ASA, Sulfa, PCN, milk		CHF	
DATE	TIME	ORDERS	PHYSICIAN'S SIG.
10/30/2015		Norepinephrine 8 mg/250 mL	
		D₅W over 24 hours	
			Thu Singh, M.D.

15. The label below is received in the IV room. If the nurse administers this IVPB using tubing with a drop factor of 10, how many drops per minute will be administered?

IV Piggyback

Memorial Hospital

Name: Geist, Polly   Room: PICU
Pt. ID#: KKU882799   Rx#: 66729937

Tobramycin 40 mg
Dextrose 5% in water (D_5W) 25 mL
Rate: over 60 min

Expires _____
RPh _____
Tech _____

Keep refrigerated – warm to room temperature before use.

16. The following label is received in the IV room. If the nurse administers it using microdrip tubing, how many milliequivalents will be administered with each drop?

Large-Volume Parenteral

Memorial Hospital

Name: Briggs, Jennifer   Room: NICU
Pt. ID#: H68YY7   Rx#: 6638927

$D_{10}W$ 500 mL
Potassium acetate 10 mEq
Rate: 5 mL/hr

Expires _____
RPh _____
Tech _____

Keep refrigerated – warm to room temperature before use.

Self-check your work in Appendix A.

Chapter Summary

- A solution is a mixture of two or more substances, which may be in the form of a gas, liquid, or solid.
- A solution is comprised of a solute (the substance dissolved in a liquid) and a solvent (the liquid).
- The concentration of one substance dissolved in another substance may be expressed as either a percentage strength or a ratio strength.
- The percentage strength of a solution refers to the number of grams/100 mL and can be classified as a solid in a liquid (weight in volume) or two liquids (volume in volume).
- The IV flow rate, also called the IV rate or administration rate, indicates how many milliliters of fluid the patient will receive every hour.

- Pharmacy technicians can determine how long an IV bag will last by dividing the total volume by the IV flow rate.
- Technicians can determine how many milliliters will be administered to the patient by dividing the total volume by the number of hours over which it will be administered.
- An IV set is identified by the number of drops it takes to make 1 mL.
- Macrodrip IV tubing is typically used for adult patients and comes in the following drop factors: 10, 15, and 20.
- Microdrip IV tubing—also known as a mini-drip set—is typically used for pediatric patients and has a drop factor of 60 gtts/mL.
- Pharmacy technicians sometimes use a tubing's drop factor to calculate the amount of drug that will be administered over a certain period.

Formulas for Success

To determine the percentage strength of a w/v solution:

$$\text{percentage strength of w/v solution} = \frac{\text{g of active ingredient}}{100 \text{ mL of solution}} \times 100$$

To determine the percentage strength of a v/v solution:

$$\text{percentage strength of v/v solution} = \frac{\text{mL of active ingredient}}{100 \text{ mL of solution}} \times 100$$

To determine the number of grams in a solution using the ratio-proportion method:

$$\frac{\text{number of grams}}{100 \text{ mL}} = \frac{x \text{ g}}{\text{total volume of solution}}$$

To determine how long an IV bag will last:

$$\frac{\text{volume}}{\text{flow rate}} \times \text{number of hours a single IV bag will last}$$

To determine IV drip rate:

$$\text{IV drip rate} = \frac{\text{IV flow rate}}{60 \text{ min/hr}} \times \text{drop factor}$$

Key Terms

drop factor the number of drops an IV set takes to make 1 mL; also called *drip set*

flow rate the rate, expressed in milliliters per hour or drops per minute, at which medication is flowing through an IV line; also called *infusion rate* and *rate of infusion*

mini-drip set a drop set at a rate of 60 gtts/mL

solute the substance dissolved in the liquid solvent in a solution

solution a mixture of two or more substances

solvent the liquid that dissolves the solute in a solution

volume in volume (v/v) the number of milliliters of a drug (solute) in 100 mL of the final product (solution)

weight in volume (w/v) the number of grams of a drug (solute) in 100 mL of the final product (solution)

Chapter Review

Additional Practice Questions

Assessing Comprehension

To check your comprehension of this chapter's key concepts, read the following multiple-choice questions and then record your answers on a separate sheet of paper. Write your answers as modeled in these examples: 1d; 2c; 3b; *etc.*

1. In a solution, the substance dissolved in the liquid is called the
   a. solvent.
   b. solute.
   c. diluent.
   d. dilution.

2. In a solution, the liquid substance is called the
   a. solvent.
   b. solute.
   c. diluent.
   d. dilution.

3. In general, when comparing two solutions containing the same components, the solution containing the smaller amount of solute is considered to be
   a. dilute.
   b. viscous.
   c. concentrated.
   d. stable.

4. The term *weight in volume (w/v)* refers to
   a. the number of milligrams of drug per 100 mL of the final solution.
   b. the number of milligrams of drug per 1000 mL of the final solution.
   c. the number of grams of drug per 100 mL of the final solution.
   d. the number of grams of drug per 1000 mL of the final solution.

5. The term *volume in volume (v/v)* refers to
   a. the number of grams of drug per 100 mL of the final solution.
   b. the number of grams of drug per 1 mL of the final solution.
   c. the number of milliliters of drug per 100 mL of the final solution.
   d. the number of milliliters of drug per 1 mL of the final solution.

6. The _____ is a term that is synonymous with the infusion rate.
   a. IV concentration rate
   b. IV dilution rate
   c. IV flow rate
   d. dimensional analysis rate

7. Which of the following explanations accurately describes drop factor related to IV tubing?
   a. the number of drops to make 1 mL
   b. the number of drops to make 100 mL
   c. the number of milliliters per drop
   d. the number of milligrams per drop

8. Which of the following drop factors is indicative of microdrip tubing?
   a. a drop factor of 10 (10 gtts/mL)
   b. a drop factor of 15 (15 gtts/mL)
   c. a drop factor of 20 (20 gtts/mL)
   d. a drop factor of 60 (60 gtts/mL)

9. What is the concentration of dextrose in the IV solution D_5W?
   a. 5 mg/mL
   b. 5 mg/100 mL
   c. 5 grams/mL
   d. 5 grams/100 mL

10. What is the percentage strength of an IV solution with 900 mg of sodium per liter?
    a. 0.9%
    b. 9%
    c. 90%
    d. none of the above

Finding Solutions

To gain practice in handling challenging situations in the workplace, consider the following real-world scenarios and then use the guiding questions to help you formulate your responses.

Scenario A: You have just received the following medication order in the pharmacy. Answer the questions below based on this medication order.

ID#: KU88399	Memorial Hospital
Name: Barker, Wally	
DOB: 10/09/45	
Room: 1018	Physician's
Dr: Marshall Rutz, M.D.	Medication Order

ALLERGY OR SENSITIVITY		DIAGNOSIS	
Bactrim, EES		hypokalemia	
DATE	TIME	ORDERS	PHYSICIAN'S SIG.
5/22/2017	3:51 PM	Potassium chloride 20 mEq/L D5NS	
		@ 125 mL/hr	
			Marshall Rutz, M.D.

1. How many mEq of KCl will the patient receive in 24 hours?

2. How many grams of dextrose will the patient receive in 24 hours?

3. How many grams of sodium chloride will the patient receive in 24 hours?

Scenario B: The following IV label was received in the IV room. Answer the questions below based on this IV label.

Large-Volume Parenteral
Memorial Hospital
Name: Vaughn, Perry   **Room:** TCU
Pt. ID#: YHYTELLL **Rx#:** 2299388
Aminophylline 1 gram
D_5W 500 mL
Rate: 20 mL/hr
Expires _____
RPh _____
Tech _____
Keep refrigerated—warm to room temperature before use.

4. How many grams of dextrose will the patient receive in 24 hours?

5. How many milligrams of aminophylline will the patient receive in 24 hours?

6. How many milliliters of fluid will the patient receive in 24 hours?

Sampling the Certification Exam

To provide you with practice for the Certification Exam, read the following questions that have been patterned after the test format and then record your answers on a separate sheet of paper. Write your answers as modeled in these examples: 1d; 2c; 3b; *etc.*

1. What is the percent strength of normal saline?
   a. 0.9%
   b. 9%
   c. 90%
   d. none of the above

2. What is the percent strength of D_5W?
   a. 0.5%
   b. 5%
   c. 50%
   d. none of the above

3. How many grams of dextrose are in 1L of D_5NS?
   a. 5
   b. 50
   c. 0.9
   d. 9

4. The prescriber has ordered $D_{10}W$ 500 mL with potassium acetate 2 mEq/100 mL of IV fluid. How many mEq of potassium acetate will be added to this IV bag?
   a. 2 mEq
   b. 5 mEq
   c. 10 mEq
   d. 20 mEq

5. The prescriber has ordered vancomycin 1 gram in 250 mL of 0.45% sodium chloride IVPB to be administered over 60 minutes using IV tubing with a drop factor of 10. What is the infusion rate in gtts/min?
   a. 41 gtts/min
   b. 42 gtts/min
   c. 43 gtts/min
   d. 44 gtts/min

To put your pharmacy calculation skills to the test, read the following questions and then record your answers on a separate sheet of paper.

Note: *Questions 23–30 have accompanying handouts that must be obtained from your instructor.*

Express the components of the following solutions.

1. the components of betaxolol ophthalmic solution 0.25% as a v/v solution.

2. the components of hexachlorophene 3% emulsion as a w/v solution.

Perform calculations to answer the following questions.

3. If there are 500 mg in a 5 mL dose, what percentage strength is this?

4. If there are 80 g of dextrose in a 1 L IV bag, what is the percentage strength?

Calculate the percentage strength of drug in the following drug formulations.

5. After reconstitution, the medication shown below will have a concentration of 10 g/100 mL. What is the percentage strength?

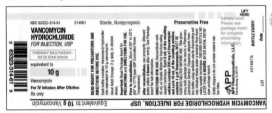

6. What is the percentage strength of the medication shown below?

Calculate the amount of medication in the following doses.

7. How many grams of sodium chloride are in 3 L of NS?

8. How many milligrams are in 10 mL of an 8% drug product?

Perform calculations to answer the following questions.

9. An IV fluid is running at 125 mL/hr. How long will 1 L last?

10. A 1000 mL bag is to be administered at 150 mL/hr. If it is started at 7 AM, what time will it run out?

11. If 125 mL is to be given over 15 minutes, what is the rate of infusion in milliliters per minute?

12. A patient is receiving NS at 100 mL/hr. If a 1 L bag is started at 10 AM, what time will it run out?

Interpret the following medication orders and provide the requested rates.

13. Medication: vancomycin 2 g
    Fluid volume: 250 mL
    Time of infusion: over 90 min

    a. How many milliliters per hour?_____

    b. How many milligrams per hour? _____

14. Medication: aminophylline 1 g
    Fluid volume: 500 mL
    Time of infusion: 8 hr

    a. How many milliliters per hour? _____

    b. How many milligrams per hour? _____

15. Medication: nitroprusside 50 mg
    in 250 mL D$_5$W
    Dose: 5 mcg/kg/min
    Patient weight: 143 lb

    a. How many milliliters per hour?

    b. How many milligrams per hour?

Perform calculations to answer the following questions.

16. A child is receiving an IV @ 20 mL/hr via microdrip tubing. How many drops per minute are administered?

17. An IV is to be administered at 60 mL/hr using an IV tubing with a drop factor of 10. How many drops per minute are administered?

18. A physician orders 750 mg of a drug in a 100 mL bag over 30 minutes. Using a 10 drop set, how many drops per minute is that?

19. If there is a flow rate of 24 gtts/min using a 15 drop set, how many liters will be administered over 24 hours?

20. If the IV flow rate is 30 gtts/min and a 10 drop set is used, how long will a 1 L bag last?

Determine the infusion rates in drops per minute for the following orders.

21. Administer 150 mL over 30 minutes using a 10 drop set.

22. Give 100 mL over 15 minutes using a 10 drop set.

Calculate the following doses in milliliters and then determine the infusion rate.

23.

IV Piggyback

Memorial Hospital

Name: James, Irene   **Room:** 628
Pt. ID#: HUY552662   **Rx#:** 55663882

Famotidine 40 mg
Dextrose 5% in water (D$_5$W) 50 mL
Rate: over 30 min

Expires _____
RPh _____
Tech _____

Keep refrigerated—warm to room temperature
before use.

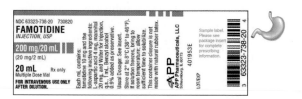

The medication you have on hand is:

a. How many milliliters of famotidine are needed for one dose? On the handout that you obtained from your instructor, indicate the correct volume on the correct measuring device.

b. What is the infusion rate in milliliters per hour?

24.

IV Piggyback

Memorial Hospital

Name: James, Irene   **Room:** 628
Pt. ID#: HUY552662   **Rx#:** 55663885

Furosemide 100 mg
Dextrose 5% in water (D$_5$W) 250 mL
Rate: over 60 min

Expires _____
RPh _____
Tech _____

Keep refrigerated—warm to room temperature
before use.

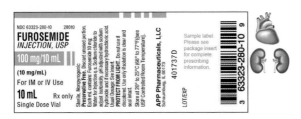

The medication you have on hand is:

a. How many milliliters of furosemide are needed for one dose? On the handout that you obtained from your instructor, indicate the correct volume on the correct measuring device.

b. What is the rate in drops per minute using microdrip tubing?

25.

IV Piggyback

Memorial Hospital

Name: Belika, Samantha   **Room:** 340

Pt. ID#: 7000388XX   **Rx#:** 99828388

Azithromycin 500 mg
Dextrose 5% in water (D$_5$W) 250 mL
Rate: over 60 min

Expires _____
RPh _____
Tech _____

Keep refrigerated – warm to room temperature before use.

The medication you have on hand is:

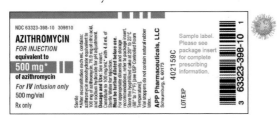

a. How many milliliters of azithromycin are needed for one dose? On the handout that you obtained from your instructor, indicate the correct volume on the correct measuring device.

b. What is the rate in drops per minute using a 20 drop set?

26.

IV Piggyback

Memorial Hospital

Name: Harden, James   **Room:** 426

Pt. ID#: DUW6310791   **Rx#:** 66735428

Gentamicin 120 mg
Dextrose 5% in water (D$_5$W) 150 mL
Rate: over 90 min

Expires _____
RPh _____
Tech _____

Keep refrigerated – warm to room temperature before use.

In this scenario, there is no adult-strength gentamicin available. The medication you have on hand is:

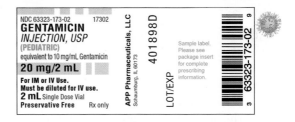

a. How many milliliters of gentamicin are needed for one dose? On the handout that you obtained from your instructor, indicate the correct volume on the correct measuring device.

b. What is the infusion rate in milliliters per hour?

27.

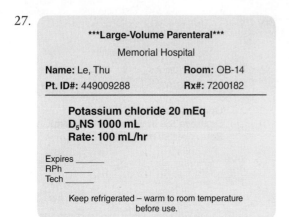

The medication you have on hand is:

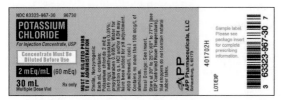

a. How many milliliters of potassium chloride are needed for one dose? On the handout that you obtained from your instructor, indicate the correct volume on the correct measuring device.

b. What is the rate in drops per minute using a 20 drop set?

28.

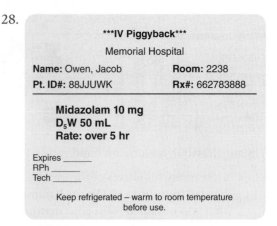

The medication you have on hand is:

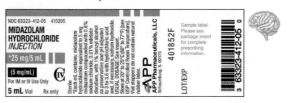

a. How many milliliters of midazolam are needed for one dose? On the handout that you obtained from your instructor, indicate the correct volume on the correct measuring device.

b. What is the rate in drops per minute using microdrip tubing?

29.

IV Piggyback

Memorial Hospital

Name: Grimaldi, Menor   **Room:** 851

Pt. ID#: M8837LLKY   **Rx#:** 1778280

     Amiodarone 150 mg
     D₅W 100 mL
     Rate: over 10 min

Expires _____
RPh _____
Tech _____

     Keep refrigerated – warm to room temperature
     before use.

The medication you have on hand is:

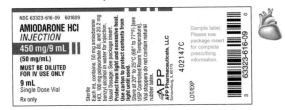

a. How many milliliters of amiodarone are needed for one dose? On the handout that you obtained from your instructor, indicate the correct volume on the correct measuring device.

b. What is the rate in drops per minute using a 10 drop set?

30.

IV Piggyback

Memorial Hospital

Name: Wright, Melissa   **Room:** 239

Pt. ID#: GYYI8872   **Rx#:** 78829993

     Vancomycin 1 g
     D₅W 250 mL
     Rate: 10 mL/hr (continuous infusion)

Expires _____
RPh _____
Tech _____

     Keep refrigerated – warm to room temperature
     before use.

The medication you have on hand is:

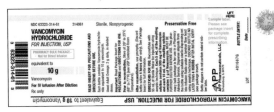

a. How many milliliters of vancomycin are needed for one dose? On the handout that you obtained from your instructor, indicate the correct volume on the correct measuring device.

b. What is the rate in milligrams per hour?

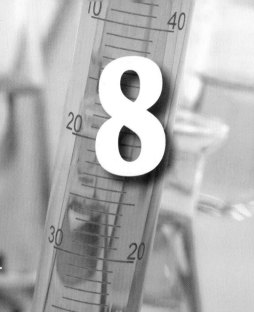

Using Special Calculations in Compounding

Lisa McCartney, BAAS, CPhT, PhTR

Learning Objectives

- Calculate the amount of each ingredient needed to enlarge a formula or recipe.

- Calculate the amount of each ingredient needed to reduce a formula or recipe.

- Compute the amount of two strengths of active ingredient needed to prepare a product whose concentration lies between the two extremes.

- Determine the amount of two ingredients using the weight-in-weight formula.

- Determine the amount of concentrate and diluent needed to prepare a special dilution.

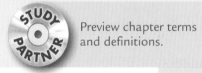

Preview chapter terms and definitions.

8.1 Compound Formulas

Compounding is the process of using raw ingredients and/or other prepared ingredients to create a drug product for a patient. This process is similar to making a cake from scratch by using ingredients such as butter, sugar, eggs, flour, and baking powder.

Safety in Numbers

Pharmacies that produce mass quantities have come under scrutiny due to contaminated products that resulted in serious illness and death. The FDA is currently reviewing the inspection process for these types of pharmacies.

A **formula**, or recipe, is a written document prepared by the pharmacist that lists the ingredients and instructions needed to prepare a compound. Some formulas are intended to prepare a single prescription, whereas others are intended to prepare a **compounded stock preparation**, or a large amount to be divided for individual prescription orders later. Commonly used compounds can be made in advance to have on hand as needed.

Some pharmacies routinely prepare compounded products for physicians who prescribe these special preparations on a regular basis. A pharmacy that prepares these compounds will often have a recipe for making a large amount to have on hand over the coming days or weeks. It is not uncommon to prepare a compound that can be divided and dispensed to as many as 20 patients. This is sometimes referred to as "batch compounding." Preparing compounds in advance can result in cost savings by reducing the labor needed to make the product and can also save time in providing the compound to the patient. Although the Food and Drug Administration (FDA) prohibits retail pharmacies from mass manufacturing compounded medications, anticipatory compounding is permitted in small quantities when a particular pharmacy is located near a physician's office that routinely orders certain compounded prescriptions.

Pharmacies store formulas in many ways. They may be maintained as a computerized file system or informally in a card file or binder. This is often called the pharmacy "recipe book." Some pharmacies also have different formulas for different prescribers, as each prescriber may prefer a slightly different version of a compound.

Enlarging or reducing formulas involves taking the recipe for a particular compounded medication and adjusting the amount of the ingredients to meet the needs of the pharmacy's order. This practice is similar to doubling the ingredients in a recipe for cookies to make twice as many cookies. Retaining the correct proportion of each ingredient in this process is critical. A cookie made from a doubled batch should have the same ratio of ingredients as a cookie made from a single batch. The same should be true when a formula is doubled in the compounding pharmacy.

Accurate records and documentation of mathematical calculations used in reducing or enlarging a formula are essential. All amounts should be calculated and recorded before weighing, measuring, and mixing. The final prepared product must match the concentration and amount ordered by the prescriber.

To accurately compound a prescription, pharmacy technicians must determine the **current formula**, which is the formula that is kept on hand in the pharmacy recipe book. In addition, technicians will need to know the **desired formula**, which is the amount that has been ordered by the prescriber.

The following examples will demonstrate the calculations for reducing or enlarging formulas.

Example 8.1.1

A prescriber has ordered a patient to receive 100 mL of a commonly used topical iodine solution. The pharmacy's recipe book lists a formula to prepare 1000 mL of the solution. Determine how much of each ingredient will be needed to prepare 100 mL of the solution.

Step 1. Determine the ratio to compare the desired formula with the current formula.

Desired formula requires you to provide 100 mL of the solution.

Current formula provides 1000 mL of the solution.

$$\frac{100}{1000} = \frac{1}{10}$$

So, you will need ¹⁄₁₀ (i.e., 100 mL desired/1000 mL formula) of the amount of each ingredient listed in the current recipe. Therefore, you will divide each ingredient amount by 10, as shown in Step 2.

Step 2. Calculate the amount of each ingredient.

Current Formula (for 1000 mL):

Iodine	30 g
Sodium iodide	25 g
Purified water	QSAD to 1000 mL

Desired Formula (for 100 mL):

Iodine	30 g / 10 = 3 g
Sodium iodide	25 g / 10 = 2.5 g
Purified water	QSAD to 1000 mL / 10 = 100 mL

You will need 3 g of iodine, 2.5 g of sodium iodide, and 100 mL of purified water.

Example 8.1.2

You need to prepare 16 oz of coal tar ointment for a patient. The pharmacy's recipe book lists a formula to prepare 4 oz of the ointment. Determine how much of each ingredient will be needed to prepare 16 oz of the ointment.

Step 1. Determine the ratio to compare the desired formula with the current formula.

Desired formula requires you to provide 16 oz of the ointment.

Current formula provides 4 oz of the ointment.

$$\frac{16}{4} = \frac{4}{1}$$

So, you will need four times (i.e., 16 desired/4 current = 4) the amount of each ingredient listed in the current formula. Therefore, you will multiply each ingredient amount by 4, as shown in Step 2.

Step 2. Calculate the amount of each ingredient.

Current Formula (for 4 oz):

Coal tar	4 g
Salicylic acid	1 g
Triamcinolone 0.1%	15 g
Aqua-base ointment	100 g

Desired Formula (for 16 oz):

Coal tar	4 g × 4 = 16 g
Salicylic acid	1 g × 4 = 4 g
Triamcinolone 0.1%	15 g × 4 = 60 g
Aqua-base ointment	100 g × 4 = 400 g

You will need 16 g of coal tar, 4 g of salicylic acid, 60 g of triamcinolone 0.1%, and 400 g of aqua-base ointment.

8.1 Problem Set

1. The following pharmacy recipe provides a formula that yields 120 g of coal tar ointment. You are to prepare a 30 g jar of coal tar ointment. State how much of each ingredient you will need.

Coal tar	4 g
Salicylic acid	1 g
Triamcinolone 0.1% ung	15 g
Aqua-base ointment	100 g

2. The following pharmacy recipe provides a formula that yields 30 vaginal suppositories. You are to prepare 150 vaginal suppositories. State how much of each ingredient you will need.

Progesterone	2.4 g
Polyethylene glycol 3350	30 g
Polyethylene glycol 1000	90 g

3. The following pharmacy recipe provides a formula that yields 20 mL of solution. You are to prepare 120 mL of the solution. State how much of each ingredient you will need.

Podophyllum resin	25%
Benzoin tincture	QSAD 20 mL

4. The following pharmacy recipe provides a formula that yields 8 oz of solution. You are to prepare 120 mL of the solution. State how much of each ingredient you will need.

Pharmacy Stock Formula (yields 8 oz)	
Tetracycline 500 mg capsules	16 capsules
Hydrocortisone suspension	15 mL
Lidocaine oral suspension	30 mL
Mylanta suspension	QSAD 240 mL

5. The following pharmacy recipe provides a formula to prepare one 30 mL dropper bottle of Oticaine. You are to prepare four 15 mL dropper bottles of Oticaine. State how much of each ingredient you will need to prepare the entire batch.

Pharmacy Stock Formula (yields 30 mL)	
Antipyrine	1.8 g
Benzocaine	0.5 g
Glycerin	QSAD 30 mL

Self-check your work in Appendix A.

8.2 Alligations

Occasionally, a prescriber will write a prescription for a medication strength that is not commercially available, or that is not kept on hand in the pharmacy. In these instances, the pharmacy may be required to mix two different strengths of the same active ingredient of a drug or solution to make the desired strength. A higher-percent strength (i.e., the more concentrated ingredient) of a drug or solution is mixed with a lower-percent strength (i.e., the less concentrated ingredient) of a drug or solution to make the desired strength, which falls somewhere between the two extremes. This scenario requires you to employ a calculation called the **alligation method**, or simply *alligation*. Alligations are rarely performed by pharmacy technicians, but you may need to carry out this kind of calculation from time to time. To understand how to set up an alligation problem, refer to Figure 8.1. Use this grid as your template for the scenario that follows.

FIGURE 8.1 Tic-Tac-Toe Alligation Grid

Safety in Numbers

As a means of checking to see that you have set up your grid properly, your desired % should always be a value in between the two concentrations you are combining.

A (higher %)		D (parts of higher %; the difference of B – C)
	B (desired %)	
C (lower %)		E (parts of lower %; the difference of A – B)

KEY

A = higher concentration or strength (stated as a percent [%])

B = desired concentration or strength (stated as a percent [%])

C = lower concentration or strength (stated as a percent [%])

Example 8.2.1

The compounded sterile preparation (CSP) label shown below indicates that the prescriber has ordered 250 mL of dextrose 7% in water (D_7W). In your pharmacy, you have both dextrose 5% in water (D_5W) and dextrose 70% in water ($D_{70}W$). Since the value of 7 falls between 5 and 70, you can use these two strengths to make the 7% you need. How much D5% and D70% must be combined to make an intravenous (IV) solution with a dextrose concentration of 7% (D_7W) and a total volume of 250 mL for infusion?

IV Solution – LVP

Mercy Hospital

Pt. Name: Werekela, Francis   **Room:** PICU-4

ID#: 543678   **Rx#:** 420883

Dextrose 7% in Water (D_7W) 250 mL
Rate: 10 mL/hr

Keep refrigerated – warm to room temperature
before administration.

Expiration Day/Time: _____ Tech _____ RPh _____

Step 1. Identify the variables by determining the component concentrations. The desired concentration (B%) is what the prescriber has written on the medication order and, therefore, is indicated on the CSP label. The higher concentration (A%) and lower concentration (C%) are determined by the stock IV base solution strengths on hand in your pharmacy. In this case, the desired concentration is 7%; the higher concentration is 70%; and the lower concentration is 5%.

For Good Measure

When using the tic-tac-toe grid, pharmacy technicians should be sure to place the desired % in the center square, the higher % in the upper left-hand square, and the lower % in the bottom left-hand square. It is also important to remember that subtraction is performed diagonally but that the "parts" are read horizontally or across the grid.

Step 2. Using the alligation template from Figure 8.1, fill in the concentration strengths (given as percentages) in the Key section below the tic-tac-toe grid. Place those same strengths in their designated squares on the grid.

A (higher %) 70		D (parts of higher %; the difference of B − C)
	B (desired %) 7	
C (lower %) 5		E (parts of lower %; the difference of A − B)

Key:
A% = 70
B% = 7
C% = 5
D (parts of 70% solution) =
E (parts of 5% solution) =

Step 3. To find the value of D in the upper right-hand square, set up the equation B − C = D.

Then fill in the values for B and C (found in Step 2) in the equation, as shown below:

7 − 5 = D
D = 2 (or the number of parts of 70% dextrose)

Record the number 2 in the key and in the upper right-hand square.

Step 4. To find the value of E in the lower right-hand square, set up the equation A − B = E.

Then fill in the values for A and B (found in Step 2) in the equation, as shown below:

70 − 7 = E
E = 63 (or the number of parts of 5% dextrose)

Record the number 63 in the key and in the lower right-hand square.

Step 5. Check that your completed grid now resembles the grid shown below:

A (higher %) 70		D (parts of higher %) 2
	B (desired %) 7	
C (lower %) 5		E (parts of lower %) 63

Key:
A% = 70
B% = 7
C% = 5
D (parts of 70% solution) = 2
E (parts of 5% solution) = 63

Step 6. Set up a ratio using the values of D and E as shown in the right-hand column of your completed grid:

$$\frac{D}{E} = \frac{2}{63}$$

This ratio indicates that to prepare the desired concentration (in this case, a D7% solution), dextrose 70% ($D_{70}W$) and dextrose 5% (D_5W) must be mixed in a 2:63 ratio: 2 parts of D70% and 63 parts of D5%.

Step 7. Using the ratio from Step 6, add together D and E to obtain the total number of parts (TP):

$$D + E = TP$$

$$2 + 63 = TP$$

$$65 = TP$$

Step 8. Now you need to determine the exact volume of each component needed to prepare 250 mL of D_7W. Because you already know the ratio in which the parts must be combined and the total number of parts, you can set up a ratio-proportion problem.

To find the volume of $D_{70}W$ needed for the CSP, use the following formula:

$$\frac{D}{TP} = \frac{x}{TV}$$

D = parts of the higher % solution
TP = total number of parts
TV = total volume of desired concentration

$$\frac{2}{65} = \frac{x}{250 \text{ mL}}$$

Cross multiply: 2 × 250 = 500; then divide 500/65 = x

$$x = 7.69 \text{ mL (rounded to 7.7 mL) of } D_{70}W$$

Step 9. To find the volume of D$_5$W needed for the CSP, use the following formula:

$$\frac{E}{TP} = \frac{x}{TV}$$

E = parts of the lower % solution
TP = total number of parts
TV = total volume of desired concentration

$$\frac{63}{65} = \frac{x}{250 \text{ mL}}$$

Cross multiply: $63 \times 250 = 15750$; then divide $15750/65 = x$

$x = 242.31$ mL (rounded to 242.3 mL) of D$_5$W

Step 10. To verify the volume of each component (determined in Steps 8 and 9), add the volumes of the two components. Your answer should equal the total volume of the desired concentration.

7.7 mL (D$_{70}$W) + 242.3 mL (D$_5$W) = 250 mL (total volume of desired concentration)

Example 8.2.2

The prescriber has ordered an IV infusion of 500 mL of dextrose 7%. You have stock concentrations of 5% dextrose and 70% dextrose on hand in the pharmacy. How much D70% and D5% must be combined to make an IV solution with a dextrose concentration of 7% (D$_7$W) and a total volume of 500 mL for infusion?

Step 1. Identify the variables. Determine the component concentrations (also called the strength or percent) by identifying the desired concentration (in this case, 7%); the higher concentration (in this case, 70%); and the lower concentration (in this case, 5%):

A (higher %) = 70
B (desired %) = 7
C (lower %) = 5

Note: The desired concentration (B%) is what the prescriber has written on the medication order, and it is also listed on the CSP label. The higher concentration (A%) and lower concentration (C%) are determined by the stock IV base solution strengths that you have on hand in your pharmacy.

Step 2. Set up a tic-tac-toe grid.

A (higher %) 70		D (parts of higher %; the difference of B − C)
	B (desired %) 7	
C (lower %) 5		E (parts of lower %; the difference of A − B)

Step 3. Determine the number of parts of each component (higher % and lower %).

a. Subtract the center number in the tic-tac-toe grid from the number in the upper left-hand square of the tic-tac-toe grid (A − B); place this number in the lower right-hand square of the grid (E).

$$A − B = E; 70 − 7 = 63$$

b. Subtract the number in the lower left-hand square of the tic-tac-toe grid from the number in the center of the grid (B − C); place this number in the upper right-hand square of the grid (D).

$$B − C = D; 7 − 5 = 2$$

D = 2 (parts of 70% dextrose)
E = 63 (parts of 5% dextrose)

Step 4. Set up a ratio using the information you determined in Step 3.

$$\frac{D}{E} = \frac{2}{63}$$

This indicates that to prepare the desired concentration (in this case, a D7% solution), dextrose 70% ($D_{70}W$) and dextrose 5% (D_5W) must be mixed in a 2:63 ratio; in other words, 2 parts of D70% and 63 parts of D5%.

Step 5. Determine the total number of parts in the ratio.

$$D + E = \text{total number of parts}$$

$$2 + 63 = 65 \text{ (total number of parts)}$$

Step 6. Determine the volume of each component.

a. Determine the volume of dextrose 70% ($D_{70}W$) needed for the CSP:

total volume (TV) of desired concentration = 500 mL
parts of $D_{70}W$ (D) = 2
total number of parts (TP) = 65

$$\frac{D}{TP} = \frac{x}{TV}$$

$$\frac{2}{65} = \frac{x}{500 \text{ mL}}$$

Cross multiply: $2 \times 500 = 1000$;
then divide $1000/65 = 15.38$, rounded to 15.4 mL

15.4 mL of $D_{70}W$

b. Determine the volume of dextrose 5% (D_5W) needed for the CSP:

total volume (TV) of desired concentration = 500 mL
parts of D_5W (D) = 63
total number of parts (TP) = 65

$$\frac{D}{TP} = \frac{x}{TV}$$

$$\frac{63}{65} = \frac{x}{500 \text{ mL}}$$

Cross multiply: $63 \times 500 = 31500$;
then divide $31500/65 = 484.62$, rounded to 484.6 mL

484.6 mL of D_5W

Therefore, to make D7% (D_7W) 500 mL, mix 15.4 mL of dextrose 70% ($D_{70}W$) with 484.6 mL of dextrose 5% (D_5W).

Step 7. Verify your answer.

The volume of each component (determined in Steps 6a and 6b) when added together should equal the total volume of the desired concentration:

volume of $D_{70}W$ = 15.4 mL
volume of D_5W = 484.6 mL

15.4 mL + 484.6 mL = 500 mL

The alligation method may also be used in extemporaneous compounding situations that require you to mix two strengths of an active ingredient to compound a product whose desired strength lies between the two extremes.

Example 8.2.3

The prescriber has ordered a topical preparation of 1.25% hydrocortisone cream 120 g. The pharmacy carries hydrocortisone cream in the following concentrations: 2.5% and 1%. Determine how much of the 2.5% cream and how much of the 1% cream will be needed to prepare 120 g of the desired 1.25% concentration.

Safety in Numbers

Technicians should always document calculations before compounding.

Step 1. Identify the variables.

A (higher %) = 2.5%
B (desired %) = 1.25%
C (lower %) = 1%

Step 2. Set up the tic-tac-toe grid.

2.5		
	1.25	
1		

Step 3. Determine the number of parts of each component.

A − B = E
2.5 − 1.25 = 1.25

B − C = D
1.25 − 1 = 0.25

Step 4. Fill in the values for D and E on the tic-tac-toe grid.

2.5		0.25
	1.25	
1		1.25

Step 5. Set up a ratio using the parts you determined in Step 3.

$$\frac{D}{E} = \frac{0.25}{1.25}$$

Step 6. Determine the total number of parts.

$$D + E = 0.25 + 1.25 = 1.5$$

Step 7. Determine the amount of each component.

$$\frac{0.25}{1.5} = \frac{x}{120}$$

Cross multiply: 0.25 × 120 = 30;
then divide 30/1.5 = 20 g of 2.5% hydrocortisone cream

$$\frac{1.25}{1.5} = \frac{x}{120}$$

Cross multiply: 1.25 × 120 = 150;
then divide 150/1.5 = 100 g of 1% hydrocortisone cream

Step 8. Verify your answer.

$$20 \text{ g} + 100 \text{ g} = 120 \text{ g}$$

8.2 Problem Set

Use the alligation method to answer the following problems.

1. Prepare 200 mL of 7.5% dextrose solution using D_5W and $D_{10}W$. How many milliliters of each solution will be needed?

2. Prepare 400 mL of D_8W using D_5W and $D_{20}W$. How many milliliters of each solution will be needed?

3. Prepare 500 mL of $D_{12.5}W$. You have on hand $D_{70}W$ and D_5W. How many milliliters of each solution will be needed?

4. You must prepare a 250 mL solution of 6% dextrose (D_6W). You have $D_{10}W$ and D_5W on hand. How many milliliters of each solution will be needed?

5. Prepare a total volume of 500 mL of $D_{7.5}W$. You have D_5W and $D_{50}W$ on hand. How many milliliters of each solution will be needed?

6. Prepare 250 mL of 8% dextrose from D_5W and $D_{20}W$. How many milliliters of each solution will be needed?

7. Prepare 300 mL of 7.5% dextrose using D_5W and $D_{20}W$. How many milliliters of each solution will be needed?

8. Prepare 500 mL of 12.5% dextrose using $D_{10}W$ and $D_{20}W$. How many milliliters of each solution will be needed?

9. Prepare 150 mL of 7.5% dextrose from D_5W and $D_{10}W$. How many milliliters of each solution will be needed?

10. A physician has ordered 250 mL of $D_{12.5}W$. You have $D_{10}W$ and $D_{20}W$ available. How many milliliters of each solution will be needed?

11. Prepare 60 g of a 3% cream from a 1% cream and a 10% cream. How many grams of each cream will be needed?

12. Prepare 30 g of a 7.5% cream from a 5% cream and a 15% cream. How many grams of each cream will be needed?

13. The pharmacy has received an order that requires the batch preparation of four 30 g jars of hydrocortisone 3% cream. The pharmacy has a 1% hydrocortisone cream and a 5% hydrocortisone cream on hand. How many grams of each cream will be needed to prepare the entire batch?

14. Prepare 45 g of 10% zinc oxide using a 5% zinc oxide ointment and a 20% zinc oxide ointment. How many grams of each ointment will be needed?

15. Prepare 100 g of an 8% cream from a 5% cream and a 10% cream. How many grams of each cream will be needed?

Self-check your work in Appendix A.

8.3 Weight-in-Weight (w/w) Calculations

When compounding two solid ingredients—an **active ingredient** and an **inactive ingredient**—the weight-in-weight (w/w) formula is sometimes used to determine the amount of each ingredient needed for the preparation. The **weight-in-weight (w/w) formula**, often signified by the abbreviation *w/w*, identifies the number of grams of drug per 100 g of the product. This concentration can be expressed as a fraction, as shown in the following:

$$\text{weight-in-weight (w/w)} = \frac{x \text{ g drug}}{100 \text{ g product}}$$

When determining **percentage strength**, the unknown (designated by an *x*) will always be placed over 100. The term *percentage strength* means *parts of 100* or *percent of the whole* (with the "whole" meaning 100%). Additionally, percentage strength signifies the number of grams of a drug per 100 g of the product. The following formula may be used to determine the percentage strength of w/w preparations:

$$\text{percentage strength of w/w preparation} = \frac{\text{g of active ingredient}}{100 \text{ g of product}} \times 100$$

Example 8.3.1

You have a compound with a concentration of 5 g hydrocortisone powder in 100 g of petrolatum. Determine the percentage strength of this compound.

$$\frac{5 \text{ g drug}}{100 \text{ g product}} \times 100$$

$$5/100 = 0.05; 0.05 \times 100 = 5$$

The percentage strength of a compound with 5 g hydrocortisone powder in 100 g of petrolatum is 5%.

When the percentage strength of the product is known, the w/w formula may also be used to determine how many grams of an active ingredient are in a defined amount of an inactive ingredient. Apply the ratio-proportion method to determine the number of grams of active ingredient needed to compound the preparation.

Example 8.3.2

If the compounded preparation has a percentage strength of 3%, how many grams of drug are in 50 g of the preparation?

$$3\% = 3 \text{ g}/100 \text{ g}$$

$$\frac{3 \text{ g}}{100 \text{ g}} = \frac{x \text{ g}}{50 \text{ g}}$$

Cross multiply: $3 \times 50 = 150$; then divide $150/100 = 1.5$

There are 1.5 g of drug in 50 g of the preparation.

Use the w/w method to solve the following problems.

1. Prepare a compound of hydrocortisone cream in petrolatum with a concentration of 2%. How many grams of hydrocortisone are contained in 75 g of the cream?

2. Prepare a compound of zinc oxide using 8 g of zinc oxide powder in 454 g of aqua-base ointment. What is the percentage strength of this compounded preparation?

3. Prepare a compound of 100 g of acyclovir cream 2.5%. How many grams of acyclovir will be needed for this preparation?

4. Prepare a compound that mixes 10 g of acyclovir with 50 g of petrolatum. What is the percentage strength of this compounded preparation?

5. The pharmacy has received a prescription for 30 g of a 2% triamcinolone ointment. How many grams of triamcinolone will be needed to prepare this prescription?

6. The pharmacy has received the following prescription:

> Todd Jackson, MD
> Anita Johnson, MD
> Kunal Gupta, MSN, FCNP
> 5730 Congress Avenue
> Boise, ID 83702
> (208) 555-1212 fax (208) 555-1313
>
> DOB _October 18, 1978_ DEA# _____
> Pt. Name _Lily Nguyen_ Date _02/12/2015_
> Address _____ 2934 Anderson Lane _____
> _____ Boise, ID 83722 _____
>
> _Elocon (mometasone fumarate) 0.1% cream_
> _aaa tid prn_
> _Disp. 15 g_
>
> Refill _5_ times (no refill unless indicated)
> _____ Anita Johnson _____ MD
> _____ N0972 _____ License #

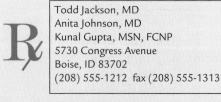

How many grams of mometasone fumarate will be needed to prepare this prescription?

7. The pharmacy has received an order to compound a batch preparation of progesterone suppositories. You will need to prepare 100 suppositories, each containing 200 mg.

   a. How many grams of progesterone will be needed for the entire batch of suppositories?

   b. What is the percentage strength of each suppository?

8. The pharmacy has received the following prescription:

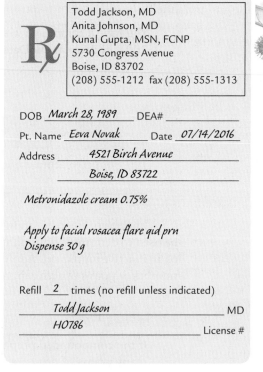

> Todd Jackson, MD
> Anita Johnson, MD
> Kunal Gupta, MSN, FCNP
> 5730 Congress Avenue
> Boise, ID 83702
> (208) 555-1212 fax (208) 555-1313
>
> DOB _March 28, 1989_ DEA# _____
> Pt. Name _Eeva Novak_ Date _07/14/2016_
> Address _____ 4521 Birch Avenue _____
> _____ Boise, ID 83722 _____
>
> _Metronidazole cream 0.75%_
>
> _Apply to facial rosacea flare qid prn_
> _Dispense 30 g_
>
> Refill _2_ times (no refill unless indicated)
> _____ Todd Jackson _____ MD
> _____ H0786 _____ License #

How many grams of metronidazole will be needed to prepare this prescription?

9. The pharmacy has received the following medication order:

ID#: HYII897			Memorial Hospital
Name: Bishop, Walter			
DOB: 01/25/71			
Room: 717a			Physician's
Dr: Michal Nikolai, MD			Medication Order

ALLERGY OR SENSITIVITY		DIAGNOSIS	
ceftazidime		cellulitis	

DATE	TIME	ORDERS	PHYSICIAN'S SIG.
03/15/2019	5:14 PM	Clindamycin topical gel 1%	
		Apply 1 g to acne bid ut. dict.	
		Dispense 30 g tube	
			Michal Nikolai, MD

How many grams of clindamycin will be needed to prepare this prescription?

10. The pharmacy has received the following medication order:

ID#: 7882993ZZ			Memorial Hospital
Name: Ellings, Grace			
DOB: 09/02/17			
Room: ICU-2			Physician's
Dr: Audrea Carter, MD			Medication Order

ALLERGY OR SENSITIVITY		DIAGNOSIS	shingles,
NKA			exacerbation of COPD

DATE	TIME	ORDERS	PHYSICIAN'S SIG.
10/09/2017	0633	Acyclovir 10% ointment 50 g tube	
		Apply 1 g tid ut. dict.	
			Audrea Carter, MD

a. How many grams of acyclovir will be needed to prepare this prescription?

b. How many doses are contained in this prescription?

Self-check your work in Appendix A.

8.4 Special Dilutions

For Good Measure

Typically, the ratio-proportion method is preferred over the dimensional analysis method to solve special dilution problems because it is easier to identify the parts of the equation.

Physicians often prescribe concentrations of medications that are not commercially available, and these prescriptions must be compounded in the pharmacy. Often this is accomplished by mixing a concentrated stock solution with a diluent. Calculations of this type were discussed in Chapters 6 and 7. However, there are times when pharmacy technicians are presented with more complex compounding scenarios, such as mixing pediatric **compounded sterile preparations (CSPs)**. In general, pediatric CSPs are compounded by diluting adult formulations of medications with a diluent such as sterile water or sterile normal saline. However, there are times when the high concentrations of adult-strength medications make reduction to child-sized doses difficult. In these situations, the pediatric doses are such small volumes that they are hard to draw up accurately in a syringe.

To provide accurate parenteral medication dosing for neonates or other particularly small patients, pharmacy technicians may be called upon to prepare a custom-made CSP or **special dilution**. To prepare this type of CSP, technicians will need to perform a series of calculations, as demonstrated in the following examples.

Example 8.4.1

Prepare a special dilution of gentamicin with a total volume of 4 mL and a concentration of 5 mg/mL. Use a stock solution of gentamicin 10 mg/mL and sterile water to prepare this special dilution.

Step 1. Determine the total number of milligrams in the desired special dilution.

desired final product = 5 mg/mL
total volume (TV) = 4 mL

Use the ratio-proportion method to determine the number of milligrams needed for the special dilution.

$$\frac{5 \text{ mg}}{1 \text{ mL}} = \frac{x \text{ mg}}{4 \text{ mL}}$$

Cross multiply: $5 \times 4 = 20$; then divide $20/1 = 20$

total number of milligrams of gentamicin needed for the special dilution = 20 mg

Step 2. Determine the number of milliliters of stock solution (10 mg/mL) needed to prepare the special dilution.

$$\frac{10 \text{ mg}}{1 \text{ mL}} = \frac{20 \text{ mg}}{x \text{ mL}}$$

Cross multiply: $20 \times 1 = 20$; then divide $20/10 = 2$

total number of milliliters of gentamicin stock solution (10 mg/mL) needed to prepare the special dilution = 2 mL

Step 3. Determine the number of milliliters of diluent (sterile water) needed to prepare the special dilution.

total volume (TV) − drug volume (DV) = volume of diluent

TV = 4 mL
DV = 2 mL
$4 - 2 = 2$
volume of diluent = 2 mL

The pharmacy technician must draw up 2 mL of the gentamicin 10 mg/mL stock solution and 2 mL of the sterile water diluent. Both syringes will be aseptically injected into a sterile, empty vial, and the resulting 4 mL special dilution will be gentamicin with a concentration of 5 mg/mL.

There are times when a pharmacy technician will need to prepare a special dilution of an IV dextrose infusion that has a percentage strength that is not commercially available. In most cases, this special dilution will be prepared by mixing a concentrated dextrose solution with sterile water to create the percentage strength ordered by the prescriber. The following example will demonstrate the three-step formula for solving this type of problem.

Example 8.4.2

Using a stock solution of dextrose 70% ($D_{70}W$) and sterile water, prepare a 1000 mL IV with a percentage strength of $D_{10}W$.

Key:
TV = total volume of the IV solution ordered by prescriber
stock % = percentage strength of the solution that is stocked in the pharmacy
desired % = percentage strength of the solution ordered by the prescriber
mL = number of milliliters of that solution needed to prepare the IV solution

Step 1. Calculate the volume of concentrated dextrose solution.

Identify the variables:
TV = 1000 mL
stock % = 70
desired % = 10

Formula used to calculate amount of concentrated dextrose solution needed:

(TV/stock %) × desired % = number of milliliters

(1000/70) × 10 = 142.86 mL, rounded to 142.9 mL

amount of dextrose needed = 142.9 mL

Step 2. Calculate the volume of sterile water by subtracting the amount determined in Step 1 from the total volume ordered by the prescriber.

1000 − 142.9 = 857.1

amount of sterile water needed = 857.1 mL

Step 3. Verify the accuracy of your calculations. Add together the volumes that you determined in Step 1 and Step 2 above. If you have performed each of the calculations correctly, they should equal the total volume ordered by the physician—in this case, 1000 mL.

Put Down Roots

The word *parenteral* comes from the Greek roots *para*, meaning "beside," and *enteron*, meaning "intestine." Therefore, a parenteral preparation refers to a product that bypasses—or goes "beside" rather than through—the gastrointestinal tract.

Occasionally, pharmacy technicians will need to prepare a special dilution known as **total parenteral nutrition (TPN)**. This large-volume IV solution is comprised of multiple solutions, such as dextrose, amino acids, fat emulsion, and sterile water. This combination of solutions is called the **TPN base solution**. In addition, most TPN solutions contain multiple electrolyte and vitamin **additives**. Additives are substances such as medications, electrolytes, or other ingredients added to another product. The following examples will demonstrate the five-part procedure for solving typical TPN problems.

Example 8.4.3

Prepare a 2000 mL TPN with the base solution and additives shown below.

Base Solution
Dextrose 15%
Aminosyn (amino acid solution) 3.5%
Liposyn (fat emulsion) 5%
Sterile water QSAD to 2000 mL

Additives
Sodium chloride 40 mEq
Potassium chloride 10 mEq
Potassium phosphate 6 mM
Multiple vitamin (MVI) 10 mL

Prepared Using the Following Pharmacy Stock Solutions (i.e., concentrations kept on hand in the pharmacy)
Dextrose 70%
Aminosyn 10%
Liposyn 20%
Sodium chloride 4 mEq/mL
Potassium chloride 2 mEq/mL
Potassium phosphate 3 mM/mL
MVI 10 mL

Key:
TV = total volume of TPN ordered by prescriber
stock % = percentage strength of the solution that is stocked in the pharmacy
desired % = percentage strength of the solution ordered by the prescriber
mL = number of milliliters of that solution needed to prepare the TPN solution

Formula used to calculate TPN base solution component:

(TV/stock %) × desired % = number of milliliters

Note: A separate calculation must be performed to determine the volume of each TPN component.

Step 1. Calculate the volume of the TPN base components—dextrose, Aminosyn, and Liposyn. (*Note:* The sterile water volume will be calculated in Step 4.)

a. Start by determining the amount of dextrose needed. Identify the variables:

TV = 2000 mL
stock % = 70
desired % = 15
(2000/70) × 15 = 2000/70 = 28.57; 28.57 × 15 = 428.57, rounded to 429
amount of dextrose needed = 429 mL

b. Next, determine the amount of Aminosyn needed.

Identify the variables:
TV = 2000 mL
stock % = 10
desired % = 3.5
(2000/10) × 3.5 = 2000/10 = 200; 200 × 3.5 = 700
amount of Aminosyn needed = 700 mL

c. Next, determine the amount of Liposyn needed.

Identify the variables:
TV = 2000 mL
stock % = 20
desired % = 5
(2000/20) × 5 = 2000/20 = 100; 100 × 5 = 500
amount of Liposyn needed = 500 mL

Step 2. Calculate the volume of each additive based on the following formula:

$$D/H = x$$

Key:
D = desired dose (the dose ordered by the prescriber)
H = concentration on hand (the concentration or strength of the drug
    per milliliter)
x = unknown volume of drug needed to be drawn up for the prepara-
    tion of the additive

a. Start by determining the amount of sodium chloride needed.

Identify the variables:
D = 40
H = 4
x = ?
40/4 = 10
amount of sodium chloride needed = 10 mL

b. Next, determine the amount of potassium chloride needed.

Identify the variables:
D = 10
H = 2
x = ?
10/2 = 5
amount of potassium chloride needed = 5 mL

c. Then, determine the amount of potassium phosphate needed.

Identify the variables:
$D = 6$
$H = 3$
$x = ?$
$6/3 = 2$
amount of potassium phosphate needed = 2 mL

d. Finally, determine the amount of MVI needed. (*Note:* Because the prescriber has ordered a specific volume of MVI, you will simply draw up the ordered volume.)

amount of MVI needed = 10 mL

Step 3. Add each of the volumes you determined in Steps 1 and 2 above.

$$
\begin{array}{r}
429 \\
700 \\
500 \\
10 \\
5 \\
2 \\
+\ 10 \\
\hline
1656
\end{array}
$$

Step 4. Determine the amount of sterile water needed to QSAD to 2000 mL. Subtract the total determined in Step 3 (the volume of base solution and additives) from the total volume of the TPN solution.

$$
\begin{array}{r}
2000 \\
-1656 \\
\hline
344
\end{array}
$$

amount of sterile water needed = 344 mL

Step 5. Verify the accuracy of your calculations by adding together all of the volumes. If you have performed each of the calculations correctly, they should equal the total volume ordered by the physician—in this case, 2000 mL.

$$
\begin{array}{r}
429 \\
700 \\
500 \\
10 \\
5 \\
2 \\
10 \\
+\ 344 \\
\hline
2000
\end{array}
$$

1. Prepare a special dilution of acyclovir with a total volume of 10 mL and a concentration of 10 mg/mL. To create this special dilution, use a stock solution of acyclovir with a concentration of 100 mg/mL and sterile water.

    a. How many milligrams of acyclovir will be needed for this special dilution?

    b. How many milliliters of the acyclovir stock solution will need to be drawn up for this special dilution?

    c. How many milliliters of sterile water will need to be drawn up for this special dilution?

2. Prepare a special dilution of tobramycin with a total volume of 5 mL and a concentration of 10 mg/mL. To create this special dilution, use a stock solution of tobramycin with a concentration of 40 mg/mL and sterile water.

    a. How many milligrams of tobramycin will be needed for this special dilution?

    b. How many milliliters of the tobramycin stock solution will need to be drawn up for this special dilution?

    c. How many milliliters of sterile water will need to be drawn up for this special dilution?

3. Prepare a special dilution of vancomycin with a total volume of 10 mL and a concentration of 10 mg/mL. To create this special dilution, use a stock solution of vancomycin with a concentration of 500 mg/5 mL and sterile water.

    a. How many milligrams of vancomycin will be needed for this special dilution?

    b. How many milliliters of the vancomycin stock solution will need to be drawn up for this special dilution?

    c. How many milliliters of sterile water will need to be drawn up for this special dilution?

4. Prepare a special dilution of dexamethasone with a total volume of 5 mL and a concentration of 1 mg/mL. To create this special dilution, use a stock solution of dexamethasone with a concentration of 4 mg/mL and sterile water.

    a. How many milligrams of dexamethasone will be needed for this special dilution?

    b. How many milliliters of the dexamethasone stock solution will need to be drawn up for this special dilution?

    c. How many milliliters of sterile water will need to be drawn up for this special dilution?

5. Prepare a special dilution of gentamicin with a total volume of 10 mL and a concentration of 1 mg/mL. To create this special dilution, use sterile water and the following gentamicin stock solution.

    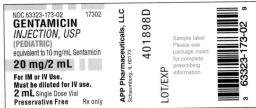

    a. How many milligrams of gentamicin will be needed for this special dilution?

    b. How many milliliters of the gentamicin stock solution shown above will need to be drawn up for this special dilution?

    c. How many milliliters of sterile water will need to be drawn up for this special dilution?

For questions 6–10, determine how much of each solution will be needed to make the preparation.

6. Prepare 500 mL of $D_{15}W$ using dextrose 70% and sterile water.

7. Prepare 2000 mL of $D_{10}W$ using dextrose 50% and sterile water.

8. Prepare 1000 mL of $D_{10}W$ using $D_{50}W$ and sterile water.

9. Prepare 750 mL of D_8W using $D_{50}W$ and sterile water.

10. Prepare 250 mL of D7.5% using $D_{70}W$ and sterile water.

11. The pharmacy has received the TPN order shown below. Use the TPN order, along with the various pharmacy stock solutions carried by your pharmacy, to determine the volume of each base solution and additive.

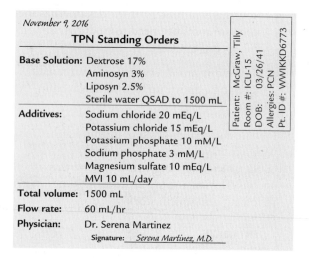

November 9, 2016

TPN Standing Orders

Base Solution: Dextrose 17%
Aminosyn 3%
Liposyn 2.5%
Sterile water QSAD to 1500 mL

Additives: Sodium chloride 20 mEq/L
Potassium chloride 15 mEq/L
Potassium phosphate 10 mM/L
Sodium phosphate 3 mM/L
Magnesium sulfate 10 mEq/L
MVI 10 mL/day

Total volume: 1500 mL
Flow rate: 60 mL/hr
Physician: Dr. Serena Martinez
Signature: _Serena Martinez, M.D._

Patient: McGraw, Tilly
Room #: ICU-15
DOB: 03/26/41
Allergies: PCN
Pt. ID #: WWIKKD6773

The pharmacy carries the following stock solutions:

Dextrose 70%
Aminosyn 10%
Liposyn 20%
Sodium chloride 4 mEq/mL
Potassium chloride 2 mEq/mL
Potassium phosphate 3 mM/mL
Sodium phosphate 3 mM/mL
Magnesium sulfate 4.06 mEq/mL
MVI 10 mL

Determine the volume of each of the following:

a. Dextrose =

b. Aminosyn =

c. Liposyn =

d. Sodium chloride =

e. Potassium chloride =

f. Potassium phosphate =

g. Sodium phosphate =

h. Magnesium sulfate =

i. MVI =

j. Sterile water =

k. Total volume =

Self-check your work in Appendix A.

Chapter Summary

- The mixing of various pharmaceutical ingredients, a process called *compounding*, is a task frequently performed by technicians in hospital and compounding pharmacies and, occasionally, in the community pharmacy setting.
- Compounding requires strict adherence to a recipe or formula.
- Technicians are often required to perform a series of calculations to reduce or enlarge an existing formula (known as the *current formula*) into the new, prescribed strength or amount (known as the *desired formula*).
- One way to reduce or enlarge a recipe is to compare the current formula with the desired formula by creating a ratio. The technician then either divides by that amount to reduce the formula, or multiplies by that amount to enlarge the formula.
- Occasionally, a technician may be required to mix two strengths of a particular ingredient to prepare a medication with a final strength whose concentration lies somewhere between the higher-strength and lower-strength ingredients.
- When working with an alligation problem, the *desired strength* should be placed in the center of the tic-tac-toe grid; the *higher strength* (stronger concentration) should be placed in the upper-left corner of the tic-tac-toe grid; and the *lower strength* (weaker

concentration) should be placed in the lower-left corner of the tic-tac-toe grid.
- When working with an alligation problem, remember to subtract diagonally, and read across to determine the parts of the higher-strength and lower-strength concentrations: A − B = E (parts of higher %); B − C = D (parts of lower %).
- When using an alligation to determine the amount of each ingredient, use the following formulas:

$$\frac{D \text{ (higher \% solution)}}{TP \text{ (total \# of parts)}} = \frac{x \text{ mL}}{TV \text{ (total volume of desired concentration)}}$$

$$\frac{E \text{ (lower \% solution)}}{TP \text{ (total \# of parts)}} = \frac{x \text{ mL}}{TV \text{ (total volume of desired concentration)}}$$

Cross multiply then divide to solve for x.
- The weight-in-weight (w/w) formula identifies the number of grams per 100 g of product.
- A special dilution is a type of compounded sterile preparation that is prepared to provide a pediatric dosage of an injectable medication that is only commercially available in an adult-strength formulation.

Formulas for Success

Alligation Tic-Tac-Toe Grid		
A (higher %)		D (parts of higher %; the difference of B − C)
	B (desired %)	
C (lower %)		E (parts of lower %; the difference of A − B)

Calculation for Percentage Strength of W/W Preparations

$$\text{percentage strength of w/w preparation} = \frac{\text{g of active ingredient}}{100 \text{ g of product}} \times 100$$

Key Terms

active ingredient the component of a pharmaceutical preparation or medication that exerts pharmacological activity designed to treat or prevent disease

additive a pharmaceutical substance, such as a medication, electrolyte, or other ingredient, that is added to another product, such as a compounded sterile preparation, in order to be easily administered to a patient

alligation method the mathematical calculation used to determine the amounts of two or more dilutions of differing strengths that will be mixed to prepare a product of a desired strength and quantity

compounded sterile preparation (CSP) the mixing of one or more sterile parenteral products using aseptic technique

compounded stock preparation a solution that is prepared in a large amount and kept in stock in the pharmacy to be divided for individual prescriptions

compounding the process of using raw ingredients and/or other prepared ingredients to create a drug product for a patient

current formula a standard pharmaceutical recipe that is commonly used in pharmacy compounding; a recipe often used to prepare compounded stock preparations

desired formula a specialized pharmaceutical recipe that may be ordered by the prescriber and that results from altering various components of the current formula

formula a written document listing the ingredients and instructions needed to prepare a compound

inactive ingredient an inert ingredient that is used as a base, or vehicle, to deliver the active ingredient in a compounded preparation; for example, petrolatum is used as a base in many topical preparations

percentage strength a mathematical formula or expression used to identify the number of grams of active ingredient per 100 mL of solution (or per 100 g of solid); may be referred to as *percent strength*

special dilution a custom-made CSP that provides accurate dosage of a medication prepared according to a desired recipe or formula; a term often associated with certain neonatal or pediatric CSPs

total parenteral nutrition (TPN) IV administration of total nutrient requirements to patients who require a long-term alternative to enteral feeding

TPN base solution components of the TPN solution that provide the primary volumetric source of hydration and calories, often comprised of a combination of dextrose, amino acids, fat emulsion, and sterile water

weight-in-weight (w/w) formula the number of grams of a drug (solid) in 100 g of the final product (solid)

Chapter Review

Assessing Comprehension

To check your comprehension of this chapter's key concepts, read the following multiple-choice questions and then record your answers on a separate sheet of paper. Write your answers as modeled in these examples: 1d; 2c; 3b; *etc.*

1. The process of using raw or prepared ingredients in the preparation of a drug product for a patient is called
   a. diluting.
   b. reconstituting.
   c. compounding.
   d. dispensing.

2. With regard to pharmacy compounding, which of the following terms has the same meaning as the term *formula?*
   a. recipe
   b. prescription
   c. concentration
   d. dilution

3. The term *percentage strength* is commonly used to describe which of the following?
   a. the number of grams/mL
   b. the number of grams/100 mL
   c. the number of milligrams/mL
   d. the number of milligrams/100 mL

4. What method does a pharmacy technician use when performing calculations for a prescription that requires mixing two different strengths of a drug (a higher-percent strength and a lower-percent strength) to make the desired strength?
   a. alligation
   b. ratio-proportion
   c. dimensional analysis
   d. dilution analysis

5. What does the acronym *CSP* mean?
   a. compounded sterile product
   b. compounding sterile personnel
   c. compounded sterile preparation
   d. compounding sterile procedures

6. An inert ingredient that is used as a base or vehicle to deliver the active ingredient in a compounded preparation is called an _____ ingredient.
   a. active
   b. activated
   c. inactive
   d. inactivated

7. Determine the amount of dextrose and sterile water needed to make the following solution:

   > $D_{12}W$ 500 mL using $D_{70}W$ and sterile water (SW)

   a. dextrose 70% 85.7 mL; SW 413.3 mL
   b. dextrose 70% 41.7 mL; SW 458.3 mL
   c. dextrose 70% 7.1 mL; SW 492.9 mL
   d. dextrose 70% 1.7 mL; SW 498.3 mL

8. Determine the amount of dextrose, Aminosyn (AA), and SW needed to make the following solution:

   > TPN solution with D18%, AA 3%, and SW QSAD to 2L
   > Stock solutions: $D_{70}W$, AA 10%

   a. dextrose 70% 514.3 mL; AA 600 mL; SW 885.7 mL
   b. dextrose 70% 777.7 mL; AA 666.6 mL; SW 555.7 mL
   c. dextrose 70% 720 mL; AA 120 mL; SW 1160 mL
   d. dextrose 70% 514.3 mL; AA 85.7 mL; SW 1400 mL

9. Determine the amount of sodium chloride needed to make the following solution:

> TPN solution with D18%, AA 3%, SW QSAD to 2L
> Additive: NaCl 15 mEq per liter
> Stock solutions: $D_{70}W$, AA 10%, NaCl 4 mEq/mL

a. 3.5 mL
b. 3.75 mL
c. 7.5 mL
d. 10 mL

10. Determine the amount of dextrose, sterile water, and potassium chloride needed to make the following solution:

> TPN solution with D15%, AA 3.5%, SW QSAD to 1500 mL
> Additives: NaCl 20 mEq, KCl 10 mEq, KPh04 12 mM
> Stock solutions: $D_{70}W$, AA 10%, NaCl 4 mEq/mL, KCl 2 mEq/mL, KPh04 3 mM/mL

a. dextrose 70% 321.4 mL; SW 639.6 mL; NaCl 5 mL
b. dextrose 70% 639.6 mL; SW 321.4 mL; NaCl 5 mL
c. dextrose 70% 321.4 mL; SW 639.6 mL; NaCl 10 mL
d. dextrose 70% 10 mL, SW 321.4 mL, NaCl 639.6 mL

Finding Solutions

To gain practice in handling challenging situations in the workplace, consider the following real-world scenarios and then use the guiding questions to help you formulate your responses.

Scenario A: You have just received the following medication order in the pharmacy. Answer the accompanying questions based on this medication order.

ID#: PPIKIEI88929	Memorial Hospital
Name: Seaholm, Brinkley	
DOB: 07/04/81	
Room: 1124	
Dr: Sarai Gupta, M.D.	Physician's Medication Order

ALLERGY OR SENSITIVITY			DIAGNOSIS	
NKA			dehydration	
DATE	TIME	ORDERS		PHYSICIAN'S SIG.
5/5/2017	3:57 P.M.	Potassium chloride 20 mEq/L		
		in D12% 1000 mL		
		@ 125 mL/hr		
				Sarai Gupta, M.D.

Pharmacy Stock Solutions:

Dextrose 50%

Potassium chloride 2 mEq/mL

1. How many mEq of KCl will be needed for one IV bag?

2. How many IV bags will the patient need for 24 hours?

3. How many milliliters of dextrose will be needed to prepare one IV bag?

4. How many milliliters of sterile water will be needed to prepare one IV bag?

5. How many milliliters of IV fluid will the patient receive in 24 hours?

Scenario B: The following TPN label was received in the IV room. Answer the accompanying questions based on this label.

TPN Solution

Memorial Hospital

Name: Burge, April   **Room:** 2284
Pt. ID#: HHUSY0068   **Rx#:** 7728829

Dextrose 15%
Aminosyn 5%
Liposyn 2.5%
SW QSAD
NaCl 10 mEq/L
KCl 10 mEq/L
MgSO$_4$ 2.5 mEq/L
Regular insulin 20 units/L
MVI 10 mL

Rate: 150 mL/hr

Expires _____
RPh _____
Tech _____

Keep refrigerated – warm to room temperature before use.

Pharmacy Stock Solutions:

D$_{70}$W

AA 10%

Liposyn 10%

NaCl 4 mEq/mL

KCl 2 mEq/mL

MgSO$_4$ 4.06 mEq/mL

Regular insulin 100 units/mL

MVI 10 mL

6. The TPN rate is 150 mL/hr. What is the total volume that will be needed for 24 hours? (*Note:* This will be the TPN total volume—the QSAD amount that should be used to determine SW volume.)

7. How much dextrose will be needed?

8. How much Aminosyn (AA) will be needed?

9. How much Liposyn will be needed?

10. How much sodium chloride will be needed?

11. How much potassium chloride will be needed?

12. How much magnesium sulfate will be needed?

13. How much regular insulin will be needed?

14. How much MVI will be needed?

15. How much sterile water will be needed?

Sampling the Certification Exam

To provide you with practice for the Certification Exam, read the following questions that have been patterned after the test format and then record your answers on a separate sheet of paper. Write your answers as modeled in these examples: 1d; 2c; 3b; *etc.*

1. What is the final concentration of a special dilution of gentamicin if you are required to draw up 1 mL of gentamicin stock solution (concentration 40 mg/mL) to prepare a special dilution with a total volume of 10 mL?
   a. 0.4 mg/mL
   b. 4 mg/mL
   c. 40 mg/mL
   d. 400 mg/mL

2. Which of the following vancomycin stock solutions and amounts would you use to prepare a special dilution that has a final concentration of 10 mg/mL and a total volume of 10 mL?
   a. vancomycin 10 mg/mL; 1 mL
   b. vancomycin 100 mg/mL; 1 mL
   c. vancomycin 1000 mg/mL; 1 mL
   d. vancomycin 1 mg/mL; 10 mL

3. What is the percentage strength of a solution that contains dextrose 8 g/100 mL?
   a. 0.8%
   b. 8%
   c. 80%
   d. 800%

4. How much $D_{50}W$ and $D_{10}W$ would be needed to prepare 2 L of $D_{15}W$?
   a. $D_{50}W$ = 1750 mL; $D_{10}W$ = 250 mL
   b. $D_{50}W$ = 875 mL; $D_{10}W$ = 125 mL
   c. $D_{50}W$ = 125 mL; $D_{10}W$ = 875 mL
   d. $D_{50}W$ = 250 mL; $D_{10}W$ = 1750 mL

5. How many grams of dextrose are contained in a TPN solution with the following base components?

Dextrose 15%
Aminosyn 5%
Liposyn 5%
Sterile water QSAD 2.5 L

   a. 15 g
   b. 37.5 g
   c. 150 g
   d. 375 g

Chapter Practice Test

Additional Practice Questions

To put your pharmacy calculation skills to the test, read the following questions and then record your answers on a separate sheet of paper.

Note: *Questions 1, 2, 3, and 5 have accompanying handouts that must be obtained from your instructor.*

1. Prepare a special dilution of hydrocortisone with a total volume of 8 mL and a concentration of 5 mg/mL. Use a stock solution of hydrocortisone with a concentration of 100 mg/2 mL and sterile water to prepare this special dilution.
   a. How many milligrams of hydrocortisone are needed for this special dilution?
   b. How many milliliters of hydrocortisone stock solution will need to be drawn up for this special dilution? On the handout that you obtained from your instructor, indicate the correct volume on the correct measuring device.
   c. How many milliliters of sterile water will need to be drawn up for this special dilution? On the handout that you obtained from your instructor, indicate the correct volume on the correct measuring device.

2. Prepare a special dilution of dopamine with a total volume of 5 mL and a concentration of 5 mcg/mL. Use a stock solution of dopamine with a concentration of 50 mcg/mL and sterile water to prepare this special dilution.
   a. How many micrograms of dopamine are needed for this special dilution?
   b. How many milliliters of dopamine stock solution will need to be drawn up for this special dilution? On the handout that you obtained from your instructor, indicate the correct volume on the correct measuring device.
   c. How many milliliters of sterile water will need to be drawn up for this special dilution? On the handout that you obtained from your instructor, indicate the correct volume on the correct measuring device.

3. Prepare a special dilution of dexamethasone with a total volume of 10 mL and a concentration of 1 mg/mL. Use sterile water and the stock solution below to prepare this special dilution.

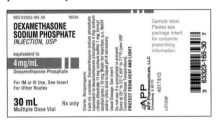

   a. How many milligrams of dexamethasone are needed for this special dilution?
   b. How many milliliters of dexamethasone stock solution will need to be drawn up for this special dilution? On the handout that you obtained from your instructor, indicate the correct volume on the correct measuring device.
   c. How many milliliters of sterile water will need to be drawn up for this special dilution? On the handout that you obtained from your instructor, indicate the correct volume on the correct measuring device.

4. Once the special dilution described in question 3 is prepared, it will have a concentration of 1 mg/mL. What is the total number of milligrams of dexamethasone in the special dilution?

5. The physician has prescribed a dose of dexamethasone 2.5 mg IV q12h. How many milliliters of the special dilution described in question 3 will need to be drawn up for a single dose? On the handout that you obtained from your instructor, indicate the correct volume on the correct measuring device.

6. The following pharmacy recipe provides a formula that yields 50 g of coal tar ointment. You are to prepare a 30 g jar of coal tar ointment. State how much of each ingredient you will need.

Coal tar	2 g
Salicylic acid	0.5 g
Triamcinolone 0.1% ung	7.5 g
Aqua-base ointment	QSAD 50 g

7. The following pharmacy recipe provides a formula that yields 30 vaginal suppositories. You are to prepare 10 vaginal suppositories. State how much of each ingredient you will need.

Progesterone	2.4 g
Polyethylene glycol 3350	30 g
Polyethylene glycol 1000	90 g

8. The following pharmacy recipe provides a formula that yields 100 mL of solution. You are to prepare 250 mL of the solution. State how much of each ingredient you will need.

| Podophyllum resin | 25% |
| Benzoin tincture | QSAD to 100 mL |

9. The following pharmacy recipe provides a formula that yields 500 mL of solution. You are to prepare 200 mL of the solution. State how much of each ingredient you will need.

Iodine	30 g
Sodium iodide	25 g
Purified water	QSAD to 500 mL

10. The following pharmacy recipe provides a formula that yields 30 mL of solution. You are to prepare 120 mL of the solution. State how much of each ingredient you will need.

Antipyrine	1.8 g
Benzocaine	0.5 g
Glycerin	QSAD 30 mL

11. Prepare 400 mL of dextrose 7.5% using D_5W and $D_{10}W$. How many milliliters of each solution will be needed?

12. Prepare 800 mL of dextrose 8% from D_5W and $D_{20}W$. How many milliliters of each solution will be needed?

13. Prepare 1000 mL of dextrose 9% using D_5W and $D_{20}W$. How many milliliters of each solution will be needed?

14. Prepare 200 mL of dextrose 12% using $D_{10}W$ and $D_{20}W$. How many milliliters of each solution will be needed?

15. Prepare 500 mL of dextrose 15% using D_5W and $D_{50}W$. How many milliliters of each solution will be needed?

16. A doctor writes an order for a total of 300 mL of 20% Liposyn. You have in stock 5% Liposyn and 50% Liposyn. How many milliliters of each solution will be needed?

17. Prepare 60 g of a 30% ointment using a 2% ointment and a 50% ointment. How many grams of each ointment will be needed?

18. An order calls for 1000 mL of 60% Travasol. The pharmacy carries 40% Travasol and 70% Travasol. How many milliliters of each solution will be needed?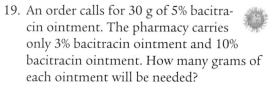

19. An order calls for 30 g of 5% bacitracin ointment. The pharmacy carries only 3% bacitracin ointment and 10% bacitracin ointment. How many grams of each ointment will be needed?

20. Prepare a compound of 30 g triamcinolone in one pound of petrolatum. What is the percentage strength of this compound?

21. Prepare 60 g of zinc oxide 10%. How many grams of zinc are contained in this compound?

22. Prepare a batch of 10 jars of zinc oxide 7.5% with each jar containing 5 g of ointment.
    a. How many grams of zinc oxide 7.5% will be needed for the batch?
    b. How many grams of zinc oxide will be in each jar?
    c. What is the percentage strength of ointment in each jar?

23. Prepare a mixture of 100 g of 8% cream into 200 g of 3% cream. What is the resulting concentration?

24. Prepare 60 g of 8.5% coal tar ointment using 5% coal tar ointment and 10% coal tar ointment. How many grams of each ointment will be needed?

25. Prepare a mixture of 300 mL of 70% alcohol and 200 mL of 95% alcohol. What is the percentage strength of the final solution?

For questions 26–30, determine how many milliliters of each solution are needed. Each question requires three answers: higher-strength dextrose volume, lower-strength dextrose volume, and sterile water volume.

26. Prepare 2 L of $D_{20}W$ using $D_{70}W$ and sterile water.

27. Prepare 1 L of D_9W using $D_{70}W$ and sterile water.

28. Prepare 500 mL of D12% using D50% and sterile water.

29. Prepare 600 mL of D11% using $D_{50}W$ and sterile water.

30. Prepare 350 mL of dextrose 4% using D_5W and sterile water.

31. Prepare a TPN solution with the following components:

Dextrose 16%
Aminosyn 4%
Liposyn 3%
Sterile water QSAD to 1000 mL
Sodium chloride 15 mEq
Potassium chloride 30 mEq
Sodium phosphate 10 mM
MVI 10 mL
Insulin 50 units

Use the following pharmacy stock solutions:

Dextrose 70%
Aminosyn 10%
Liposyn 20%
Sodium chloride 4 mEq/mL
Potassium chloride 2 mEq/mL
Sodium phosphate 3 mM/mL
MVI 10 mL
Insulin 100 units/mL

Determine the volume of each of the following:
a. Dextrose =
b. Aminosyn =
c. Liposyn =
d. Sodium chloride =
e. Potassium chloride =
f. Sodium phosphate =
g. MVI =
h. Insulin =
i. Sterile water =
j. Total volume =

Using Business Math in the Pharmacy

9

Lisa McCartney, BAAS, CPhT, PhTR

Learning Objectives

- Describe overhead and calculate overhead cost.
- Understand the distinction between net profit and gross profit.
- Calculate markup and the markup rate.
- Compute discounts.

- Apply average wholesale price to profit calculations.
- Calculate inventory turnover.
- Determine depreciation.

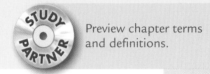 Preview chapter terms and definitions.

9.1 Calculations Related to Business

Like other types of business, pharmacies must perform certain accounting operations on a regular basis. In the hospital or institutional setting, pharmacy personnel closely monitor their inventory of medication and supplies to determine if the facility is staying within its allotted annual budget. In the retail setting, it is important for the pharmacy to make a profit. In general, a **profit** is the financial gain made when the amount earned is greater than the amount spent during a specified period. To make a profit and stay in business, retail pharmacies must effectively manage markup, discounts, and sales, as well as inventory and overhead. **Income** refers to the money or equivalent received from the sale of a medication, supply item, or equipment. To gain a better understanding of these business concepts, refer to the following sections.

Overhead

A pharmacy's **overhead** is its general cost of doing business. This overall cost includes personnel salaries, equipment, and operating expenses such as rent, taxes, and utilities. Overhead also includes the dollar value of the medications and supply items that are maintained in the pharmacy inventory.

In the simplest terms, a pharmacy's **base profit** is determined by subtracting the total overhead amount from the total income.

Example 9.1.1

The River City Apothecary Shop has an annual income of $850,000.00. The pharmacy's annual overhead expenses include:

salary of pharmacist	$120,000.00
salaries of two pharmacy technicians ($31,500 each)	$63,000.00
rent	$14,400.00
utilities	$5,000.00
pharmacy software maintenance	$2,200.00
liability insurance	$3,500.00
business insurance	$4,000.00
pharmacy inventory amount	$550,000.00
total pharmacy overhead amount	$762,100.00

With that in mind, determine the pharmacy's base profit by subtracting the total pharmacy overhead amount from the pharmacy's annual income.

Based on the income and overhead amounts above, determine the pharmacy's base profit.

income	$850,000.00
overhead	− $762,100.00
base profit	$87,900.00

Therefore, the base profit of the River City Apothecary Shop is $87,900.00.

A pharmacy manager often sets goals for the pharmacy's annual profit. To do this, the manager must know the pharmacy's current income, overhead, and base profit amounts. The **current percentage of profit** is determined by dividing the base profit by income and then multiplying that quotient by 100. Once the pharmacy manager knows the current percentage of profit, he or she can determine the desired percentage of profit. The **desired percentage of profit** is the percentage of profit the pharmacy intends to make after the overall cost is subtracted from the selling price. Establishing the desired percentage of profit can, in turn, help the pharmacy manager determine the amount of annual income needed to achieve this goal. These business calculations provide the manager with the necessary information to establish a pharmacy's budget and to set sales goals.

To provide practice in calculating percentage of profit and annual profit, see the examples on the next page. Note that converting the desired percentage of profit to a decimal allows for easier calculation.

Example 9.1.2

Determine the River City Apothecary Shop's current percentage of profit based on the annual income and base profit information calculated in Example 9.1.1.

$$\frac{\text{base profit}}{\text{annual income}} \times 100 = \text{current percentage of profit}$$

$$\frac{\$87,900.00}{\$850,000.00} \times 100 = 10.34, \text{ rounded to } 10\%$$

The River City Apothecary Shop has a current percentage of profit of 10%.

Example 9.1.3

The River City Apothecary Shop has set a goal of a 25% profit. Based on the overhead and income amounts provided in Example 9.1.1, what annual income must the pharmacy have to meet this goal?

$$\text{overhead} \times \text{desired percentage of profit} = \text{desired amount of profit}$$
$$\$762,100.00 \times 0.25 = \$190,525.00$$

$$\text{overhead} + \text{desired amount of profit} = \text{desired income goal}$$
$$\$762,100.00 + \$190,525.00 = \$952,625.00$$

Therefore, to meet the 25% profit goal (the desired percentage of profit), the pharmacy's income must reach $952,625.00.

Net Profit

In pharmacy practice, profit is influenced by the selling prices of drugs. For each drug, the **net profit** is the difference between the selling price and the overall cost. The **overall cost** is the sum of the cost to purchase the drug from the wholesaler or manufacturer (known as the pharmacy's purchase price) and the cost to dispense the drug. The cost to dispense a drug is based on factors such as pharmacy overhead, professional handling, prescription processing and recording, and patient consultation and counseling. The pharmacy will decide on a selling price for a medication or supply item based on the desired percentage of profit. The **selling price** is the amount that the pharmacy charges for a particular drug or product. Selling price is often used to determine the amount due from a customer to the pharmacy for the sale of drugs and other products; this is sometimes referred to as *accounts receivable*. As mentioned earlier, the desired percentage of profit is the percentage of profit the pharmacy intends to make on the product after the overall cost is subtracted from the selling price. To easily calculate the selling price, convert the desired percentage of profit to a decimal. If the pharmacy has correctly set the selling price, the net profit should yield the desired percentage of profit.

$$\text{pharmacy's purchase price} + \text{cost to dispense} = \text{overall cost}$$

$$(\text{overall cost} \times \text{desired percentage of profit}) + \text{overall cost} = \text{selling price}$$

$$\text{selling price} - \text{overall cost} = \text{net profit}$$

Example 9.1.4

The pharmacy purchase price of a pint bottle of Nystatin Oral Suspension is $20.25. After considering the various factors that influence pharmacy costs, it is determined that the pharmacy's cost to dispense this item is $5.10. Determine the overall cost for this item. If the pharmacy has a desired percentage of profit of 20% for this product, what should the selling price be?

$$\text{pharmacy's purchase price} + \text{cost to dispense} = \text{overall cost}$$
$$\$20.25 + \$5.10 = \$25.35$$

$$(\text{overall cost} \times \text{desired percentage of profit}) + \text{overall cost} = \text{selling price}$$
$$(\$25.35 \times 0.2) + \$25.35 = \$30.42$$

$$\text{selling price} - \text{overall cost} = \text{net profit}$$
$$\$30.42 - 25.35 = \$5.07$$

The overall cost for a pint bottle of Nystatin Oral Suspension is $25.35. To yield a net profit of $5.07 or 20%, the selling price of the product must be $30.42.

Example 9.1.5

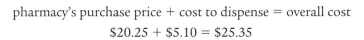

The pharmacy purchased a 100-count bottle of propranolol 10 mg tablets at a price of $3.96. A customer presents a prescription that requires you to dispense a total of 30 tablets. The pharmacy charges a dispensing fee of $4.25 for each prescription it fills. The total charge to the customer for this prescription is $8.59. Calculate the net profit that the pharmacy made on the sale of this prescription.

For Good Measure

In pharmacy practice, the term *count* refers to the number of pills, doses, or units in a single container.

Step 1. Pharmacy cost/count = cost per tablet

$$\$3.96/100 = \$0.0396, \text{ rounded to } \$0.04 \text{ per tablet}$$

Step 2. Determine the pharmacy cost of the customer's prescription.

cost per tablet $\times$ amount dispensed = overall cost of prescription

$$\$0.04 \times 30 = \$1.20$$

Step 3. Calculate the pharmacy's net profit for this prescription.

selling price − overall cost = net profit

$$\$8.59 − \$1.20 = \$7.39$$

The pharmacy made a net profit of $7.39 on the sale of this prescription.

Gross Profit, Net Profit, and Markup Rate

The difference between the selling price and the pharmacy's **purchase price** (the price that it costs for the pharmacy to purchase the drug from the manufacturer or drug wholesaler) is called the **gross profit**. Gross profit is the difference between sales and cost of sales; however, this relationship between purchasing and selling goods does not take into account the cost of preparing and dispensing the drug. Thus, the gross profit will always be more than the net profit. Net profit is what remains after all expenses and taxes have been paid.

Gross profit and net profit are similar to gross pay and net pay. Gross pay is your pay before taxes and other deductions are taken out. Net pay is the amount you "take home." For example, you may earn $400.00 per week (gross pay), but your take-home pay may be $325.00 per week (net pay) after all taxes and deductions are applied.

Using the example of the Nystatin Oral Suspension from Example 9.1.4, the gross profit would be $10.17.

selling price − pharmacy's purchase price = gross profit

$$\$30.42 − \$20.25 = \$10.17$$

The **profit margin** is the difference between the cost of doing business (the pharmacy's purchase price, overhead, and preparation costs) and the selling price of a drug or product. A loss—sometimes called a *negative profit*—occurs when the selling price or receipts for a product are less than the cost of presenting that product for sale.

Like all businesses, pharmacies purchase their products (drugs or supply items) at one price from the manufacturer or **wholesaler**, and then sell them at a higher price. Although pharmacies are subject to governmental laws and regulations regarding the sale of drugs, markup plays a significant role in the pharmacies' pricing systems and, ultimately, their profit margins.

The markup amount is computed as:

selling price − pharmacy's purchase price = markup amount

The **markup rate** is expressed as a percentage and is computed as:

$$\frac{\text{markup amount}}{\text{pharmacy's purchase price}} \times 100 = \text{markup rate}$$

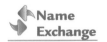

Name Exchange

The generic drug metformin is also known by the brand name Glucophage.

Example 9.1.6

A 30-day supply of the antidiabetic agent metformin has a selling price of $45.00. The pharmacy's purchase price is $30.00. What is the markup amount? What is the markup rate?

$$\text{selling price} - \text{pharmacy's purchase price} = \text{markup amount}$$

$$\$45.00 - \$30.00 = \$15.00$$

$$\frac{\text{markup amount}}{\text{pharmacy's purchase price}} \times 100 = \text{markup rate}$$

$$\frac{\$15.00}{\$30.00} \times 100 = 50\%$$

The markup amount on a 30-day supply of metformin is $15.00. The markup rate is 50%.

Markup rates on brand name drug products are typically lower than markup rates on generic drugs. If a pharmacy marks up a $100.00 brand name drug by 5%, the pharmacy's selling price (the cost to the consumer) would be $105.00. The markup rate for generic medications is typically much higher, but the selling prices of generic drugs are generally less. As a result of these markup practices, the percentage of profit from selling generic drugs is often higher than the percentage of profit for the corresponding brand name products. For example, a pharmacy may mark up a $15.00 generic drug by 33%, which would result in a selling price of $20.00, and a $5.00 profit for the pharmacy. The corresponding brand name drug may have a purchase price of $30.00 and a markup of 5%, which would result in a selling price of $31.50, and a $1.50 profit for the pharmacy.

In general, both the pharmacy and the patient receive financial benefit in using generic medications: The patient purchases the medication at a much lower cost, and the pharmacy receives a larger profit. Although the pharmacy's percentage of profit from selling a generic drug is generally higher than the percentage of profit for the corresponding brand name drug, the actual money made from the sale of an individual drug may not be particularly significant due to a relatively low selling price of the generic drug.

A growing trend in retail pharmacies is to sell generic drugs to customers at a flat dollar rate, such as $4.00 or $7.00, regardless of the cost of the drug, which fluctuates over time. A **flat rate** is a low pharmacy selling price for a certain amount of medication, a supply designed to last a specific number of days—for example, a 30-day or 90-day supply. The types of medications that are available to customers at a flat rate are typically generic medications with low pharmacy purchase prices. Because the medications are inexpensive for the pharmacy to purchase, the pharmacy is still able to make a profit on the drugs while generating additional sales from nonpharmacy sales, over-the-counter (OTC) products, or other prescriptions that the patient may purchase at the same time. Table 9.1 lists examples of medications that are often included in a flat-rate listing.

TABLE 9.1   Flat-Rate Medications

Medication	Indication
amoxicillin	bacterial infections
atenolol	hypertension or heart conditions
estradiol	hormone replacement therapy
fluoxetine	depression
levothyroxine	thyroid disorders
loratadine	allergies
metformin	diabetes
naproxen	pain and inflammation
triamcinolone	skin disorders

The following example applies the formulas for markup amount and markup rate to a flat-rate prescription to illustrate how profitable such rates can be for the pharmacy.

Example 9.1.7

A retail pharmacy has advertised a $4.00 flat-rate price for generic prescriptions. If the pharmacy's purchase price for #30 amoxicillin 250 mg capsules is $1.20, what is the percentage of profit on this prescription when it is sold for the flat-rate price?

The markup amount is

$$\text{selling price} - \text{pharmacy's purchase price} = \text{markup amount}$$
$$\$4.00 - \$1.20 = \$2.80$$

The markup rate is

$$\frac{\text{markup amount}}{\text{pharmacy's purchase price}} \times 100 = \text{markup rate}$$
$$\frac{\$2.80}{\$1.20} \times 100 = 233.3\%$$

The percentage of profit of amoxicillin sold for the flat rate is 233.3%. Note that although the markup rate is high, the gross profit is still relatively low due to the drug's low cost.

Math Morsels

When working with percents, pharmacy technicians should change the discount rate from a percent to a decimal.

Discount

Sometimes, a manufacturer or supplier offers an item at a lower price to a pharmacy. This reduced price is a **discount**. Similarly, a pharmacy may offer consumers a discount, or a reduction from what is normally charged, as an incentive to purchase an item. The **discount rate** is the percent that the price is reduced from the regular selling price. When working with percents, it is helpful to change the discount rate from a percent to a decimal.

$$\text{regular selling price} \times \text{discount rate} = \text{discount amount}$$

$$\text{regular selling price} - \text{discount amount} = \text{discounted selling price}$$

Discounts are one of the easiest business-related math calculations, probably because you use them nearly every time you go shopping or buy something on sale. For example, a sale that offers 50% off means that the sales item(s) may be purchased at one-half of the regular selling price. In such a scenario, the sales price is calculated by multiplying the regular price by 0.5 (50% = 0.5). The sales price may also be calculated by dividing the regular price by two.

Example 9.1.8

A retail pharmacy has announced a 40%-off sale on all headache products during the two weeks leading up to the tax-filing deadline. The following products are on sale:

Tylenol 325 mg tablets; 100 count; selling price $6.99

Excedrin Migraine tablets; 100 count; selling price $7.89

Advil 250 mg tablets; 100 count; selling price $7.29

If a customer purchases one bottle of each item at the sales price, how much will he or she pay for each drug? How much will the customer pay for the entire purchase?

Step 1. Calculate the discount amount on Tylenol.

$$\text{regular selling price} \times \text{discount rate} = \text{discount amount}$$
$$\$6.99 \times 0.4 = \$2.796, \text{rounded to } \$2.80$$

Step 2. Determine the amount the customer saved on Tylenol.

$$\text{regular selling price} - \text{discount amount} = \text{discounted selling price}$$
$$\$6.99 - \$2.80 = \$4.19$$

Step 3. Calculate the discount amount on Excedrin Migraine.

$$\text{regular selling price} \times \text{discount rate} = \text{discount amount}$$
$$\$7.89 \times 0.4 = \$3.156, \text{rounded to } \$3.16$$

Step 4. Determine the amount the customer saved on Excedrin Migraine.

$$\text{regular selling price} - \text{discount amount} = \text{discounted selling price}$$
$$\$7.89 - \$3.16 = \$4.73$$

Step 5. Calculate the Advil sale price.

$$\text{regular selling price} \times \text{discount rate} = \text{discount amount}$$
$$\$7.29 \times 0.4 = \$2.916, \text{ rounded to } \$2.92$$

Step 6. Determine the amount the customer saved on Advil.

$$\text{regular selling price} - \text{discount amount} = \text{discounted selling price}$$
$$\$7.29 - \$2.92 = \$4.37$$

Step 7. Calculate the amount the customer will pay for the entire purchase by adding the discounted selling price of each item.

$$\$4.19 + \$4.73 + \$4.37 = \$13.29$$

Consequently, the customer will pay $4.19 for Tylenol, $4.73 for Excedrin Migraine, and $4.37 for Advil. For the entire purchase, the customer will pay $13.29.

Example 9.1.9

Assume the pharmacy purchases five cases of hydrocortisone cream at $100.00 per case. If the account is paid in full within 30 days, the wholesaler will give a 15% discount on the purchase. How much money will the pharmacy save if it pays the account in full within 30 days?

Step 1. Calculate the regular selling price.

$$\text{quantity of product} \times \text{purchase price per unit} = \text{regular selling price}$$
$$5 \text{ cases} \times \$100.00 \text{ per case} = \$500.00$$

Step 2. Determine the discount amount.

$$\text{regular selling price} \times \text{discount rate} = \text{discount amount}$$
$$\$500.00 \times 0.15 = \$75.00$$

Step 3. Calculate the discounted sales price.

$$\text{regular selling price} - \text{discount amount} = \text{discounted selling price}$$
$$\$500.00 - \$75.00 = \$425.00$$

If the pharmacy pays the account in full within 30 days, it will pay $425.00, thus saving $75.00 off of the regular wholesaler price.

9.1 Problem Set

Birch Lake Pharmacy has the following overhead expenses. Use this information to answer questions 1 through 3.

pharmacist salary	$135,000.00
technician salary	52,000.00
rent	23,000.00
utilities	6,000.00
computer maintenance	4,000.00
software subscriptions	2,000.00
liability insurance	4,000.00
business insurance	4,000.00
drug purchases	750,000.00

1. If an 18% profit is desirable, what must the pharmacy's income be to meet this goal?

2. If the pharmacy's income is $1,401,489.00, what is its percentage of profit?

3. If the pharmacy's income is $1,191,692.00, what is its percentage of profit?

Summit Avenue Pharmacy has the following overhead expenses. Use this information to answer questions 4 through 6.

pharmacist salary	$72,000.00
technician salary	52,000.00
rent	13,000.00
utilities	5,500.00
computer maintenance	2,000.00
software subscriptions	1,500.00
liability insurance	4,000.00
business insurance	3,500.00
drug purchases	50,000.00

4. If a 20% profit is desirable, what must the pharmacy's income be to meet this goal?

5. If the pharmacy's income is $991,982.00, what is its percentage of profit?

6. If the pharmacy's income is $1,248,301, what is its percentage of profit?

7. The pharmacy determines that its income for the week was $54,617.53 and that the net profit was $3700.83. What was the overhead for the week?

8. Martelli's Pharmacy has a weekly overhead of $13,033.06. If this pharmacy is to make a 22% profit, what must its sales of goods and services amount to each week?

For items 9–15, calculate the dollar amount of net profit and the markup rate for the following prescription drug items (round to whole percents). The pharmacy charges a $4.25 dispensing fee for each prescription.

9. Medication: propranolol 10 mg
   Pharmacy's purchase price: $3.96
   Count: 100 tablets
   Amount dispensed: 50 tablets
   Pharmacy's selling price: $8.59

10. Medication: amoxicillin 250 mg
    Pharmacy's purchase price: $8.50
    Count: 500 capsules
    Amount dispensed: 30 capsules
    Pharmacy's selling price: $14.80

11. Medication: paroxetine 20 mg
    Pharmacy's purchase price: $118.50
    Count: 100 tablets
    Amount dispensed: 30 tablets
    Pharmacy's selling price: $45.50

12. Medication: furosemide 40 mg
    Pharmacy's purchase price: $83.50
    Count: 500 tablets
    Amount dispensed: 100 tablets
    Pharmacy's selling price: $23.16

13. Medication: levothyroxine 0.1 mg
    Pharmacy's purchase price: $41.20
    Count: 100 tablets
    Amount dispensed: 90 tablets
    Pharmacy's selling price: $41.70

14. Medication: promethazine cough syrup
    Pharmacy's purchase price: $37.50
    Count: one 16 oz bottle (480 mL)
    Amount dispensed: 8 oz
    Pharmacy's selling price: $25.34

15. Medication: Loestrin oral contraceptive
    28-day pack
    Pharmacy's purchase price: $62.30
    Count: six 28-day packs
    Amount dispensed: one 28-day pack
    Pharmacy's selling price: $17.90

The pharmacy is selling the items listed in questions 16–23 at a discount this week. Calculate the discounted selling price for each.

16. cough syrup: regular selling price, $5.89; discounted 20%

17. facial tissues: regular selling price, $1.19; discounted 15%

18. hair color kit: regular selling price, $7.29; discounted 30%

19. body lotion: regular selling price, $5.69; discounted 15%

20. baby shampoo: regular selling price, $3.89; discounted 25%

21. antacid liquid: regular selling price, $4.26; discounted 30%

22. acetaminophen tablets: regular selling price, $8.70; discounted 50%

23. toothpaste: regular selling price, $2.99; discounted 40%

For questions 24–29, perform the necessary calculations and state the answer in dollars or percentages as indicated.

24. Antiviral ointment costs a pharmacy $12.50 per tube. The standard markup is 30%. What is the total selling price of a box of 12 tubes?

25. Eyedrops with antihistamine are purchased from the manufacturer in cases of 36 drop-dispenser bottles. The pharmacy desires a markup of $1.75 per bottle. The pharmacy's purchase price is $111.60 per case. What is the selling price per bottle?

26. Identify the markup and the selling price of an oral antibiotic suspension that costs the pharmacist $15.60 per bottle if the markup rate is 25%.

27. An asthma tablet costs the pharmacy $24.80 for a month's supply, and the selling price is $30.75. Calculate the markup rate.

28. Calculate the gross profit from a medication that costs the pharmacy $520.00 for 1000 tablets and sells for $650.00.

29. The cost of dispensing the medication in question 28 is $2.05 per 100 tablets. Calculate the net profit for selling one tablet.

The pharmacy where you work has received a shipment of medications and supplies from its wholesaler. Calculate the pharmacy's markup amount and selling price for each item listed in questions 30–36.

	Drug		Count/ Quantity	Pharmacy's Purchase Price	Markup Rate	Pharmacy's Markup Amount	Pharmacy's Selling Price
30.	Augmentin oral solution		1200 mL	$120.50	25%		
31.	triamcinolone foot powder		12 containers	$24.00	15%		
32.	ibuprofen		2000 tablets	$200.00	27%		
33.	Band-Aids		10 boxes	$27.50	21%		
34.	Neosporin antibiotic ointment		18 tubes	$67.50	18%		
35.	birth control 28-day packs		24 packs	$840.00	32%		
36.	DiaBeta		600 tablets	$550.00	30%		

37. Calculate the total amount that the pharmacy spent on the shipment above. Then determine the total amount the pharmacy made upon selling all of the items. Finally, calculate the overall markup rate for the entire shipment.

Self-check your work in Appendix A.

9.2 Insurance Reimbursements for Prescriptions

Reimbursement for prescription and pharmacy services is largely controlled by contracts with insurance companies and is often brokered through a large prescription processing service called a **pharmacy benefits manager (PBM)**. PBMs use a pharmacy benefits management system that determines the amount of money that will be paid to pharmacies in insurance reimbursement for prescriptions.

Prescription reimbursement may be calculated based on the pharmacy's purchase price, or the average wholesale price of a medication. Prescription reimbursement may also be established by a set contract for an approved list of preferred drugs. The amount of money paid by the PBM for a particular prescription is calculated and approved by the PBM's computer system, or by the pharmacy's computer system via an Internet connection with the PBM. Rarely is this cost calculated by personnel in the pharmacy. Nevertheless, it is helpful to understand the reimbursement process and the methods used to calculate the reimbursement amount for medications. Patients are likely to ask questions about charges and reimbursements, so having a basic understanding of this process, which is sometimes referred to as *reconciliation*, is essential.

Some claims will be reconciled by an individual pharmacy, but most will pass electronically through a PBM or similar type of clearinghouse that is responsible for processing and settling insurance claims. These businesses bill the insurance companies under contract and then reimburse the pharmacy periodically for a batch of prescriptions. Batch reimbursements may be made daily, weekly, or monthly. Some large chain pharmacies may receive a single reimbursement payment that covers a large number of stores. In these instances, the individual store does not receive a check from the PBM, but rather an invoice or a memo indicating the amount of money that the company is being reimbursed.

One of the most challenging aspects of working in the retail pharmacy setting can occur when prescription drug charges are rejected or denied. In such instances, the customer must pay out-of-pocket for the prescriptions. Because of the cost of the prescriptions, some customers may be unable to pay for the medications and, therefore, become upset with pharmacy personnel. Occasionally, a prescription drug claim is rejected outright; however, some rejections or denials will come back to the pharmacy when the batch reimbursement is processed. It is not uncommon to receive an initial online approval for a prescription and then later to receive a rejection or denial of the charge once the batch is processed.

When considering profit on an individual prescription, the overall cost of the medication is compared with the amount the pharmacy receives for the dispensed drug. In this situation, the term *profit* refers only to the pharmacy's purchase price of the drug and does not include the cost of materials, labor, or overhead. The amount that is charged over and above the pharmacy's purchase price for a medication is referred to as the **dispensing fee**. The dispensing fee is meant to cover all costs related to filling a prescription, beyond the purchase price of the drug. This includes any actual profit that is gained.

Average Wholesale Price

A pharmacy may potentially receive payment from several different sources. Historically, patients have been responsible for paying for their own medications. However, beginning in the mid-1970s, health maintenance organizations (HMOs) and health insurers began to assume a portion of the responsibility for healthcare costs, including patient medications. More recently, HMOs and health insurers have become major players in determining the cost of health care, including the cost of prescriptions. The very survival of a pharmacy depends on its ability to contain costs.

The **average wholesale price (AWP)** of a drug refers to an average price at which drugs are purchased at the wholesale level, or the average value at which wholesalers sell a particular drug to pharmacies. Usually, third parties, such as PBMs, reimburse a pharmacy based upon a percentage of the AWP. Therefore, the pharmacy has an incentive to purchase a drug below its AWP whenever possible. Wholesalers may sell drugs below AWP in some situations, such as when volume discounts, contract prices, or rebates from drug manufacturers are available.

Each third-party reimbursement system (insurance company or PBM) has a predetermined prescription reimbursement amount for each drug. The formula that determines the amount of prescription reimbursement varies depending on the current AWP for that drug, the percentage or markup (which may be either positive or negative depending on the agreement with the third party), and the individual pharmacy's dispensing fee. In practice, you will often hear terms such as "AWP plus _____ %" or "AWP less _____ %." Note that when the term *AWP less* is used, it has the same meaning as *AWP minus* _____%.

$$\text{prescription reimbursement} = \text{AWP} \pm \text{percentage} + \text{dispensing fee}$$

The amount that an insurance company or patient is charged for a prescription is generally predetermined by PBMs and is done automatically through the pharmacy's computer system. Pricing information is preloaded into the PBM's computer system based on the insurance company contracts with the pharmacy. Pharmacy personnel access that pricing information via direct Internet connection between the pharmacy computer and the PBM or insurance company. The following examples illustrate one of the methods used to calculate the amount billed, which is similar to the calculation for prescription reimbursement shown above.

Example 9.2.1

A pharmacy has three drugs with the following AWPs:

Drug A, AWP $120.00

Drug B, AWP $80.00

Drug C, AWP $25.00

The pharmacy has a markup of 5% and a dispensing fee of $4.00 for each of these drugs. If a patient presents a prescription for each of these drugs, what will be the total billed?

Begin by calculating the amount billed to the patient for each of the individual drugs.

Drug A

$$\text{AWP} + \text{percentage} + \text{dispensing fee} = \text{amount billed}$$
$$\$120.00 + (\$120.00 \times 0.05) + \$4.00 =$$
$$\$120.00 + \$6.00 + \$4.00 = \$130.00$$

Drug B

$$\text{AWP} + \text{percentage} + \text{dispensing fee} = \text{amount billed}$$
$$\$80.00 + (\$80.00 \times 0.05) + \$4.00 =$$
$$\$80.00 + \$4.00 + \$4.00 = \$88.00$$

Drug C

$$\text{AWP} + \text{percentage} + \text{dispensing fee} = \text{amount billed}$$
$$\$25.00 + (\$25.00 \times 0.05) + \$4.00 =$$
$$\$25.00 + \$1.25 + \$4.00 = \$30.25$$

Next, determine the total amount billed by adding the amounts billed for the three drugs.

$$\$130.00 + \$88.00 + \$30.25 = \$248.25$$

The total billed is $248.25.

Example 9.2.2

A certain tablet comes in a quantity of 60 and has an AWP of $100.00. The pharmacy has an agreement with the supplier to purchase the drug at the AWP minus 15%. The insurer is willing to pay AWP plus 5% plus a $2.00 dispensing fee. A patient on this insurer's plan purchases 30 tablets for $54.50. How much profit does the pharmacy make on this prescription?

Begin by calculating the amount of the discount.

$$\$100.00 \times 0.15 = \$15.00$$

Then calculate the pharmacy's purchase price of the drug.

$$\$100.00 - \$15.00 = \$85.00$$

Therefore, the pharmacy can purchase this drug at $85.00 per 60 tablets. The insurance company will pay the pharmacy AWP + 5%.

$$\$100.00 + (\$100.00 \times 0.05) =$$
$$\$100.00 + \$5.00 = \$105.00$$

At that price, the amount the insurance company will pay to fill a prescription for 30 pills is

$$(\$105.00 \div 2) + \$2.00 \text{ (dispensing fee)} =$$
$$\$52.50 + \$2.00 = \$54.50$$

Compare this amount with the pharmacy's cost of 30 tablets.

$$\$85.00 \div 2 = \$42.50$$

Therefore, the pharmacy's profit on 30 tablets is

$$\$54.50 - \$42.50 = \$12.00$$

The pharmacy will make a profit of $12.00 on 30 tablets.

Example 9.2.3

Two hundred capsules are purchased at AWP minus 20%, where AWP is $125. The insurer allows a charge of AWP plus 3% per 200 capsules. What is the highest charge per capsule allowed by the insurer? What will be the profit per capsule?

The pharmacy's discounted purchase price of 200 capsules is

$$\$125.00 - (\$125.00 \times 0.20) =$$
$$\$125.00 - \$25.00 = \$100.00$$

Thus, the cost per capsule to the pharmacy is

$$\$100.00 \div 200 = \$0.50/\text{capsule}$$

The insurance company will pay the pharmacy AWP plus 3% per 200 capsules.

$$\$125.00 + (\$125.00 \times 0.03) =$$
$$\$125.00 + \$3.75 = \$128.75$$

Therefore, the pharmacy would be wise to charge patients

$$\$128.75 \div 200 \text{ capsules} = \$0.64/\text{capsule}$$

thereby making a profit of

$$\text{selling price} - \text{pharmacy's purchase price} = \text{profit}$$
$$\$0.64/\text{capsule} - \$0.50/\text{capsule} = \$0.14/\text{capsule}$$

The pharmacy can charge $0.64/capsule and, therefore, earn a profit of $0.14/capsule.

Capitation Fee

Some insurers use a prescription reimbursement plan in which the pharmacy is paid a monthly fee, called a **capitation fee**, for some patients. The insurer pays the pharmacy the monthly fee whether or not the patients on the plan receive prescriptions during that month. Under this type of plan, the pharmacy must dispense the patients' prescriptions, even if the pharmacy's purchase price of the medications and the dispensing fees are more than the monthly reimbursement amount. Under plans that use capitation fees, pharmacies are not allowed to charge a dispensing fee unless the contract between the pharmacy and the third-party payer specifically states that a dispensing fee is allowed.

> ### Example 9.2.4
>
> **O'Rourke's Drug Store receives a monthly capitation fee of $250.00 for Paul Arcand. During April, Paul fills three prescriptions totaling $198.75. How much profit does the capitation fee provide?**
>
> In this case, the monthly fee exceeds the sum of the pharmacy's purchase price, yielding a profit for the pharmacy.
>
> $$\$250.00 - \$198.75 = \$51.25$$
>
> The capitation fee provides O'Rourke's Drug Store with a profit of $51.25.

Example 9.2.5

Cindy Carver has the same insurance plan as Paul Arcand, with the same capitation fee. During April, Cindy fills four prescriptions at the Willow Creek Pharmacy for a total of $301.25. What is the profit margin?

In this case, the pharmacy wasn't so fortunate: The pharmacy's purchase price of the prescriptions exceeds the monthly fee, which costs the pharmacy money (expressed as a negative number).

$$\$250.00 - \$301.25 = -\$51.25$$

The Willow Creek Pharmacy had a negative profit.

Example 9.2.6

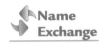

The cardiovascular drug amlodipine is known among pharmacy personnel by the trade name Norvasc.

The pharmacy purchased a 100-count bottle of amlodipine 10 mg tablets at the AWP of $118.00. A patient presents a prescription that requires you to dispense 30 tablets. The patient's insurance plan does not allow the pharmacy to charge a dispensing fee. If the plan calls for the pharmacy to be reimbursed at AWP less 10%, what is the pharmacy's reimbursement on this prescription?

Step 1. Calculate the pharmacy's cost of the prescription.

$$\begin{pmatrix} \text{pharmacy's purchase} \\ \text{price/count} \end{pmatrix} \times \begin{matrix} \text{amount} \\ \text{dispensed} \end{matrix} = \begin{matrix} \text{pharmacy's cost of} \\ \text{prescription} \end{matrix}$$

$$(\$118.00/100) \times 30 = \$35.40$$

Step 2. Determine the amount based on %.

$$\text{pharmacy's cost of prescription} \times \% = \text{amount based on percent}$$
$$\$35.40 \times 0.10 = \$3.54$$

Step 3. Calculate the pharmacy's reimbursement on this prescription. *Note:* If the instructions say "AWP less" (or "AWP minus"), you must *subtract* the amount based on percent from the pharmacy's cost of the prescription.

$$\begin{matrix} \text{pharmacy's cost of} \\ \text{prescription} \end{matrix} - \begin{matrix} \text{amount based} \\ \text{on percent} \end{matrix} = \begin{matrix} \text{pharmacy's reimbursement} \\ \text{amount} \end{matrix}$$

$$\$35.40 - \$3.54 = \$31.86$$

The pharmacy's reimbursement on this prescription is $31.86.

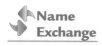
Example 9.2.7

The pharmacy purchased a 250-count bottle of esomeprazole 40 mg capsules at AWP. The insurance plan reimburses at AWP + 4% and allows a $5.00 dispensing fee on this prescription. If the AWP is $82.00 and the patient receives a prescription for 90 capsules, what is the amount that the pharmacy will submit for reimbursement? What is the pharmacy's profit?

Step 1. Calculate the pharmacy's cost of the prescription.

$$\begin{array}{ccc} \text{(pharmacy's purchase} & \times & \text{amount} \\ \text{price/count)} & & \text{dispensed} \end{array} = \begin{array}{c} \text{pharmacy's cost of} \\ \text{prescription} \end{array}$$

$$(\$82.00/250) \times 90 = \$29.52$$

Step 2. Determine the reimbursement amount based on %.

$$\text{pharmacy's cost of prescription} \times \% = \text{amount based on percent}$$
$$\$29.52 \times 0.04 = \$1.18$$

Step 3. Calculate the pharmacy's reimbursement on this prescription. *Note:* If the instructions say "AWP plus," you must *add* the amount based on percent to the pharmacy's cost of the prescription.

$$\begin{array}{c} \text{pharmacy's cost of} \\ \text{prescription} \end{array} + \begin{array}{c} \text{amount based} \\ \text{on percent} \end{array} + \begin{array}{c} \text{dispensing} \\ \text{fee} \end{array} = \begin{array}{c} \text{pharmacy's} \\ \text{reimbursement} \\ \text{amount} \end{array}$$

$$\$29.52 + \$1.18 + \$5.00 = \$35.70$$

Step 4. Determine the pharmacy's profit.

$$\text{amount of reimbursement} - \text{pharmacy's cost of prescription} = \text{profit}$$
$$\$35.70 - \$29.52 = \$6.18$$

The pharmacy will submit $35.70 for reimbursement and will earn a $6.18 profit on this prescription.

9.2 Problem Set

For problems 1–3, calculate the amount that the pharmacy will submit for reimbursement on each prescription based on AWP less 13%. The pharmacy is not permitted to charge a dispensing fee on these prescriptions.

1. AWP $48.90 per 60 tablets and dispense 20 tablets

2. AWP $84.07 per 100 tablets and dispense 30 tablets

3. AWP $30.25 per 1000 tablets and dispense 100 tablets

For problems 4–6, calculate the amount that the pharmacy will submit for reimbursement on each prescription based on AWP plus 4%. The pharmacy charges a $6.25 dispensing fee for each prescription.

4. AWP $120.68 per 500 tablets and dispense 30 tablets

5. AWP $39.78 per 100 capsules and dispense 60 capsules

6. AWP $317.50 per 30 tablets and dispense 20 tablets

7. The pharmacy purchased 100 tablets at $71.35. The insurer will pay AWP plus 3.5% and a $4.50 dispensing fee.

   a. If the pharmacy dispenses a prescription of 50 tablets, what is the pharmacy's cost of the prescription?

   b. What is the total amount that the pharmacy will submit to the insurance company for reimbursement on this prescription?

   c. How much profit will the pharmacy make on this prescription?

8. The pharmacy purchased five metered-dose inhalers (MDIs) at a cost of AWP less 3%. The third-party payer will reimburse at AWP plus 5% and does not allow a dispensing fee. The AWP is $36.35 per inhaler.

   a. If the pharmacy dispenses a single prescription of two MDIs, what is the pharmacy's cost of the prescription?

   b. What is the amount that the pharmacy will submit to the third-party payer for reimbursement on this prescription?

   c. How much profit will the pharmacy make on this prescription?

9. The pharmacy purchased a 30-count bottle of tadalafil (Cialis) tablets for AWP of $302.35. The PBM will pay AWP less 3% and allows a $7.00 dispensing fee per prescription.

   a. If the pharmacy dispenses a prescription for 10 tablets, what is the pharmacy's cost of the prescription?

   b. What is the amount that the pharmacy will submit to the PBM for reimbursement on this prescription?

   c. How much profit will the pharmacy make on this prescription?

10. The pharmacy purchased 50 tablets of atorvastatin (Lipitor) for $117.35. The insurance company will reimburse at AWP plus 3% and a $4.00 dispensing fee.

    a. If the pharmacy dispenses 30 tablets, what is the pharmacy's cost of the prescription?

    b. What is the amount that the pharmacy will submit to the insurance company for this prescription?

    c. How much profit will the pharmacy make on this prescription?

11. The pharmacy purchased an 80 g bulk jar of triamcinolone (Kenalog) cream at a cost of $85.35. The PBM will reimburse at AWP plus 4.5% but does not allow a dispensing fee.

    a. If the pharmacy dispenses a prescription for 15 g of the cream, what is the pharmacy's cost of the prescription?

    b. What is the amount that the pharmacy will submit to the insurance company for this prescription?

    c. How much profit will the pharmacy make on this prescription?

12. Mountain HMO pays a per patient capitation fee of $310.00 per month. Six patients on this plan have prescriptions filled in July. The pharmacy's drug costs for the prescriptions are as follows:

Patient #1: $15.75, $106.50, $27.80
Patient #2: $210.00
Patient #3: $47.50, $105.25, $160.00, $52.00
Patient #4: $150.00, $210.00, $76.00
Patient #5: $10.50, $28.00, $62.50
Patient #6: $210.00, $210.00, $17.00

a. What is the total amount that the HMO reimbursed the pharmacy for capitation fees?

b. What is the pharmacy's drug cost for all of the prescriptions on this plan?

c. Did the pharmacy make a profit or lose money?

d. If the pharmacy made a profit, what was the amount? If the pharmacy took a loss, what was the amount?

13. Valley HMO pays AWP plus 3% and a $2.00 dispensing fee for each prescription dispensed. Six patients on this plan have prescriptions filled in July. The pharmacy paid AWP drug costs for the prescriptions as follows:

Patient #1: $15.75, $106.50, $27.80
Patient #2: $210.00
Patient #3: $47.50, $105.25, $160.00, $52.00
Patient #4: $150.00, $210.00, $76.00
Patient #5: $10.50, $28.00, $62.50
Patient #6: $210.00, $210.00, $17.00

a. What is the pharmacy's drug cost for all of the prescriptions on this plan?

b. What is the amount that the pharmacy will submit for insurance reimbursement on this plan?

c. Did the pharmacy make a profit or lose money?

d. If the pharmacy made a profit, what was the amount? If the pharmacy took a loss, what was the amount?

e. Compare your answers for question 13 with your answers for question 12. Did the pharmacy make more money under the Mountain HMO's capitation plan, or under the Valley HMO's plan?

f. How much more or less?

14. Jackson HMO pays a per patient capitation fee of $275.00 per month to Healthy Pharmacy. Healthy Pharmacy contracts with Jackson HMO to serve 10 of Jackson's clients. Five of the Jackson HMO clients get prescriptions filled during the month of June; the other five patients do not get any prescriptions filled in June. The pharmacy's drug costs for these prescriptions are as follows:

Patient #1: $89.63
Patient #2: $126.54 (total cost for two prescriptions)
Patient #3: $420.45 (total cost for five prescriptions)
Patient #4: $117.50
Patient #5: $46.75

a. What is the total amount that the HMO reimbursed the pharmacy for capitation fees?

b. What is the pharmacy's drug cost for all of the prescriptions on this plan?

c. Did the pharmacy make a profit or lose money?

d. If the pharmacy made a profit, what was the amount? If the pharmacy took a loss, what was the amount?

15. Baker HMO pays a per patient capitation fee of $275.00 per month to Healthy Pharmacy. Healthy Pharmacy contracts with Baker HMO to serve 12 of Baker's clients. Five of the Baker HMO clients get prescriptions filled during the month of May; the other seven clients did not get any prescriptions filled in May. The pharmacy's drug costs for these prescriptions are as follows:

Patient #1: $78.26, $75.23, $25.48

Patient #2: $128.46, $21.86

Patient #3: $61.89, $41.20

Patient #4: $16.59, $5.80, $3.87, $21.67

Patient #5: $58.24

a. What is the total amount that the HMO reimbursed the pharmacy for capitation fees?

b. What is the pharmacy's drug cost for all of the prescriptions on this plan?

c. Did the pharmacy make a profit or lose money?

d. If the pharmacy made a profit, what was the amount? If the pharmacy took a loss, what was the amount?

16. Blue Care HMO pays a per patient capitation fee of $225.00 per month to Key Pharmacy. Key Pharmacy contracts with Blue Care HMO to serve 40 of Blue Care's clients. Twelve of the Blue Care HMO clients get prescriptions filled during the month of August; the other 28 clients did not get any prescriptions filled in August. The pharmacy drug costs for all of the Blue Care prescriptions filled in August are $1867.50. The contract with Blue Care HMO allows the pharmacy to bill for a single charge of $60.00 for dispensing fees for the month.

a. Taking into consideration the allowable dispensing fees, what is the total amount that the HMO reimbursed the pharmacy for the month of August?

b. Did the pharmacy make a profit or lose money?

c. If the pharmacy made a profit, what was the amount? If the pharmacy took a loss, what was the amount?

17. Wellness Insurance Company pays a per patient capitation fee of $210.00 per month to Apple Pharmacy. Apple Pharmacy contracts with Wellness to serve 42 of the Wellness Insurance Company's clients. During the month of September, 39 of the Wellness Insurance Company's clients had 54 prescriptions filled. Apple Pharmacy's drug costs for all of the Wellness Insurance Company prescriptions filled in September are $9634.73. The contract with Wellness Insurance Company allows the pharmacy to bill $4.25 in dispensing fees for each filled prescription.

a. Taking into consideration the allowable dispensing fees, what is the total amount that the insurance company reimbursed the pharmacy for the month of September?

b. Did the pharmacy make a profit or lose money?

c. If the pharmacy made a profit, what was the amount? If the pharmacy took a loss, what was the amount?

Self-check your work in Appendix A.

9.3 Pharmacy Inventory

An **inventory** is a listing of all of the items that are available for sale in a business. **Inventory value** is defined as the total value of all of the drugs and merchandise in stock on a given day. Pharmacies must maintain a record of all of the drugs, supplies, and merchandise purchased and sold to know when to reorder from the wholesaler to restock, or resupply, their shelves. Pharmacies continually adjust their inventory levels based on how quickly items are being sold.

Space must be properly allocated to maintain adequate inventory. Other considerations include shelving design and available refrigeration space. Keeping medications on the shelf is a cost to a pharmacy, and a large inventory can hinder cash flow. To minimize the shelf space needed and control inventory costs, pharmacy personnel should try to manage their pharmacy's inventory so that medications are readily available when needed, but do not sit on the shelves for an extended period. Pharmacy personnel generally try to manage their inventory so that medications arrive from the wholesaler shortly before they are dispensed and sold. However, there are instances when a pharmacy may need to stock some slow-moving drugs as a service to a small number of customers that require those medications.

Managing Inventory

In the past, pharmacy personnel kept track of inventory by maintaining handwritten records of all pharmacy purchases and sales. Today, this labor- and time-intensive inventory system has been replaced by inventory records that are computerized. Each time drugs or other merchandise is purchased from the wholesaler and received in the pharmacy, the quantity and price are entered into the pharmacy's computer database. As customers make purchases from the pharmacy, the computer system automatically adjusts the inventory record for the item purchased.

A pharmacy usually establishes an inventory range for each item, sometimes called a **par level**. The par level indicates the minimum and maximum number of units—packages, bottles, boxes, or containers—to have in pharmacy stock for each inventory item. When the inventory item drops to the predetermined minimum par level (sometimes called the *reorder point*), the item is purchased from the wholesaler to restock the pharmacy's supply. The reorder points and reorder quantity for each inventory item are predetermined based on the historical use of the item and the time it takes to get the reorder shipment from the pharmacy's wholesaler.

In general, reorder quantities are set to replenish the inventory item back up to at least the minimum par level. However, it may be more economical to order enough of the drug to bring the par level to the maximum level if ordering a larger package size saves the pharmacy money. In addition, there are circumstances that dictate a reorder quantity that exceeds the maximum par level. For example, during cold and flu season, an unusually high number of customers receives prescriptions for the same medications. Consequently, a pharmacy will typically keep a larger supply of anti-infective, antiviral, and OTC cold remedies in stock than it would at other times of the year.

Drug manufacturers typically supply medications in containers that hold various quantities, known as package sizes, or counts. For example, the anti-infective drug ampicillin, 250 mg capsules, is available in the following quantities: 50, 100, 250, 500, and 1000 count containers. The package size a pharmacy orders when replenishing inventory depends on how much of the drug the facility is using, how quickly the drug is being used, the package size that is typically ordered, and the price. Often, it is more economical to order a larger package size because both the drug manufacturer and the wholesaler usually offer lower prices on bulk package sizes.

These inventory reorder decisions are typically made by pharmacy personnel who have extensive experience in this area. However, pharmacy technicians should have a basic understanding of the calculations involved in inventory management. The following examples will illustrate some of the scenarios encountered in inventory management, and their possible solutions.

Name Exchange

Zantac is a brand name for the generic drug ranitidine, which is used to reduce the amount of acid that the stomach produces.

Example 9.3.1

The inventory of Zantac 150 mg is to be maintained at a minimum of 240 tablets and a maximum of 300 tablets. If 15 tablets are left on the shelf at the end of the day, how many bottles will be ordered to meet the inventory minimum? Zantac 150 mg is commercially available in a bottle containing 60 tablets.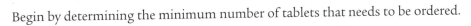

Begin by determining the difference between the current inventory and the minimum inventory.

$$240 \text{ tablets} - 15 \text{ tablets} = 225 \text{ tablets}$$

Therefore, it will take at least 225 tablets to bring the inventory up to the minimum level for Zantac 150 mg. But the tablets must be ordered in bottles of 60.

$$225 \text{ tablets} \div 60 \text{ tablets/bottle} = 3.75 \text{ bottles, rounded up to 4 bottles}$$

Therefore, four bottles of Zantac must be ordered.

Name Exchange
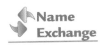

The generic drug propranolol, a beta blocker, is commonly known among pharmacy personnel as the brand name Inderal.

Example 9.3.2

The inventory of propranolol 10 mg is to be maintained at a minimum of 300 tablets and a maximum of 1500 tablets. If 212 tablets are left on the shelf at the end of the day, how many bottles will you order to meet the inventory minimum? Propranolol is available in bottles containing 100 tablets, 500 tablets, and 1000 tablets. You typically order the largest-size bottle.

Begin by determining the minimum number of tablets that needs to be ordered.

$$300 \text{ tablets} - 212 \text{ tablets} = 88 \text{ tablets}$$

Although either of the smaller-sized bottles will work, it is common business practice to order the same package size. Therefore, even though it significantly surpasses the minimum, you will order one 1000 count bottle of propranolol. The resulting inventory will still be within the acceptable range and will not exceed 1500 tablets.

Example 9.3.3

You would like to replenish the lip balm that is kept on the pharmacy counter by the cash register, and you need 18 tubes to fill the container. When you look in the wholesale catalog, it states that the lip balm is $10.20/dozen. How much should you order?

You will order 2 dozen—or 24 tubes of lip balm.

As part of maintaining inventory, it is also important to economize when purchasing stock medications. A pharmacy can often save money by buying in bulk, and it is usually more economical to buy a larger rather than a smaller amount of a drug since the per-tablet price is usually lower when the package size or quantity is larger. When purchasing drugs from the wholesaler, pharmacy personnel must balance the optimal inventory level with the replenishment costs of available bulk containers (such as bottles containing 100, 500, or 1000 tablets). Because the largest containers typically have a lower cost per tablet (or other unit), it is usually cost-effective for a pharmacy to purchase these container sizes. However, this rationale may not be the case if the inventory item is used infrequently. If the item is used infrequently, a large bulk container may reach its expiration date before it is used. Since expired medications may not be dispensed, they must be destroyed, and the pharmacy loses the cost of that inventory. The following examples illustrate calculations commonly performed when comparing bulk pricing and cost per unit.

Example 9.3.4

An antibiotic is available in the following stock bottle sizes for the prices indicated.

100 capsules/bottle, $2.80

500 capsules/bottle, $12.10

1000 capsules/bottle, $25.30

Which container provides the best price per capsule, and what is the price per capsule?

Divide each amount by the number of capsules in the bulk container to determine a per capsule cost.

$2.80/bottle ÷ 100 capsules/bottle = $0.028/capsule
$12.10/bottle ÷ 500 capsules/bottle = $0.0242/capsule
$25.30/bottle ÷ 1000 capsules/bottle = $0.0253/capsule

The 500 count bottle is the best value purchase for this medication at 2.4 cents per capsule.

Example 9.3.5

In your pharmacy, the maximum par level for ampicillin 250 mg capsules is 1000; the minimum par level is 100. At the end of the day, the pharmacy computer prints a list of items that have fallen below the minimum par level and, therefore, need to be reordered. The printout shows that there are currently 75 ampicillin 250 mg capsules in the pharmacy stock. Due to a recent increase in the number of ampicillin prescriptions, the pharmacist has asked you to replenish to at least the maximum par level for this item. Given the following information, what scenario illustrates the most economical way to replenish the pharmacy's supply of ampicillin 250 mg capsules?

The wholesaler sells ampicillin 250 mg capsules in the following quantities and prices:

> Ampicillin 250 mg capsules; 1000 count bottle; $12.55 per bottle
>
> Ampicillin 250 mg capsules; 500 count bottle; $8.75 per bottle
>
> Ampicillin 250 mg capsules; 250 count bottle; $4.65 per bottle
>
> Ampicillin 250 mg capsules; 100 count bottle; $3.60 per bottle
>
> Ampicillin 250 mg capsules; 50 count bottle; $2.50 per bottle
>
> Ampicillin 250 mg capsules; 25 count bottle; $1.85 per bottle

Step 1. Calculate how many capsules will be needed to replenish this item to at least the maximum par level.

$$\frac{\text{maximum}}{\text{par level}} - \frac{\text{current}}{\text{stock level}} = \frac{\text{amount needed to bring}}{\text{to maximum par level}}$$

$$1000 - 75 = 925 \text{ capsules}$$

Step 2. Determine the possible ways to replenish this item to the maximum par level.

Solution 1: Order exactly 925 capsules by purchasing one of each of the following:

500 count bottle at	$8.75
250 count bottle at	$4.65
100 count bottle at	$3.60
50 count bottle at	$2.50
25 count bottle at	$1.85
925 capsules	$21.35

In this scenario, the cost to purchase the amount needed is $21.35.

Solution 2: Order enough stock to bring up the inventory to at least the maximum par level in the most cost-effective manner, by purchasing the following:

1000 count bottle at	$12.55
1000 capsules	$12.55

In this scenario, the cost to purchase the amount needed is $12.55.

Step 3. Determine which scenario is the most cost-effective way to replenish this item.

Solution 1 cost = $21.35

Solution 2 cost = $12.55

The most cost-effective way to replenish this item up to the maximum par level is to purchase a single, 1000 count bottle of ampicillin 250 mg capsules for $12.55.

Days' Supply

Today's retail pharmacies generally have at least $100,000.00 of inventory in the form of drugs, supplies, and other merchandise. If a large chain has 10 stores in a particular region, the amount of money in merchandise sitting on the shelves adds up very quickly. Consequently, large companies often set goals for lowering the inventory to improve cash flow.

Setting inventory goals for a pharmacy requires pharmacy personnel to attempt to keep the approximate value of inventory on a pharmacy's shelves relatively equal to the cost of all of the drugs and merchandise sold in a specified period—usually either one week (7 days) or one month (30 days). For example, if a pharmacy manager establishes a goal of "30 days' supply," the pharmacy's goal is to keep the value of its inventory approximately equal to the total cost of the drugs and merchandise sold by the pharmacy in 30 days.

The pharmacy's computer system maintains a record of the value of the inventory currently on the pharmacy's shelves. In addition, most computer systems can provide an accurate record of the pharmacy's cost for all products sold by the pharmacy in a 24-hour period. Many of these systems can print off inventory and cost records, as well as average usage and costs for a specified period.

In rare instances, smaller independent pharmacies may not have ready access to this type of inventory and cost information. In these situations, a pharmacy manager may not know the best number of days to use as a goal in calculating costs. However, the manager likely has a good estimate of the current inventory value and can easily calculate average daily cost of items sold in the pharmacy (weekly costs/7 days). With this information, he or she can then determine how many days it will take (what is referred to as "days' supply") for the average daily product costs to equal the value of the inventory on the shelves. The manager can use this information to revise the inventory goal as necessary.

$$\frac{\text{value of inventory on the shelves}}{\text{average daily cost of products sold}} = \text{number of days' supply}$$

Example 9.3.6

Toussaint's Pharmacy has a total inventory value of $103,699.00. It had sales last week of $37,546.00, and the cost to the pharmacy of the products sold was $28,837.00. What should the pharmacy's days' supply be to keep its inventory value stable?

Toussaint's Pharmacy average daily product costs were

$$\$28,837.00 \div 7 \text{ days} = \$4120.00 \text{ (rounded)}$$

Now, according to the above formula, dividing the value of the inventory by the average daily product costs approximately equals the number of days' supply:

$$\text{number of days' supply} = \frac{\$103,699.00}{\$4120.00} = 25 \text{ (rounded)}$$

Toussaint's Pharmacy will have sold products approximately equal to the value of its inventory in 25 days.

Example 9.3.7

Malaya's Pharmacy has a total inventory value of $176,989.00. Last week, it had sales of $45,813.00, and the cost to the pharmacy of the products sold came to $36,592.00. The pharmacy's goal for the number of days' supply is 29, but the facility is currently over that goal. How many days' supply is the pharmacy over, and how much inventory value does this represent?

The average daily product costs were

$$\$36,592.00 \div 7 \text{ days} = \$5227.00 \text{ (rounded)}$$

At the present time, the number of days' supply for the pharmacy is

$$\frac{\$176,989.00}{\$5227.00} = 34 \text{ (rounded)}$$

Therefore, it takes 34 days for costs to equal the inventory value. In other words, Malaya's Pharmacy is 5 days over its days' supply.

$$5 \times \$5227.00 = \$26,135.00$$

If Malaya's Pharmacy can reduce its inventory by $26,135.00, the pharmacy will have met its goal of 29 days' supply.

Turnover Rate

If a pharmacy does not maintain computerized inventory, it must perform a physical inventory—or actual count—at specified intervals, usually annually or semiannually. The physical inventory value is then used to determine the average inventory value as follows:

$$\frac{\text{value of initial inventory} + \text{value of current inventory}}{2} = \text{average annual inventory value}$$

Knowing the average inventory value allows a pharmacy to calculate the number of times its inventory was repurchased during a cycle (usually a year).

Dividing total annual purchases of inventory by the average inventory value gives the **turnover rate**, or the number of times the amount of goods in inventory was sold during the year. Turnover rate can be calculated as follows:

$$\frac{\text{annual purchases of inventory}}{\text{average inventory value}} = \text{turnover rate}$$

Turnover rate can be used to determine how quickly a particular item is being used. In addition, turnover rate can be applied more broadly to the entire pharmacy inventory, which helps the pharmacy manager know how well the pharmacy is meeting its cash flow goals. Knowing the turnover rate can help pharmacy personnel determine if the average inventory level should be increased or decreased, as extra costs may be associated with high or low inventories. Thus, if a pharmacy has an average inventory value of $25,250.00 and the cost of its annual inventory purchases is $75,000.00, the inventory will "turn over" 2.970 times, or approximately three times in a year.

$$\frac{\text{annual purchases of inventory}}{\text{average inventory value}} = \text{turnover rate}$$

$$\frac{\$75,000.00}{\$25,250.00} = 2.970$$

Example 9.3.8

A pharmacy does a quarterly inventory and has an average inventory value of $100,000.00. The pharmacy's annual inventory purchases are $500,000.00. What is the pharmacy's turnover rate?

$$\frac{\text{annual purchases of inventory}}{\text{average inventory value}} = \text{turnover rate}$$

$$\frac{\$500,000.00}{\$100,000.00} = 5$$

The pharmacy's inventory will "turn over" five times in a year.

Depreciation

Depreciation is an allowance made to account for the decreasing value of a fixed asset. Properties, furnishings, and equipment owned by the pharmacy are called fixed assets, or simply *assets*. **Assets** are generally put into two broad categories: current and long-term assets. The assets that can be consumed or converted into cash within one year—such as drugs and OTC products—are current assets; those that cannot, such as buildings and high-dollar equipment, are considered long-term assets. Depreciation and asset amounts are used by the pharmacy to prepare its annual taxes.

Most fixed assets gradually lose value due to use, obsolescence, and the passage of time. The straight-line method of calculating depreciation uses the total cost, the estimated life of the property (in years), and the **disposal value** of the item, or the value of an item should it be sold or otherwise disposed of at the end of its useful life. Below is the depreciation formula:

(total cost − disposal value)/estimated life in years = annual depreciation

Example 9.3.9

Rafael's Pharmacy buys a used, compact car for drug deliveries to local customers. The cost of the car is $9000.00. Its estimated useful life is five years, and the disposal value is $1200.00. What is the annual depreciation?

(total cost − disposal value)/estimated life in years = annual depreciation

($9000.00 − $1200.00) /5 = $1560.00

The annual depreciation of the car is $1560.00.

9.3 Problem Set

For items 1–9, the number of units that need to be reordered for each item based on the current inventory and the number of units or packages needed to bring the drug up to at least the minimum par level.

Drug		Count/ Package Size	Minimum Par Level	Maximum Par Level	Current Inventory	Reorder Amount
1.	tetracycline 250 mg cap	500	120	700	80	
2.	amoxicillin 500 mg cap	100	300	400	118	
3.	amoxicillin 250 mg cap	500	240	1000	180	
4.	cefaclor 500 mg tab	60	20	120	35	
5.	cefprozil 250 mg tab	100	40	150	28	
6.	cefprozil 500 mg tab	50	20	75	24	
7.	metronidazole 500 mg tab	50	30	120	12	
8.	azithromycin 250 mg cap	30	18	60	36	
9.	doxycycline 50 mg cap	50	30	150	42	

The inventory of topical products, which are often dispensed as "partial containers" (i.e., 1 oz from a 16 oz jar), is checked frequently due to multiple compounding needs, manufacturer back orders, and poor computer tracking of dispensed partial containers of topical products. For this reason, reordering of topical products must be closely monitored, even with computer-generated orders.

Consider the following scenario: It is a Friday afternoon and Monday is a holiday; therefore, the pharmacy is expected to be very busy over the weekend. Because the pharmacy won't be able to get an order from its wholesaler until at least Tuesday, a pharmacy technician decides to order enough to bring the item up to at least the maximum par level. For questions 10–14, calculate the number of packages that need to be ordered to bring the item up to at least the maximum par level.

Drug		Count/ Package Size	Minimum Par Level	Maximum Par Level	Current Inventory	Reorder Amount
10.	triamcinolone 0.25% cream	15 g	2	4	1	
		80 g	2	4	0	
11.	triamcinolone 0.1% ung	15 g	1	2	1	
		60 g	1	2	1	
		80 g	1	2	0	
12.	triamcinolone 0.1% lotion	60 mL	1	2	1	

Drug		Count/ Package Size	Minimum Par Level	Maximum Par Level	Current Inventory	Reorder Amount
13. fluocinolone 0.025% cream		15 g	1	2	1	
		60 g	1	2	1	
14. fluocinolone 0.025% ung		60 g	1	2	0 tubes and 1 order waiting	

For items 15–36, calculate the number of units that need to be reordered for each item based on the current inventory and the number of units or packages that are needed to bring the item up to at least the minimum par level.

Drug		Count/ Package Size	Minimum Par Level	Maximum Par Level	Current Inventory	Reorder Amount
15. desoximetasone 0.25% cream		15 g	1	2	0	
		60 g	1	2	0	
		4 oz	1	2	1	
16. desoximetasone 0.05% gel		15 g	1	1	0 on shelf and 1 order waiting	
		60 g	1	1	0	
17. halobetasol 0.05% cream		15 g	1	2	1	
		45 g	1	2	1	
18. fluocinonide 0.05% cream		15 g	1	2	1	
		30 g	2	4	1	
		60 g	2	4	2	
		120 g	1	2	0	
19. fluocinonide 0.05% gel		15 g	1	1	1	
		30 g	1	3	2	
		60 g	1	3	0	
20. fluocinonide 0.05% ung		15 g	1	2	1	
		30 g	1	2	1	
		60 g	1	2	1 partial	
		120 g	1	2	1	
21. fluocinonide 0.05% soln		20 mL	1	1	0	
		60 mL	1	3	1 partial	
22. ramipril 5 mg cap		100	120	240	64	
23. verapamil 120 mg SR		100	80	240	52	
24. verapamil 240 mg SR		100	120	360	30	

Drug		Count/ Package Size	Minimum Par Level	Maximum Par Level	Current Inventory	Reorder Amount
25. nicardipine 60 mg SR		60	120	240	20	
26. captopril 50 mg tab		100	150	300	76	
27. furosemide 40 mg tab		1000	240	1500	134	
28. doxazosin 2 mg tab		100	80	240	83	
29. atenolol 50 mg tab		1000	240	1500	107	
30. atenolol 100 mg tab		100	150	300	111	
31. nifedipine 60 mg tab		300	120	625	12, and two Rx for 60 pending	
32. nifedipine 90 mg tab		100	120	300	63	
33. lisinopril 5 mg tab		100	90	260	110	
34. lisinopril 10 mg tab		1000	240	1500	146	
35. lisinopril 20 mg tab		100	180	250	145	
36. lisinopril 40 mg tab		100	90	220	152	

37. Review John's Drug Shop inventory below and calculate the number of units that needs to be reordered for each item based on the current inventory and the number of units or packages needed to bring the item up to at least the maximum par level.

Drug		Count/ Package Size	Minimum Par Level	Maximum Par Level	Current Inventory	Reorder Amount
a. Eucerin cream		100 g jars	3 jars	10 jars	3 jars	
b. ampicillin 250 mg caps		1000 capsule	1000 caps	5000 caps	2400 caps	
c. NS Nasal Spray		30 mL spray bottle	12 bottles	24 bottles	4 bottles	
d. Nystatin Oral Suspension		pint bottle (480 mL)	1 bottle	4 bottles	720 mL	
e. NS Nasal Spray		100 mL bottle	3 bottles	12 bottles	1 bottle	

38. Grimm's Pharmacy has a total inventory value of $183,445.00. Last week, the pharmacy had sales of $47,293.00, and the cost to the pharmacy for the products sold came to $38,207.00. The pharmacy's goal is to have a days' supply of 28 days.

    a. How many days' supply does Grimm's Pharmacy have?

    b. How much is the pharmacy over or under its goal in dollars?

39. Corbin's Pharmacy has a total inventory value of $123,490.00. Last week, the pharmacy had sales of $34,829.00, and the cost to the pharmacy for the products sold came to $26,504.00. Corbin's goal is to have a days' supply of 26 days.

    a. How many days' supply does Corbin's Pharmacy have?

    b. How much is the pharmacy over or under its goal in dollars?

40. Singh's Pharmacy has $147,210.00 in inventory. The pharmacy is currently at its goal of 24 days' supply. What was the approximate cost of products sold last week?

41. Scott's Pharmacy had sales of $51,280.00 last week. What must the pharmacy's daily sales average be this week in order to make $5000.00 more than last week?

42. Jethwani's Pharmacy has an inventory of $213,840.00. Last week's sales were $63,910.00. What was the percentage of profit if the cost of last week's sales was $48,891.00?

43. Rubio's Pharmacy has an inventory of $164,590.00. Last week's sales, which totaled $58,223.00, brought in a 21% profit. Now the pharmacy has set a days' supply goal of 31 days.

    a. What was the cost to the pharmacy of the product sold last week?

    b. What is the pharmacy's days' supply?

    c. How much is the value of the days' supply above or below the goal in dollars?

44. Amina's Pharmacy has an inventory of $184,520.00. The pharmacy's cost of sales last week was $28,223.00, and the facility made a 26% profit. The days' supply goal is 34 days.

    a. What was the amount sold last week?

    b. What is the pharmacy's days' supply?

    c. How much is the value of the days' supply above or below goal in dollars?

45. If a pharmacy's average inventory for the past year was $132,936.00 and the annual cost total was $1,612,000.00, what was the turnover rate?

46. If a pharmacy's average inventory for the past year was $156,200.00 and the annual cost total was $1,768,000.00, what was the turnover rate?

For items 47–51, calculate the turnover rate for the following drugs sold at Ming's Pharmacy.

Drug		Average Inventory	Annual Purchases	Turnover Rate
47. metformin 500 mg		$520.00	$20,800.00	
48. divalproex 250 mg		$178.00	$5760.00	
49. citalopram 40 mg		$360.00	$7213.00	
50. raloxifene 60 mg		$320.00	$5060.00	
51. montelukast chewtab 4 mg		$385.00	$6000.00	

52. Nadia's Drug Shop purchases $52,500.00 of antibiotics annually. The pharmacy does an inventory count twice annually, and its average inventory of antibiotics is $5000.00. What is the pharmacy's turnover rate for antibiotics?

53. A pharmacy has a new cash register system. The system costs $8294.00 and should last six years. Its disposal value is $2138.00. What is the annual depreciation?

54. A hospital pharmacy just purchased two new biological safety cabinets at $18,350.00 each. Each cabinet should last 12 years if maintained properly. The disposal value is $1567.00 each. What is the annual depreciation amount for both cabinets?

Self-check your work in Appendix A.

Chapter Summary

- Pharmacies must consider both income and overhead when calculating actual profit and when setting goals for desired percentage of profit.
- The net profit of an item is based upon the percentage of profit that the pharmacy intends to make and is determined by subtracting the overall cost of an item from the item's selling price.
- Pharmacies have contracts with wholesalers who provide drugs and supply items from the manufacturer to the pharmacy.

- Pharmacies have contracts with pharmacy benefits managers (PBMs) who broker insurance reimbursement claims.
- Pharmacy personnel must be familiar with the average wholesale price and capitation fees that affect the profitability of the facility.
- Pharmacy technicians are actively involved in managing pharmacy inventory, determining days' supply, establishing the turnover rate, and replenishing stock to the desired par level.

Key Terms

assets properties, furnishings, inventory, supplies, and equipment owned by the pharmacy; may be put into two categories: current, or short-term, assets and long-term assets

average wholesale price (AWP) an average price at which drugs are purchased at the wholesale level, or the average value at which wholesalers sell a particular drug to pharmacies

base profit the amount of profit determined by subtracting the total pharmacy overhead amount from the pharmacy's income

capitation fee a monthly fee paid by some insurance plans to a pharmacy under a specific prescription reimbursement plan

current percentage of profit the amount of profit that is determined by dividing the base profit by income and then multiplying that quotient by 100; often used to determine the desired percentage of profit

depreciation an allowance made to account for the decreasing value of a fixed asset; properties, furnishings, and equipment owned by the pharmacy are called *fixed assets*, or simply *assets*

desired percentage of profit the percentage of profit the pharmacy intends to make on the product after the overall cost is subtracted from the selling price

discount a price that is reduced from what is typically charged

discount rate the percent that the discounted price is reduced from the regular selling price

dispensing fee the amount that is charged over and above the pharmacy's purchase price for a medication; this amount is meant to cover all costs related to filling a prescription, beyond the purchase price of the drug

disposal value the value of an item should it be sold or disposed of at the end of its useful life

flat rate a low pharmacy selling price for a certain amount of medication, a supply designed to last a specific number of days

gross profit the difference between the pharmacy's selling price and purchase price

income the money or equivalent received from the sale of medications, supply items, or equipment

inventory a listing of all of the items that are available for sale in a business

inventory value the total value of all of the drugs and merchandise in stock on a given day

markup rate a percentage amount that is determined by subtracting the pharmacy's purchase price for an item from the pharmacy's selling price for that item

net profit the difference between the selling price and the overall cost

overall cost the sum of the cost to purchase the drug from the manufacturer (known as the pharmacy's purchase price) and the cost to dispense the drug

overhead the pharmacy's cost of doing business; this cost includes personnel salaries, equipment, and operating expenses such as rent, taxes, and utilities

par level an average inventory range for an item, which generally includes the minimum and maximum stock levels for the item

pharmacy benefits manager (PBM) a large prescription processing service that contracts with insurance companies and pharmacies to process insurance reimbursement

profit the financial gain made when the amount earned is greater than the amount spent during a specified period

profit margin the difference between the cost of doing business (the pharmacy's purchase price, overhead, and preparation costs) and the selling price of a drug or product

purchase price the cost to purchase the drug from the wholesaler or manufacturer

selling price the amount that the pharmacy charges for a particular drug or product; sometimes referred to as *accounts receivable*

turnover rate the number of times the amount of goods in inventory was sold during the year

wholesaler a company that sells and distributes a large number of goods such as medications and supply items to a pharmacy; a company that acts as a go-between for pharmacies and manufacturing companies such as drug manufacturers

Chapter Review

Assessing Comprehension

To check your comprehension of this chapter's key concepts, read the following multiple-choice questions and then record your answers on a separate sheet of paper. Write your answers as modeled in these examples: 1d; 2c; 3b; *etc.*

1. Which of the following terms refers to the money or equivalent received from the sale of a medication, supply item, or equipment?
   a. overhead
   b. profit
   c. net profit
   d. income

2. Which of the following items is considered overhead in pharmacy practice?
   a. personnel salaries and some employee benefits
   b. inventory and equipment
   c. rent, utilities, and taxes
   d. all of the above

3. Which of the following terms is used to describe the difference between the selling price and the overall cost?
   a. profit
   b. net profit
   c. gross profit
   d. percentage of profit

4. Which of the following terms is used to describe the difference between the selling price and the pharmacy's purchase price?
   a. profit
   b. net profit
   c. gross profit
   d. percent profit

5. What is the meaning of the acronym *PBM*?
   a. Personnel Benefits Manager
   b. Personnel Benefits Management
   c. Pharmacy Benefits Manager
   d. Pharmacy Benefits Management

6. What is the meaning of the acronym *AWP*?
   a. average wholesale price
   b. annual wholesale price
   c. average wholesale product
   d. annual wholesale product

7. Some third-party payers use a system that reimburses the pharmacy a flat, _____ fee each month for each contracted client regardless of whether the client has a prescription filled that month.
   a. capital
   b. capitalization
   c. capitation
   d. none of the above

8. Which of the following terms describes all of the drugs, supply items, and merchandise on hand in a pharmacy?
   a. pharmacy stock
   b. pharmacy overhead
   c. pharmacy inventory
   d. pharmacy supply

9. What term is used to describe the minimum and maximum inventory range for a pharmacy item?
   a. markup level
   b. PBM level
   c. AWP level
   d. par level

10. What term refers to a common method used to establish an inventory range for each pharmacy item?
    a. days' supply
    b. depreciation
    c. gross profit
    d. markup rate

Finding Solutions

To gain practice in handling challenging situations in the workplace, consider the following real-world scenarios and then use the guiding questions to help you formulate your responses.

Note: *To indicate your answers for Scenario A (Questions 1–3) and Scenario B (Questions 4–7), ask your instructor for the corresponding handouts.*

Scenario A: In your pharmacy, the minimum par level for ampicillin 250 mg capsules is 500; the maximum par level is 2000. At the end of the day, the pharmacy computer prints a list of items that have fallen below the minimum par level and, therefore, need to be reordered. The printout shows that there are currently 350 ampicillin 250 mg capsules in the pharmacy stock. Given the information below, determine the most economical way to replenish the pharmacy's supply of ampicillin 250 mg capsules up to at least the minimum par level.

The wholesaler sells ampicillin 250 mg capsules in the following quantities and prices:

Ampicillin 250 mg capsules; 1000 count bottle; $10.00 per bottle

Ampicillin 250 mg capsules; 500 count bottle; $8.75 per bottle

Ampicillin 250 mg capsules; 250 count bottle; $4.65 per bottle

Ampicillin 250 mg capsules; 100 count bottle; $3.60 per bottle

Ampicillin 250 mg capsules; 50 count bottle; $2.50 per bottle

Ampicillin 250 mg capsules; 25 count bottle; $1.85 per bottle

For Questions 1–3, record your answers on the handout that you obtained from your instructor.

1. What size/quantity bottle(s) will you order?

2. How many of each bottle will you order?

3. What will the final cost be for this order?

Scenario B: Beneficial HMO pays a per-client capitation fee of $149.00 per month to the Georgetown Pharmacy. The pharmacy is contracted to serve 127 of the HMO's clients and their families. During the month of December, 21 of these clients and/or their family members had a total of 52 prescriptions filled at the pharmacy. The pharmacy's total drug cost for these prescriptions was $6283.24. The contract allows the pharmacy to bill a $3.50 dispensing fee for each filled prescription.

For Questions 4–7, record your answers on the handout that you obtained from your instructor.

4. What is the total amount that the HMO reimbursed the pharmacy for capitation fees?

5. What is the pharmacy's drug cost for all of the prescriptions on this plan?

6. Did the pharmacy make a profit or lose money?

7. If the pharmacy made a profit, what was the amount? If the pharmacy took a loss, what was the amount?

Sampling the Certification Exam

To provide you with practice for the Certification Exam, read the following questions that have been patterned after the test format and then record your answers on a separate sheet of paper. Write your answers as modeled in these examples: 1d; 2c; 3b; etc.

1. What is the percentage of profit if the pharmacy has a base profit of $110,000.00 and an annual income of $500,000.00?
   a. 0.22%
   b. 2.2%
   c. 22%
   d. 220%

2. What should the selling price be for an item that the pharmacy purchased for $25.00 and that costs the pharmacy $5.00 to dispense if the pharmacy wishes to have a 20% profit?
   a. $24.00
   b. $25.00
   c. $36.00
   d. $37.00

3. The pharmacy purchased a 100 count bottle of medication at a price of $7.50. You dispense a prescription for 30 tablets to a customer, who paid $12.53 for the prescription. The pharmacy charges a dispensing fee of $3.50. What is the net profit on this sale?
   a. $0.92
   b. $9.23
   c. $92.30
   d. $923.30

4. Calculate the markup amount and the markup rate for the following:

> Propranolol 10 mg tablets
> Pharmacy's purchase price: $3.96
> Pharmacy's selling price: $8.59

Round the markup rate to the nearest whole percent.

a. $4.63; 117%
b. $4.63; 463%
c. $12.55; 396%
d. $12.55; 859%

5. Calculate the markup amount and the markup rate for the following:

> Amoxicillin 250 mg
> Pharmacy's purchase price: $8.50
> Pharmacy's selling price: $14.80

Round the markup rate to the nearest whole percent.

a. $6.30; 63%
b. $6.30; 74%
c. $23.30; 27.4%
d. $23.40; 274%

Chapter Practice Test

Additional Practice Questions

To put your pharmacy calculation skills to the test, read the following questions and then record your answers on a separate sheet of paper.

Use the OWL Pharmacy's expenses listed below to answer questions 1 and 2.

pharmacist salary	$126,000.00
technician salary	38,000.00
rent	12,000.00
utilities	7,000.00
computer maintenance	1,500.00
software subscriptions	1,500.00
liability insurance	2,500.00
business insurance	3,000.00
drug purchases	425,000.00

1. If a 25% profit is desirable, what must the pharmacy's income be to meet this goal?

2. If the pharmacy's income is $1,401,750.00, what is its percentage of profit?

Using the prescription drug items provided in questions 3 and 4, calculate the dollar amount of net profit and the percentage of profit (markup rate). Round to whole percents. The dispensing fee is $5.24 for each prescription.

3.

> Pepcid (famotidine) 40 mg tablets
> Cost: $84.30 per 30 tablets
> Dispense: 30 tablets
> Rx charge: $95.00

a. What is the net profit?

b. What is the percentage of profit (markup rate) rounded to the nearest whole number?

4.

> Acetaminophen/codeine #3
> Cost: $32.50 per 500 count bottle
> Dispense: 40 tablets
> Rx charge: $8.95

a. What is the net profit?

b. What is the percentage of profit (markup rate) rounded to the nearest whole percent?

For questions 5 and 6, perform the necessary calculations and state the answers in dollars and cents.

5. Bizup's Medicine Shop purchases five cases of dermatological cream at $100.00 per case. The invoice specifies a 15% discount if the account is paid in full within 15 days. What is the discounted price?

6. There are 24 tubes of cream per case in question 5. You are to mark up each tube by 20% based on the pharmacy's discounted purchase price. What will the selling price be per tube?

For questions 7–12, calculate the markup and percent profit of each of the following items. Round to whole percents.

Item	Pharmacy's Purchase Price	Selling Price	Markup	% Profit
7. amoxicillin	$0.14	$0.28		
8. nasal spray	$1.45	$2.15		
9. fungal ointment	$3.25	$4.15		
10. analgesic tablets	$0.10	$0.15		
11. contraceptive foam	$1.35	$5.75		
12. nitroglycerin tablets	$8.50	$14.95		

13. The pharmacy purchased a 120 g jar of medication at an AWP of $94.45. You must dispense a prescription for a tube of 30 g of the medication. The third-party contract will reimburse AWP less 12%. The contract allows for a $4.50 dispensing fee for each prescription. What is the reimbursement amount for this prescription?

14. The pharmacy purchased a pint bottle of medication at an AWP of $12.50. You must fill a prescription for 4 oz of the medication. The third-party contract will reimburse AWP less 12% but does not allow a dispensing fee. What is the reimbursement amount for this prescription?

15. The pharmacy purchased a 30 g tube of medication at an AWP of $21.35. You must fill a prescription for 30 g. The PBM will reimburse for AWP plus 3% and allows a $5.75 per prescription dispensing fee. What is the reimbursement amount for this prescription?

16. The pharmacy purchased a pint bottle of medication at an AWP of $90.32. You must fill a prescription for 180 mL. The PBM will reimburse for AWP plus 3% and allows a $5.75 per prescription dispensing fee. What is the reimbursement amount for this prescription?

For questions 17 and 18, calculate the pharmacy's profit based on the information provided.

17. A prescription is written for a tube of ointment. The AWP is $62.00. Khan's Pharmacy purchases the tube at AWP, and Albright's Pharmacy purchases the tube at AWP minus 10%. The insurer will reimburse at AWP plus 2% plus a $1.50 dispensing fee. How much profit does each pharmacy make?

18. A prescription is written for a bottle of cough medication. The AWP is $18.75. McDougall Pharmacy purchases the cough syrup at a cost of $4.00. The pharmacy sells the cough syrup for AWP minus 10% plus $6.00 dispensing fee. How much profit does the pharmacy make?

19. Grant County HMO pays a capitation fee of $195.00 per month to the Sun City Pharmacy. The pharmacy is contracted to serve 17 of the HMO's clients. During the month of August, 12 of these clients had prescriptions filled at the pharmacy. The pharmacy's total drug cost for these prescriptions was $867.50. The contract allows the pharmacy to bill a single charge of $60.00 for dispensing fees for the month.
   a. What is the total amount that the HMO reimbursed the pharmacy for this contract in the month of August?
   b. What is the pharmacy's drug cost for all of the prescriptions on this plan?
   c. Did the pharmacy make a profit or lose money?
   d. If the pharmacy made a profit, what was the amount? If the pharmacy took a loss, what was the amount?

20. Travis County HMO pays a per client capitation fee of $120.00 per month to the Eppley Pharmacy. The pharmacy is contracted to serve 46 of the HMO's clients. During the month of March, 28 of these clients had a total of 37 prescriptions filled. The pharmacy's total drug cost for these prescriptions was $6187.50. The contract allows the pharmacy to bill a single charge of $128.00 for dispensing fees for the month.
   a. What is the total amount that the HMO reimbursed the pharmacy for this contract in the month of March?
   b. What is the pharmacy's drug cost for all of the prescriptions on this plan?
   c. Did the pharmacy make a profit or lose money?
   d. If the pharmacy made a profit, what was the amount? If the pharmacy took a loss, what was the amount?

For questions 21–24, review the inventory list below and calculate the number of units that need to be reordered for each item based on the current inventory and the number of units or packages needed to bring the item up to at least the minimum par level.

	Drug		Count/ Package Size	Minimum Par Level	Maximum Par Level	Current Inventory	Reorder Amount
21.	nicardipine 30 mg SR		60	120	240	18	
22.	captopril 25 mg tab		100	150	300	60	
23.	metoprolol 50 mg tab		1000	120	1500	83	
24.	metoprolol 100 mg		1000	120	2000	341	

For questions 25–28, calculate the requested value.

25. Winstead's Pharmacy does inventory three times annually, and the average inventory value is $125,825.00. Annual purchases of inventory total $188,737.50. What is the turnover rate?

26. Chu's Pharmacy has an inventory program in the computer system, and the average value of the inventory is calculated daily. It is $114,900.00. Annual purchases of inventory total $546,210.00. What is the turnover rate?

27. Carroll's Drug Store has a van for home deliveries, and its total cost was $18,452.00. Its disposal value is $12,208.00. It has an estimated life of three years. What is the annual depreciation?

28. Midway Pharmacy has some lab equipment that costs $1478.00. Its disposal value is $850.00, and its estimated life is eight years. What is the annual depreciation?

Chapter 1

1.1 Problem Set

1. $\frac{1}{2}$

2. $\frac{3}{8}$

3. $\frac{2}{1}$

4. $\frac{2}{6}$

5. $\frac{1}{10}$

6. $1^{14}/_{15}$

Work

Solution 1.

Create common denominators:

$\frac{5}{6} \times \frac{10}{10} = \frac{50}{60}$, $\frac{7}{10} \times \frac{6}{6} = \frac{42}{60}$, $\frac{2}{5} \times \frac{12}{12} = \frac{24}{60}$

Add the numerators:

$\frac{50}{60} \times \frac{42}{60} = \frac{24}{60} \times \frac{116}{60}$

Simplify:

$\frac{116}{60} = \frac{156}{60} = \frac{114}{15}$

Solution 2.

Create common denominators:

$\frac{5}{6} \times \frac{5}{5} = \frac{25}{30}$, $\frac{7}{10} \times \frac{3}{3} = \frac{21}{30}$, $\frac{2}{5} \times \frac{6}{6} = \frac{12}{30}$

Add the numerators:

$\frac{25}{30} + \frac{21}{30} + \frac{12}{30} = \frac{58}{30}$

Simplify:

$\frac{58}{30} = \frac{29}{15} = 1^{14}/_{15}$

7. $1^{37}/_{96}$

Work

Create common denominators:

$\frac{21}{32} \times \frac{3}{3} = \frac{63}{96}$, $\frac{1}{12} \times \frac{8}{8} = \frac{8}{96}$, $\frac{31}{48} \times \frac{2}{2} = \frac{62}{96}$

Add the numerators:

$\frac{63}{96} + \frac{8}{96} + \frac{62}{96} = \frac{133}{96}$

Simplify:

$\frac{133}{96} = 1^{37}/_{96}$

8. $\frac{1}{4}$

9. $6^{7}/_{10}$

10. $2^{1}/_{5}$

11. $\frac{9}{10}$

12. $\frac{2}{5}$

13. $\frac{1}{12}$

Work

$126 = 12 \div 6 = 12 \times 16 = 112$

14. 0.2

15. 0.05

16. 4.5

17. 0.3

18. 0.005

19. 0.002

20. 1.8

21. 0.04

22. 0.008

23. 3 tablets

Work

Create common denominators:

$\frac{1}{4}$, $\frac{1}{2} \times \frac{2}{2} = \frac{2}{4}$, $1\frac{1}{2} = \frac{3}{2} \times \frac{2}{2} = \frac{6}{4}$, $\frac{3}{4}$

Add the numerators:

$\frac{1}{4} + \frac{2}{4} + \frac{6}{4} + \frac{3}{4} = \frac{12}{4}$

Simplify:

$\frac{12}{4} = 3$

24. 2 tablets containing $\frac{1}{100}$ grain in each tablet

Work

$2 \times \frac{1}{100} = \frac{2}{100} = \frac{1}{50}$

Because the denominator is smaller, $\frac{1}{50} > \frac{1}{150}$

25. $\dfrac{375 \text{ grains} \times 1 \text{ unit dose}}{\frac{1}{4} \text{ grain}} = 375 \times 4 = 1500$ containers

26. 3 bags

Work

Create common denominators:

$\frac{1}{2} \times \frac{10}{10} = \frac{10}{20}$, $\frac{4}{5} \times \frac{4}{4} = \frac{16}{20}$, $\frac{1}{4} \times \frac{5}{5} = \frac{5}{20}$,
$2\frac{1}{2} = \frac{5}{2} \times \frac{10}{10} = \frac{50}{20}$

Add the numerators:

$\frac{10}{20} + \frac{16}{20} + \frac{5}{20} + \frac{50}{20} = \frac{81}{20}$

Simplify:

$\frac{81}{20} = 4\frac{1}{20}$ lb sugar needed

Sugar is sold in bags of 2 lb/bag; 2 bags would = 4 lb sugar (2×2 lb = 4 lb), and we need $\frac{1}{20}$ lb more than that, so 3 bags are needed. 3 bags $\times$ 2 lb/bag = 6 lb; 6 lb total $-$ 4 $\frac{1}{20}$ lb needed = 1 $\frac{19}{20}$ lb left over.

27. 1 bag

Work

Since we need 4 $\frac{1}{20}$ lb sugar (problem 24), one 5 lb bag will provide the sugar needed.

1.2 Problem Set

1. 10
2. 5
3. 624
4. 2050
5. 48
6. XVII
7. LXVII
8. MCMXCV or MVM
9. 4.1
10. 0.6
11. 2.02
12. 0.017
13. 0
14. 6
15. 3
16. hundreds
17. hundredths
18. thousandths
19. ones
20. tenths
21. 68,000 (move decimal to the right 4 places)
22. 1,870,000 (move decimal to the right 6 places)
23. 10,300,000 (move decimal to the right 7 places)
24. 0.00084 (move decimal to the left 4 places)
25. 0.00768 (move decimal to the left 3 places)
26. 0.00006239 (move decimal to the left 5 places)
27. 3.29×10^{-9}
28. 3.9×10^{11}
29. 3.8×10^{-3}
30. 5.2×10^{16}
31. 3.779×10^{6}
32. 2.02×10^{-10}
33. 157.5 tablets (158 tablets, to the next whole tablet)
34. a. 10 grain
    b. 1 daily
    c. 100 tablets
35. a. $\frac{1}{2}$ grain
    b. 2 grains or 4 tablets daily
    c. 28 tablets
    d. 25 days
36. a. 28 tablets
    b. 7 days

37. a. 5 tablets daily

    b. 150 tablets

    c. 20 days

1.3 Problem Set

1. 784.36

2. 0.9

3. 1.88

4. 2.729

5. 14.373

6. 3.0983

7. 11.998

8. 467.42

9. 450

10. 1.846

11. 1.333

12. 3.87

13. 0.14

14. 0.08

15. 0.196

16. 0.049

17. 34.907 (34.9)

18. 1.395 (1.4)

19. a. 3 tablet/dose × 0.25 mg/tablet = 0.75 mg/dose

    b. 0.75 mg/dose × 4 doses/day = 3 mg

    c. 3 tablets/dose × 4 doses/day × 14 days = 168 tablets

    d. no; 168 tablets − 100 tablets = 68 tablets; the patient will need 68 more tablets

    e. alprazolam 0.25 mg #100/$14.95 + $7.59 = $22.54

20. a. 0.25 mg/tablet × 4 tablets /dose = 1 mg/dose

    b. $17.46 × 1.25 × $21.825, rounded to $21.83

    c. $23.87 × 0.5 = $11.935, rounded to $11.94

    d. 50 tablets × 1 day/4 tablets = 12.5 days

21. a. 1000 mL × 1 bottle/120 mL = 8.33 bottles, rounded to 8 bottles

    b. 120 mL/bottle × 8 bottles = 960 mL; 1000 mL − 960 mL = 40 mL

22. 8.5 mL/dose × 2 doses/day × 2 days = 34 mL

    5.75 mL/dose × 2 doses/day × 5 days × 57.5 mL

    34 mL + 57.5 mL = 91.5 mL

23. a. $47

    b. $15

    c. $4

24. a. $70.08

    b. $111.64

25. a. 89.5%

    b. 85.0%

    c. 92.2%

1.4 Problem Set

1. 200 + 700 + 300 + 600 = 1800; (100/2) × 4 = 200; 1800 + 200 = 2000 estimate, 1915 actual

2. 100; (100/2) × 4 = 200; 100 + 200 = 300 estimate, 275 actual

3. 10 + 10 + 10 = 30; (10/2) × 4 = 20; 30 + 20 = 50 estimate, 54.11 actual

4. 90 + 10 + 40 + 10 = 150; (10/2) × 4 = 20; 150 + 20 = 170 estimate, 170.42 actual

5. 20 estimate, 20.82 actual

6. $7 estimate, $6.38 actual

7. $12 estimate, $12.25 actual

8. $5 estimate, $5.19 actual

9. $82 estimate, $81.71 actual

10. $50 estimate, $50.58 actual

11. 56,000 estimate, 52,060.8 actual

12. 1400 estimate, 1407.3 actual

13. 1) Round to 600 and 15, ignoring the 3 decimals. 2) 600 × 15 = 9000. 3) Put 3 decimals back, so answer is 9. Actual is 8.976.

14. 1) Round to 5000 and 1, ignoring 1 decimal.
    2) 5000 × 1 × 5000. 3) Put decimal back, or
    500. Actual is 444.1068.

15. 120,000 estimate, 111,294 actual

16. 9000 estimate, 11,402.3 actual

17. 10 estimate, 10.28 actual

18. 300 estimate, 321.70 actual

19. 75 estimate, 73 actual

20. 200 estimate, 191.87 actual

21. 100/10 = 10 estimate, 8.79 actual

22. food dye $2 estimate + sugar $8 estimate
    + soda $1 estimate + cherry $2 estimate +
    bleach $2 estimate + water $4 estimate = $19
    estimate, $19.10 actual

23. 3 mL + 8 mL + 2 mL + 4 mL = 17 mL
    estimate; therefore, use 30 mL vial

24. 1720 mL IV fluids + 150 mL juice + 130 mL
    coffee = 2000 mL estimate

25. 800 mL + 200 mL + 300 mL + 3000 mL =
    4300 mL estimate

1.5 Problem Set

1. 6

2. 2

3. 2

4. 3

5. 1

6. 4

7. 2

8. 1

9. 8

10. 1

11. 42.8

12. 100.0

13. 0.0427

14. 18.4

15. 0.00392

16. 0.35, 2 significant figures

17. 0.06, 1 significant figure

18. 1.99, 3 significant figures

19. 0.01, 1 significant figure

20. 1.03, 3 significant figures

21. 63.8

22. 30

23. 163

24. a. 1.784 g to 1.78 g

    b. 3.2 g

    c. 3.2 g + 1.78 g + 2.46 g + 5.87 g = 13.31 g;
       13.31 g/0.125 g = 106.48 capsules; 0.48 of a
       capsule × 0.125 g = 0.06 g

25. a. 21.65 mg × 45 doses = 974.25 mg

    b. 5 significant figures

1.6 Problem Set

1. 07:30

2. 16:28

3. 00:45

4. 21:20

5. 02:24

6. 22:58

7. 23:50

8. 01:20

9. 00:03

10. 12:20

11. 5:30 PM

12. 11:49 PM

13. 3:22 PM

14. 12:34 AM

15. 12:04 PM

16. 3:55 AM

17. 10:45 PM

18. 5:19 PM

19. 1:00 PM

20. 1:45 AM

21. 0815; 1315; 1900

22. 0500

23. 10:00 PM

24. 6:00–7:00 PM

25. 1500; 1505; 1510

Chapter 2

2.1 Problem Set

1. $\frac{3}{7}$

2. $\frac{8}{6} = \frac{4}{3} = 1\frac{1}{3}$

3. $\frac{3}{4}$

4. $\frac{4}{6} = \frac{2}{3}$

5. $\frac{1}{7}$

6. 2:3

7. 6:8 = 3:4

8. 5:10 = 1:2

9. 1:9

10. 1:10,000

11. 30 mg:1 tablet or 1 tablet:30 mg

12. 100 mg: 1 capsule or 1 capsule:100 mg

13. 250 mg: 5 mL or 5 mL:250 mg

14. 90 mg/3 capsules

15. 200 mg/2 capsules

16. 750 mg/15 mL

17. 10 g, 1000 mL, 1 g (or x g/100 mL = 10 g/1000 mL; x g = 1 g)

18. 1 g, 100 mL, 5 g (or x g/500 mL = 1 g/100 mL; x g = 5 g)

19. 1 g, 250 mL, 4 g (or x g/1000 mL = 1 g/250 mL; x g = 4 g)

20. 1 g, 1000 mL, 0.05 g (or x g/50 mL = 1 g/1000 mL; x g = 0.05 g)

2.2 Problem Set

1. $\frac{6}{7} = 0.857$, rounded to 0.86; 0.86 × 100 = 86%

2. $\frac{5}{12} = 0.416$, rounded to 0.42; 0.42 × 100 = 42%

3. $\frac{1}{4} = 0.25$; 0.25 × 100 = 25%

4. $\frac{2}{3} = 0.666$, rounded to 0.67; 0.67 × 100 = 67%

5. $\frac{0.5}{10} = 0.05$; 0.05 × 100 = 5%

6. $\frac{2}{3} = 0.666$, rounded to 0.67; 0.67 × 100 = 67%

7. $\frac{1.5}{4.65} = 0.3225$, rounded to 0.323; 0.323 × 100 = 32.3%

8. $\frac{1}{250} = 0.004$; 0.004 × 100 = 0.4%

9. $\frac{1}{10,000} = 0.0001$; 0.0001 × 100 = 0.01%

10. $\frac{1}{6} = 0.166$, rounded to 0.17; 0.17 × 100 = 17%

11. 50% = $\frac{50}{100} = \frac{5}{10} = \frac{1}{2}$

12. 2% = $\frac{2}{100} = \frac{1}{50}$

13. 6% = $\frac{6}{100} = 0.06$

14. 12.5% = $\frac{12.5}{100} = 0.125$

15. 126% = $\frac{126}{100} = 1.26$

16. 20 × 0.05 = 1

17. 60 × 0.20 = 12

18. 63 × 0.19 = 11.97

19. 70 × 1.10 = 77

20. 50 × 0.002 = 0.1

21. 1:3, 0.33

22. $\frac{1}{40}$, 0.025

23. 50%, 1:2

24. 1%, $\frac{1}{100}$

25. $\frac{9}{10}$, 9:10

26. $\frac{2}{3}$ or $\frac{67}{100}$; 2:3 or 67:100

27. 0.2%, 0.002

28. $\frac{0.09}{20}$, 0.09:20

29. $\frac{1}{20}$, 0.05

30. 1:5, 0.2

31. $\frac{1}{10,000} = 0.0001 × 100 = 0.01\%$ solution

32. $\frac{1}{20} = 0.05 × 100 = 5\%$ solution

33. $\frac{1}{25} = 0.04 × 100 = 4\%$ solution

34. $\frac{1}{800} = 0.00125 × 100 = 0.125\%$ solution

35. $\frac{1}{10} = 0.1 × 100 = 10\%$ solution

2.3 Problem Set

1. 5

2. 0.07843, rounded to 0.08

3. 4.5

4. 0.1

5. 0.16

6. 5.7692, rounded to 5.77

7. 54.4

8. 242.6666, rounded to 242.67

9. 25.9411, rounded to 25.94

10. 16

11. 44.3571, rounded to 44.36

12. 21.3870, rounded to 21.39

13. 78.3333, rounded to 78.33

14. 10.7307, rounded to 10.73

15. 77.3636, rounded to 77.36

16. $x\%/100 = 72\%/254$; $x\% = 28.3464\%$, rounded to 28.35%

17. $x/100\% = 44/90\%$; $x = 48.8888$, rounded to 48.89

18. $x/100\% = 100/44\%$; $x = 227.2727$, rounded to 227.27

19. $x/100\% = 34/28\%$; $x = 121.4285$, rounded to 121.43

20. $x\%/100 = 24.5\%/45$; $x\% = 54.4444\%$, rounded to 54.44%

21. x g/100 mg = 1 g/1000 mg; x g = 0.1 g

22. x g/247 mg = 1 g/1000 mg; x g = 0.247 g

23. x g/1420 mg = 1 g/1000 mg; x g = 1.42 g

24. x g/495 mg = 1 g/1000 mg; x g = 0.495 g

25. x g/3781 mg = 1 g/1000 mg; x g = 3.781 g

26. x mg/0.349 g = 1000 mg/1 g; x mg = 349 mg

27. x mg/1.5 g = 1000 mg/1 g; x mg = 1500 mg

28. x mg/0.083 g = 1000 mg/1 g; x mg = 83 mg

29. x mg/0.01 g = 1000 mg/1 g; x mg = 10 mg

30. x mg/2.1 g = 1000 mg/1 g; x mg = 2100 mg

31. x kg/6.3 lb = 1 kg/2.2 lb; x kg = 2.863 kg, rounded to 2.9 kg

32. x kg/15 lb = 1 kg/2.2 lb; x kg = 6.818 kg, rounded to 6.8 kg

33. x kg/97 lb = 1 kg/2.2 lb; x kg = 44.090 kg, rounded to 44.1 kg

34. x kg/115 lb = 1 kg/2.2 lb; x kg = 52.272 kg, rounded to 52.3 kg

35. x kg/186 lb = 1 kg/2.2 lb; x kg = 84.545 kg, rounded to 84.5 kg

36. x lb/7.5 kg = 2.2 lb/1 kg; x lb = 16.5 lb

37. x lb/3.6 kg = 2.2 lb/1 kg; x lb = 7.92 lb, rounded to 7.9 lb

38. x lb/79.2 kg = 2.2 lb/1 kg; x lb = 174.24 lb, rounded to 174.2 lb

39. x lb/90 kg = 2.2 lb/1 kg; x lb = 198 lb

40. x lb/0.5 kg = 2.2 lb/1 kg; x lb = 1.1 lb

41. x mL/100 mg = 1 mL/50 mg; x mL = 2 mL

42. x tablets/375 mg = 1 tablet/125 mg; x tablets = 3 tablets

43. x mL/300 mg = 1 mL/20 mg; x mL = 15 mL

44. x folders/$15.00 = 100 folders/$7.40; x folders = 202.7 folders; 200 folders can be purchased (2 boxes of 100 folders)

45. x mL/10,000 units = 15 mL/250,000 units; x mL = 0.6 mL

46. x mL/60 mg = 2 mL/20 mg; x mL = 6 mL

47. x mL/60 mg = 4 mL/40 mg; x mL = 6 mL

48. x mL/300 mg = 10 mL/500 mg; x mL = 6 mL

49. x mL/30 mg = 1 mL/5 mg; x mL = 6 mL

50. x mL/30 mg = 1 mL/20 mg; x mL = 1.5 mL

51. x mg/5 mL = 20 mg/2 mL; x mg = 50 mg

52. x mL/80 mg = 2 mL/20 mg; x mL = 8 mL

53. x mL/50 mg = 2 mL/20 mg; x mL = 5 mL

54. x mL/12.5 mg = 2 mL/20 mg; x mL = 1.25 mL

55. x mg/3.5 mL = 20 mg/2 mL; x mg = 35 mg

2.4 Problem Set

1. 189 mg − 185 mg = 4 mg; (4 mg/185 mg) × 100 = 2.162%, rounded to 2.16%

2. 500 mg − 476 mg = 24 mg; (24 mg/500 mg) × 100 = 4.8%

3. 1507 mg − 1200 mg = 307 mg; (307 mg/1200 mg) × 100 = 25.583%, rounded to 25.58%

4. 15 mg − 12.5 mg = 2.5 mg; (2.5 mg/15 mg) × 100 = 16.666%, rounded to 16.67%

5. 415 mcg − 400 mcg = 15 mcg; (15 mcg/400 mcg) × 100 = 3.75%

6. 6.3 mL − 5 mL = 1.3 mL; (1.3 mL/5 mL) × 100 = 26%

7. 15 mL − 13 mL = 2 mL; (2 mL/15 mL) × 100 = 13.333%, rounded to 13.33%

8. 20 mL − 15 mL = 5 mL; (5 mL/15 mL) × 100 = 33.333%, rounded to 33.33%

9. 1.5 L − 1.45 L = 0.05 L; (0.05 L/1.5 L) × 100 = 3.333%, rounded to 3.33%

10. 726 mL − 700 mL = 26 mL; (26 mL/700 mL) × 100 = 3.714%, rounded to 3.71%

11. 0.03 × 3 mL = 0.09 mL; because 3 mL − 2.6 mL = 0.4 mL, the difference is *not* within a percentage of error of 3%

12. 0.03 × 12.5 mL = 0.375; because 12.5 mL − 12.1 mL = 0.4 mL, the difference is *not* within a percentage of error of 3%

13. 0.03 × 1.8 mL = 0.054 mL; because 1.8 mL − 1.5 mL = 0.3 mL, the difference is *not* within a percentage of error of 3%

14. 0.03 × 3.2 mL = 0.096 mL; because 3.2 mL − 3.29 mL = −0.09 mL, the difference is within a percentage of error of 3%

15. 0.06 × 150 mg = 9 mg; because 150 mg − 149 mg = 1 mg, the difference is within a percentage of error of 6%

16. 0.06 × 200 mg = 12 mg; because 200 mg − 192 mg = 8 mg, the difference is within a percentage of error of 6%

17. 0.06 × 30 mg = 1.8 mg; because 30 mg − 31.5 mg = −1.5 mg, the difference is within a percentage of error of 6% (or 1.5 mg < 1.8 mg)

18. 0.06 × 454 mg = 27.24 mg; because 454 mg − 450 mg = 4 mg, the difference is within a percentage of error of 6%

19. 200 mL × 0.005 = 1 mL; 200 mL − 1 mL = 199 mL; 200 mL + 1 mL = 201 mL; the acceptable range is 199 mL to 201 mL

20. 10.3 mL × 0.0075 = 0.07725 mL, rounded to 0.08 mL; 10.3 mL − 0.08 mL = 10.22 mL; 10.3 mL + 0.08 mL = 10.38 mL; the acceptable range is 10.22 mL to 10.38 mL

21. 830 mL × 0.02 = 16.6 mL; 830 mL − 16.6 mL = 813.4 mL; 830 mL + 16.6 mL = 846.6 mL; the acceptable range is 813.4 mL to 846.6 mL

22. 18 g × 0.0015 = 0.027 g, rounded to 0.03 g; 18 g − 0.03 g = 17.97 g; 18 g + 0.03 g = 18.03 g; the acceptable range is 17.97 g to 18.03 g

23. 750 mg × 0.004 = 3 mg; 750 mg − 3 mg = 747 mg; 750 mg + 3 mg = 753 mg; the acceptable range is 747 mg to 753 mg

24. 100 mg × 0.2 = 20 mg; so the range of accuracy is 80 mg (100 mg − 20 mg) to 120 mg (100 mg + 20 mg)

25. 500 mg × 0.12 = 60 mg; so the range of vitamin C contained in the tablet is 440 mg (500 mg − 60 mg) to 560 mg (500 mg + 60 mg)

Chapter 3

3.1 Problem Set

1. Number does not meet standard validity tests. J is not an appropriate initial letter for the DEA number of a medical doctor. Checksum calculation: 2 + 6 + 8 = 16; (1 + 9 + 7) × 2 = 34; 16 + 34 = 50; last digit of checksum matches last digit (0).

2. The number meets standard validity tests. M is an appropriate initial letter for the DEA number of a mid-level practitioner; G is the first letter of the prescriber's last name. Checksum calculation: 3 + 8 + 6 = 17; (0 + 1 + 5) × 2 = 12; 17 + 12 = 29; last digit of checksum matches last digit (9).

3. Number does not meet standard validity tests. B is an appropriate initial letter for the DEA number of a primary practitioner; H is the first letter of the prescriber's last name. Checksum calculation: 9 + 9 + 0 = 18; (9 + 8 + 7) × 2 = 48; 18 + 48 = 66; last digit of sum (6) does not match checksum digit (0).

4. Number does not meet standard validity tests. A is an appropriate initial letter for the DEA number of a primary practitioner; L is the first letter of the prescriber's last name. Checksum calculation: $6 + 3 + 6 = 15$; $(2 + 0 + 1) \times 2 = 6$; $15 + 6 = 21$; Last digit of sum (1) does not match checksum digit (8).

5. Number does not meet standard validity tests. The second letter (D) of the DEA number does not match the first letter of the physician's last name (L). Checksum calculation: $7 + 3 + 2 = 12$; $(6 + 8 + 2) \times 2 = 32$; $12 + 32 = 44$; last digit of checksum matches last digit (4).

6. Number meets standard validity tests. B is an appropriate initial letter for the DEA number of a primary practitioner; P is the first letter of the prescriber's last name. Checksum calculation: $4 + 1 + 2 = 7$; $(4 + 2 + 0) \times 2 = 12$; $7 + 12 = 19$; last digit of checksum matches last digit (9).

7. Number meets standard validity tests. A is an appropriate initial letter for the DEA number of a primary practitioner; P is the first letter of the prescriber's last name. Checksum calculation: $3 + 5 + 4 = 12$; $(0 + 1 + 9) \times 2 = 20$; $12 + 20 = 32$; last digit of checksum matches last digit (2).

8. Number meets standard validity tests. M is an appropriate initial letter for the DEA number of a mid-level practitioner; W is the first letter of the prescriber's last name. Checksum calculation: $2 + 6 + 2 = 10$; $(8 + 4 + 2) \times 2 = 28$; $10 + 28 = 38$; last digit of checksum matches last digit (8).

9. b. 0.25% acetic acid is correct answer. Calculation: x g/100 mL = 1 g/400 mL; x g = 0.25 g

10. c. isoproterenol 1:200 solution is correct answer. Calculation: x g/100 mL = 0.005 g/mL; x g = 0.5 g, or 0.5%, a 1:200 solution

11. Brand/trade name: Macrobid
Generic name: nitrofurantoin monohydrate
Dosage form: capsules
Strength: 100 mg
Total quantity: 100 capsules
Storage requirements: Store at controlled room temperature (59–86 °F)
Manufacturer: Almitica Pharma
NDC number: 52427-285-01

12. Brand/trade name: Prozac
Generic name: fluoxetine
Dosage form: pulvules or capsules
Strength: 20 mg
Total quantity: 100 capsules
Storage requirement(s): room temperature (59–86 °F)
Manufacturer: Eli Lilly & Company (Dista)
NDC number: 077-3105-02

13. Brand/trade name: Strattera
Generic name: atomoxetine HCl
Dosage form: capsules
Strength: 18 mg
Total quantity: 30 capsules
Storage requirements: Store at 25 °C (77 °F) excursions permitted 15–30 °C (59–86 °F)
Manufacturer: Lilly
NDC number: 0002-3238-30

14. Brand/trade name: none
Generic name: spironolactone
Dosage form: tablets
Strength: 50 mg
Total quantity: 100 tablets
Storage requirements: 20° to 25 °C (68° to 77 °F). (See USP Controlled Room Temp.) Room Temperature (68–77 °F)
Manufacturer: Mylan
NDC number: 0378-0243-01

15. Brand/trade name: Vistaril
Generic name: hydroxyzine pamoate
Dosage form: capsules
Strength: 50 mg
Total quantity: 100 capsules
Storage requirements: Store below 86 °F (30 °C)
Manufacturer: Pfizer Labs
NDC number: 0069-5420-66

16. Brand/trade name: Restoril
Generic name: temazepam
Dosage form: capsule
Strength: 7.5 mg
Total quantity: 100 capsules
Storage requirement(s): room temperature
Manufacturer: Mallinckrodt
NDC number: 0406-9915-01

17. 20 tablets; XX is Roman numeral for 20

18. 3 capsules/day × 10 days = 30 capsules

19. 48 tablets. Determine number of tablets needed for each part of the prescription: 4 tablets/dose × 2 doses/day × 2 days = 16 tablets; 3 tablets/dose × 2 doses/day × 2 days = 12 tablets; 4 tablets/dose × 1 dose/day × 2 days = 8 tablets; 3 tablets/dose × 1 dose/day × 2 days = 6 tablets; 2 tablets/dose × 1 dose/day × 2 days = 4 tablets; 1 tablet/dose × 1 dose/day × 2 days = 2 tablets. Add the subtotals to determine the total number to dispense: 16 tablets + 12 tablets + 8 tablets + 6 tablets + 4 tablets + 2 tablets = 48 tablets.

20. 1 oz/day × 7 days/week = 7 oz for a one week supply

21. 150 capsules; #CL = Roman numeral C (100) plus Roman numeral L (50)

22. 28 capsules/2 daily = 14 days

23. 90 tablets/1 daily = 90 days

24. 120 capsules/4 daily = 30 days; (every 6 hours assumes 4 daily)

25. 120 doses/2 daily = 60 days

3.2 Problem Set

1. bid = twice a day

2. DAW = dispense as written

3. IM = intramuscular

4. IV = intravenous

5. mL = milliliter

6. NKA = no known allergy

7. npo = nothing by mouth

8. q3 h = every 3 hours

9. qid = four times a day

10. tid = three times a day

11. A route of administration is the way the drug is to be given to the patient.

12. Oral, injection, rectal, topical. Additional answers may vary.

13. IM intramuscular; IV intravenous; po by mouth. Additional answers may vary.

14. bid = twice a day; qid = four times a day; q2 h = every 2 hours, etc. Additional answers may vary.

15. IM (intramuscular) administration means medication is injected into a muscle; IV (intravenous) administration means it is injected into a vein.

16. Take two capsules by mouth four times a day as needed for itching.

17. Apply one patch every night at bedtime and remove every morning.

18. Apply one half inch of ointment every six hours.

19. Take two tablets by mouth three times a day before meals.

20. Take one half tablet by mouth twice a day.

21. Instill two drops into the right eye every four hours.

22. Take one tablet by mouth each week, 30 minutes before breakfast with water

23. 6 weeks × 7 days = 42 days; 42 days × 1 capsule daily = 42 capsules should be dispensed.

24. 1 capsule × 3 daily × 10 days = 30 capsules; 10 remain; 1 daily × 10 capsules = 10 additional days. 10 days + 10 days = 20 days total.

25. Presuming that a patient would take 1 tablet in the morning, one midday, and one in the evening; 3 a day would be taken while awake. 3 tablets daily/63 tablets = 21 days

Chapter 4

4.1 Problem Set

1. mcg

2. mg

3. L

4. g

5. kg

6. m

7. cm

8. mL

9. cc

10. dL

11. 0.6 g

12. 50 kg

13. 0.4 mg

14. 0.04 L

15. 4.2 g

16. 0.005 g

17. 0.06 g

18. 2.6 L

19. 0.03 L

20. 0.02 mL

21. 13,333 doses
Work: 5 kg = 5000 g = 5,000,000 mg
5,000,000 mg available/375 mg = 13,333.33
doses, rounded to 13,333 doses

22. a. 2 tablets/dose × 2 doses/day = 4 tablets;
4 tablets + 1 tablet/dose = 5 tablets/day
5 tablets/day × 30 days = 150 tablets

   b. 150 tablets × 0.05 mg/tablet = 7.5 mg/
month

23. 0.9 g/3 doses = 0.3 g

24. a. 1.2 g/4 doses = 0.3 g
   b. Convert to milligrams, 0.3 g × 1000 mg/1 g
= 300 mg
Only the 300 mg tablets can be used.

25. a. x g/100 mL = 1 g/1000 mL, x g = 0.1 g or
0.1%

   b. August 31, 2015

4.2 Problem Set

1. x mg/1964 mcg = 1 mg/1000 mcg; x mg =
1.964 mg

2. x g/418 mg = 1 g/1000 mg; x g = 0.418 g

3. x mcg/651 mg = 1000 mcg/1 mg; x mcg =
651,000 mcg

4. x mcg/0.84 mg = 1000 mcg/1 mg; x mcg =
840 mcg

5. x mcg/0.012 g = 1,000,000 mcg/1 g; x mcg =
12,000 mcg

6. x g/9,213,406 mcg = 1 g/1,000,000 mcg; x g =
9.213406 g

7. x g/284 mg = 1 g/1000 mg; x g = 0.284 g

8. x mg/9382.5 mcg = 1 mg/1000 mcg; x mg =
9.3825 mg

9. x g/12,321 mcg = 1 g/1,000,000 mcg; x g =
0.012321 g

10. x kg/184 g = 1 kg/1000 g; x kg = 0.184 kg

11. 52 mL × 1 L/1000 mL = 0.052 L

12. 2.06 g × 1000 mg/1 g = 2060 mg

13. 16 mg × 1000 mcg/1 mg = 16,000 mcg

14. 256 mg × 1 g/1000 mg = 0.256 g

15. 2,703,000 mcg × 1 g/1,000,000 mcg = 2.703 g

16. 6.9 L × 1000 mL/1 L = 6900 mL

17. 62.5 mg × 1 g/1000 mg = 0.0625 g

18. 15 kg × 1000 g/1 kg = 15,000 g

19. 2,785,000 mcg × 1 g/1,000,000 mcg = 2.785 g

20. 8.234 mg × 1000 mcg/1 mg = 8234 mcg

21. 2 kg × 1,000,000 mg/1 kg = 2,000,000 mg;
or x mg/2 kg = 1,000,000 mg/1 kg, x mg =
2,000,000 mg

22. 21 L × 1000 mL/1 L = 21,000 mL; or x mL/21
L = 1000 mL/1 L, x mL = 21,000 mL

23. 576 mL × 1 L/1000 mL = 0.576 L;
or x L/576 mL = 1 L/1000 mL, x L = 0.576 L

24. 823 kg × 1,000,000 mg/1 kg = 823,000,000
mg; or x mg/823 kg = 1,000,000 mg/1 kg, x
mg = 823,000,000 mg

25. 27 mcg × 1 mg/1000 mcg = 0.027 mg; or
x mg/27 mcg = 1 mg/1000 mcg, x mg =
0.027 mg

26. 5000 mcg × 1 mg/1000 mcg = 5 mg; or
x mg/5000 mcg = 1 mg/1000 mcg, x mg =
5 mg

27. 20 mcg × 1 mg/1000 mcg = 0.02 mg; or
x mg/20 mcg = 1 mg/1000 mcg, x mg =
0.02 mg

28. 4.624 mg × 1000 mcg/1 mg = 4624 mcg; or x mcg/4.624 mg = 1000 mcg/1 mg, x mcg = 4624 mcg

29. 3.19 g × 1000 mg/1 g = 3190 mg; or x mg/3.19 g = 1000 mg/1 g, x mg = 3190 mg

30. 8736 mcg × 1 mg/1000 mcg = 8.736 mg; or x mg/8736 mcg = 1 mg/1000 mcg, x mg = 8.736 mg

31. 830 mL × 1 L/1000 mL = 0.83 L; or x L/830 mL = 1 L/1000 mL, x L = 0.83 L

32. 0.94 L × 1000 mL/1 L = 940 mL; or x mL/0.94 L = 1000 mL/1 L, x mL = 940 mL

33. 1.84 g × 1000 mg/1 g = 1840 mg; or x mg/1.84 g = 1000 mg/1 g, x mg = 1840 mg

34. 560 mg × 1 g/1000 mg = 0.56 g; or x g/560 mg = 1 g/1000 mg, x g = 0.56 g

35. 1200 mcg × 1 mg/1000 mcg = 1.2 mg; or x mg/1200 mcg = 1 mg/1000 mcg, x mg = 1.2 mg

36. 125 mcg × 1 mg/1000 mcg = 0.125 mg; or x mg/125 mcg = 1 mg/1000 mcg, x mg = 0.125 mg

37. 0.275 mg × 1000 mcg/1 mg = 275 mcg; or x mcg/0.275 mg = 1000 mcg/1 mg, x mcg = 275 mcg

38. 480 mL × 1 L/1000 mL = 0.48 L; or x L/480 mL = 1 L/1000 mL, x L = 0.48 L

39. 239 mg × 1 g/1000 mg = 0.239 g or x g/239 mg = 1 g/1000 mg, x g = 0.239 g

40. 1500 mg × 1 g/1000 mg = 1.5 g; or x g/1500 mg = 1 g/1000 mg, x g = 1.5 g

41. a. 2 tsp/dose × 5 mL/tsp × 2 doses/day = 20 mL/day

    b. 20 mL/day × 7 days/course of treatment = 140 mL/course of treatment

    c. 20 mL/day × 125 mg/5 mL × 1 g/1000 mg = 0.5 g

    d. Since each bottle contains 100 mL, two bottles will be needed (200 mL − 140 mL = 60 mL to be discarded).

42. (1) Convert 1.5 g to milligrams: x mg/1.5 g = 1000 mg/1 g, x mg = 1500 mg.
    (2) Determine number of capsules: 1500 mg × 1 capsule/250 mg = 6 capsules

43. a. Convert the prescribed dose to grams, 1000 mg = 1 g. Since one vial contains 10 g, there are ten 1 g doses in one vial.

    b. x days/10 doses × 1 day/2 doses, x days = 5 days

4.3 Problem Set

1. x tablets/30 mg = 1 tablet/7.5 mg, x tablets = 4 tablets

2. x mL/20 mg = 2 mL/25 mg, x mL = 1.6 mL

3. x mL/125 mg = 5 mL/100 mg, x mL = 6.25 mL, rounded to 6.3 mL

4. x mL/4 mg = 1 mL/5 mg, x mL = 0.8 mL

5. x capsules/1750 mg = 1 capsule/250 mg, x capsule = 7 capsules

6. x mL/40 mg = 5mL/100 mg; x mL = 2mL

7. x mL/400 mg = 5 mL/200 mg, x mL = 10 mL

8. a. x mL/1000 mg = 5 mL/250 mg, x mL = 20 mL

    b. x mL/75 mg = 1 mL/15 mg, x mL = 5 mL

    c. x tablets/500 mg = 1 tablet/1000 mg, x tablets = 0.5 tablet; 0.5 tablet/dose × 4 doses/day = 2 tablets/day

9. Convert 10 mg to 10,000 mcg; x mL/10,000 mcg = 1 mL/40 mcg, x mL = 250 mL

10. x mg/2 mL = 20 mg/2 mL; x mg = 20 mg

11. Convert 400 mcg to 0.4 mg; x mL/1 mg = 1 mL/0.4 mg, x mL = 2.5 mL

12. x mcg/1.2 mL = 400 mcg/1 mL, x mcg = 480 mcg

13. Convert 80 mg to 80,000 mcg; x mcg/0.63 mL = 80,000 mcg/15 mL, x mcg = 3360 mcg

14. 1.05 kg = 1050 g = 1,050,000 mg; x capsules/1,050,000 mg = 1 capsule/35 mg, x capsules = 30,000 capsules

15. x doses/880 mg = 2 doses/80 mg, x dose = 22 doses

16. Convert 1600 mg to 1,600,000 mcg; x mcg/4 mL = 1,600,000 mcg/560 mL, x mcg = 11,428.571 mcg, rounded to 11,428.6 mcg

17. Convert 10 mg to 10,000 mcg; x mL/10,000 mcg = 1 mL/40 mcg, x mL = 250 mL

18. x mL/2000 units = 1 mL/1000 units; x mL = 2 mL

19. x mL/900 mg = 1 mL/150 mg; x mL = 6 mL

20. x mg/4 mL = 150 mg/1 mL; x mg = 600 mg

21. x mg/12.5 mL = 50 mg/5 mL, x mg = 125 mg

22. x mL/100 mg = 5 mL/50 mg, x mL = 10 mL

23. x mg/0.5 mL = 10 mg/mL; x = 5 mg

24. 0.8 mL × 10 mg/1 mL; x = 8 mg

25. x mL/150 mg = 5 mL/100 mg; x mL = 7.5 mL

26. 0.5 g = 500 mg; x mL/500 mg = 5 mL/100 mg; x mL = 25 mL

27. x mL/50 mg = 1 mL/5 mg; x = 10 mL

28. x mg/0.8 mL = 5 mg/1 mL, x = 4 mg

29. x mL/100 mg = 5 mL/125 mg, x mL = 4 mL

30. x mg/7.5 mL = 125 mg/5 mL, x mg = 187.5 mg; rounded to 188 mg

31. x mL/20 mg = 5 mL/12.5 mg, x mL = 8 mL

32. x mL/50 mg = 5 mL/12.5 mg, x mL = 20 mL

33. a. Since 150 mg × 1 capsule/25 mg = 6 capsules, 150 mg × 1 capsule/50 mg = 3 capsules, and 150 mg × 1 capsule/75 mg = 2 capsules, the 75 mg/capsule product will result in the fewest capsules taken per day, 2 capsules.

   b. 2 capsules/day × 7 days/week = 14 capsules/week

34. a. 500 mg/dose × 4 doses/day = 2000 mg/day; 2000 mg × 5 mL/250 mg = 40 mL

   b. 50 mg × 1 tablet/25 mg = 2 tablets

   c. 8 mEq × 15 mL/20 mEq = 6 mL

   d. 200 mg/dose × 3 doses/day = 600 mg/day; 600 mg × 5 mL/100 mg = 30 mL

4.4 Problem Set

To view the completed Nomogram for Estimating Body Surface Area of Children for questions 1–4, turn to page 283.

1. 0.405 m², rounded to 0.41 m²

2. 0.565 m², rounded to 0.57 m²

3. 0.89 m²

4. 0.71 m²

To view the completed Nomogram for Estimating Body Surface Area of Adults for questions 5–10, turn to page 284.

5. 1.275 m², rounded to 1.28 m²

6. 1.75 m²

7. 1.72 m²

8. 1.96 m²

9. 1.49 m²

10. 2.15 m²

11. 56 kg × 0.5 mg/kg = 28 mg

12. 87 kg × 125 mg/kg = 10,875 mg per day; for each dose, 10,875 mg/6 doses = 1812.5 mg

13. 1.4 kg × 4 mL/kg = 5.6 mL

14. a. 80 kg × 0.625 mg/kg = 50 mg

   b. 50 mg/3 doses = 16.6666 mg/dose, rounded to 16.67 mg/dose

15. 6 kg × 5 mg/kg/day = 30 mg/day; 30 mg/2 doses = 15 mg/dose

16. 68.64 kg × 125 mg/kg/day = 8580 mg/day

17. 10 kg × 10 mg/kg/day = 100 mg/day; 1 day = 24 hr; 100 mg/day = 100 mg/24 hr; 100 mg/2 = 50 mg; 24 hr/2 = 12 hr; 50 mg/12 hr

18. 1.1 m² × 25 mg/m² = 27.5 mg; 27.5 mg/2 doses = 13.75 mg/dose

19. 0.67 m² × 0.75 mg/m² = 0.5025 mg, rounded to 0.50 mg

20. 0.85 m² × 100 mg/m² = 85 mg

21. 0.71 m² × 250 mg/m² = 177.5 mg

22. 0.83 m² × 3.3 mg/m² = 2.739 mg, rounded to 2.74 mg

23. $0.7 \text{ m}^2 \times 2 \text{ mg/m}^2 = 1.4$ mg. The physician has ordered a dose higher than the recommended dose. To view the completed Nomogram for Estimating Body Surface Area of Children, turn to page 285.

24. $0.48 \text{ m}^2 \times 3.3 \text{ mg/m}^2 = 1.584$ mg. The physician has ordered a dose higher than the recommended dose. To view the completed Nomogram for Estimating Body Surface Area of Children, turn to page 286.

25. $0.47 \text{ m}^2 \times 250 \text{ mg/m}^2 = 117.5$ mg. The physician has ordered a dose higher than the recommended dose. To view the completed Nomogram for Estimating Body Surface Area of Children, turn to page 287.

26. 40.9 kg × 50 mg/kg/day = 2045 mg/day is the recommended dose; order is 300 mg × 3 doses/day = 900 mg/day, which is under the recommended dose per day.

27. a. 36.4 kg × 50 mg/kg = 1820 mg

    b. 36.4 kg × 100 mg/kg = 3640 mg

    c. 250 mg × 3 doses/day = 750 mg/day, which is under the minimum recommended dose

    d. 250 mg/dose × 50 mL/500 mg = 25 mL/dose

28. a. 5.45 kg × 20 mg/kg = 109 mg

    b. 5.45 kg × 40 mg/kg = 218 mg

    c. 125 mg × 3 doses/day = 375 mg, which is higher than the maximum recommended dose

    d. 125 mg/dose × 5 mL/125 mg = 5 mL/dose

29. a. 11.8 kg × 0.5 mg/kg = 5.9 mg

    b. 11.8 kg × 1 mg/kg = 11.8 mg

    c. 10 mL × 12 mg/5 mL = 24 mg

    d. No, it is not a safe dose. It is higher than 11.8 mg, the maximum recommended dose.

30. a. 9.32 kg × 5 mg/kg = 46.6 mg; 24 hr/day × 1 dose/8 hr = 3 doses/day; 46.6 mg × 3 doses/day = 139.8 mg/day

    b. 9.32 kg × 10 mg/kg = 93.2 mg; 24 hr/day × 1 dose/6 hr = 4 doses/day; 93.2 mg × 4 doses/day = 372.8 mg/day

    c. 125 mg/dose × 3 doses/day = 375 mg/day, which is higher than the maximum recommended dose

    d. 125 mg × 5 mL/100 mg = 6.25 mL

31. a. 50 kg × 25 mg/kg = 1250 mg

    b. 50 kg × 50 mg/kg = 2500 mg

    c. 500 mg × 2 doses/day = 1000 mg/day, which is under the minimum recommended dose

    d. 500 mg × 5 mL/250 mg = 10 mL

32. a. 28.6 kg × 10 mg/kg = 286 mg

    b. 28.6 kg × 15 mg/kg = 429 mg

    c. It is within the recommended range.

    d. 325 mg × 5 mL/160 mg = 10.156 mL, rounded to 10.16 mL

33. a. [8 years/(8 years + 12 years)] × 600 mg = 240 mg

    b. 68 lb/150 lb × 600 mg = 271.99 mg, rounded to 272 mg

Chapter 5

5.1 Problem Set

1. 8 cups × 1 pt/2 cups = 4 pt

2. 3 pt × 2 cups/1 pt = 6 cups; 6 cups × 8 fl oz/1 cup = 48 fl oz

3. 1 pt × 2 cups/1 pt = 2 cups; 2 cups × 8 fl oz/1 cup = 16 fl oz; 16 fl oz × 2 tbsp/1 fl oz = 32 tbsp

4. 3 qt × 2 pt/1 qt = 6 pt; 6 pt × 2 cups/1 pt = 12 cups; 12 cups × 8 fl oz/1 cup = 96 fl oz

5. 28 tsp × 1 tbsp/3 tsp = 9.333 tbsp, rounded to 9.33 tbsp; 9.33 tbsp × 1 fl oz/2 tbsp = 4.665 fl oz, rounded to 4.67 fl oz or $4^2/_3$ fl oz

6. 1 pt × 1 qt/2 pt = 0.5 qt or $^1/_2$ qt

7. 6 cups × 8 fl oz/1 cup = 48 fl oz; 48 fl oz × 2 tbsp/1 fl oz = 96 tbsp; 96 tbsp × 3 tsp/1 tbsp = 288 tsp

8. 80 mL = 5.3 tbsp; $5^1/_3$ tbsp

9. 6 fl oz = 180 mL

10. 90 mL = 3 fl oz

11. 800 mL = 1.67 pt or 1⅔ pt

12. 53 mL = 10.6 tsp, about 10⅔ tsp

13. 35 mL = 7 tsp

14. 10 L = 10,000 mL; 10,000 mL × 1 gal/3840 mL = 2.604 gal, rounded to 2.6 gal

15. 4 tbsp = 60 mL

16. 15 mL × 1 tsp/5 mL = 3 tsp

17. 720 mL × 1 pt/480 mL = 1.5 pt, or 1½ pt

18. 30 tsp × 5 mL/1 tsp = 150 mL

19. 120 mL × 1 fl oz/30 mL = 4 fl oz

20. ½ gal = 0.5 gal × 3840 mL/1 gal = 1920 mL

21. 2 L = 2000 mL; 2000 mL × 1 pt/480 mL = 4.166 pt, rounded to 4.2 pt

22. 3 tbsp × 15 mL/1 tbsp = 45 mL

23. 1 fl oz × 30 mL/1 fl oz = 30 mL

24. 2 fl oz × 30 mL/1 fl oz = 60 mL

25. 3 fl oz × 30 mL/1 fl oz = 90 mL

26. 4 fl oz × 30 mL/1 fl oz = 120 mL

27. 5 fl oz × 30 mL/1 fl oz = 150 mL

28. 6 fl oz × 30 mL/1 fl oz = 180 mL

29. 7 fl oz × 30 mL/1 fl oz = 210 mL

30. 8 fl oz × 30 mL/1 fl oz = 240 mL

31. 12 fl oz × 30 mL/1 fl oz = 360 mL

32. 16 fl oz × 30 mL/1 fl oz = 480 mL

33. 2 oz × 30 g/1 oz = 60 g

34. 1.5 oz × 30 g/1 oz = 45 g

35. 8 oz × 30 g/1 oz = 240 g

36. 906 g × 1 lb/454 g = 1.995 lb, rounded to 2 lb

37. 30 g × 1 lb/454 g = 0.0660 lb, rounded to 0.07 lb, about 1/16 lb

38. 0.8 oz × 30 g/1 oz = 24 g

39. 3.5 lb × 1 kg/2.2 lb = 1.59 kg, rounded to 1.6 kg

40. 14 lb × 1 kg/2.2 lb = 6.364 kg, rounded to 6.4 kg

41. 42 lb × 1 kg/2.2 lb = 19.09 kg, rounded to 19 kg

42. 97 lb × 1 kg/2.2 lb = 44.09 kg, rounded to 44 kg

43. 112 lb × 1 kg/2.2 lb = 50.909 kg, rounded to 50.9 kg

44. 165 lb × 1 kg/2.2 lb = 75 kg

45. 178 lb × 1 kg/2.2 lb = 80.909 kg, rounded to 80.9 kg

46. 247 lb × 1 kg/2.2 lb = 112.27 kg, rounded to 112 kg

47. 2 pt = 960 mL and 6 fl oz = 180 mL, so total milliliters = 960 mL + 180 mL = 1140 mL; 1140 mL × 1 dose/5 mL = 228 doses

48. 3 cups = 24 fl oz; 24 fl oz = 720 mL; 720 mL × 1 dose/10 mL = 72 doses

49. 12 bottles × 16 fl oz = 192 fl oz; 192 fl oz = 5760 mL; 5760 mL × 1 dose/15 mL = 384 doses

50. 5 fl oz = 150 mL; 150 mL × 1 dose/5 mL = 30 doses

51. 1 pt = 480 mL; 480 mL × 1 dose/15 mL = 32 doses

52. 1.5 fl oz = 45 mL; 45 mL × 3 times/day = 135 mL/day

53. 8 fl oz = 240 mL; 240 mL × 1 dose/7.5 mL = 32 doses

54. ½ tsp × 5 mL/1 tsp × 10 mg/1 mL = 25 mg

55. 4 fl oz × 30 mL/1 fl oz = 120 mL; 120 mL × 10 mg/1 mL = 1200 mg; 1200 mg × 1 day/20 mg = 60 days

56. 20 mL × 3 tsp/15 mL = 4 tsp

57. 473 mL × 1 day/15 mL = 31.53 days or 31½ days

58. Conversions: 180 lb × 1 kg/2.2 lb = 81.8181 kg, rounded to 81.8 kg; 2 tsp × 5 mL/1 tsp = 10 mL
81.8 kg × 10 mL/68 kg = 12.029411 mL, rounded to 12 mL
300 mL × 1 dose/12 mL = 25 doses

59. Conversions: 52 lb × 1 kg/2.2 lb = 23.636 kg, rounded to 23.6 kg; 1 tsp × 5 mL/1 tsp = 30

5 mL; 4 fl oz $\times$ 30 mL/1 fl oz = 120 mL

23.6 kg $\times$ 5 mL/20 kg = 5.9 mL

120 mL $\times$ 1 dose/5.9 mL = 20.3389 doses, or 20 full doses

60. Conversions: 172 lb $\times$ 1 kg/2.2 lb = 78.181 kg, rounded to 78.2 kg; 2 tbsp $\times$ 15 mL/1 tbsp = 30 mL; 12 fl oz $\times$ 30 mL/1 fl oz = 360 mL

78.2 kg $\times$ 30 mL/50 kg = 46.92 mL, rounded to 46.9 mL

360 mL $\times$ 1 dose/46.9 mL = 7.6759 doses, or 7 full doses

5.2 Problem Set

1. 243 mg

2. 324 mg

3. 405 mg

4. 648 mg

5. 6 lb $\times$ 1 kg/2.2 lb = 2.727 kg, rounded to 2.73 kg; per day range is 6.6 mcg to 16.4 mcg (rounded from 6.552 mcg and 16.38 mcg)

6. 1 lb = 16 oz, so 7 lb 12 oz = (16 oz $\times$ 7) + 12 oz = 124 oz, and 124 oz / 16 oz = 7.75 lb; 7.75 lb $\times$ 1 kg/2.2 lb = 3.52 kg; per day range is 8.4 mcg (rounded from 8.448 mcg) to 21.1 mcg

7. 23 lb $\times$ 1 kg/2.2 lb = 10.454 kg, rounded to 10.45 kg; per day range is 37.6 mcg to 50.2 mcg (rounded from 50.16 mcg)

8. 18 lb $\times$ 1 kg/2.2 lb = 8.181 kg, rounded to 8.18 kg; per day range is 24.5 mcg to 29.5 mcg (rounded from 29.448 mcg)

9. 5 mL $\times$ 80 mg/15 mL = 26.67 mg

10. 60 mg $\times$ 5 mL/120 mg = 2.5 mL or ½ tsp

11. 240 mL $\times$ 24 mg/5 mL = 1152 mg or 1.152 g

12. 120 mL $\times$ 65 mg/15 mL = 520 mg

13. 10 mL $\times$ 2500 mg/60 mL = 417 mg (rounded from 416.67 mg)

14. 15 mL $\times$ 260 mg/600 mL = 6.5 mg

15. 600 mL $\times$ 25 mg/5 mL = 3000 mg = 3 g

16. 30 mg/5 mL = x mg/15 mL

15 $\times$ 30 = 450

450/5 = 90

90 mg

17. 480 mL $\times$ 40 mg/1 mL = 19,200 mg or 19.2 g

18. a. 150 mL $\times$ 1 dose/3.75 mL = 40 doses; 40 doses $\times$ 1 day/3 doses = 13.3 days

    b. 3.75 mL/dose $\times$ 3 doses/day = 11.25 mL/day $\times$ 10 days = 112.5 mL; 150 mL − 112.5 mL = 37.5 mL

19. a. 1 tsp = 5 mL; 10 mL/day $\times$ 14 days = 140 mL; 150 mL bottle selected

    b. 150 mL − 140 mL = 10 mL

20. 1 tbsp = 15 mL and 12 fl oz/bottle = 360 mL/bottle; 15 mL/dose $\times$ 3 doses/day = 45 mL/day; 360 mL/bottle $\times$ 1 day/45 mL = 8 days/bottle

21. 2 tsp = 10 mL and 1 tbsp = 15 mL, so 25 mL/1 2-day total; 300 mL $\times$ 1 2-day unit/25 mL = 12 2-day units, or 24 days

22. 600 mL $\times$ 25 mg/15 mL = 1000 mg or 1 g

23. 12 fl oz/bottle = 360 mL/bottle and 1 fl oz $\times$ 4 doses/day = 30 mL $\times$ 4 doses/day = 120 mL/day; 120 mL/day $\times$ 14 days/treatment = 1680 mL/treatment; 1680 mL/treatment $\times$ 1 bottle/360 mL = 4.666 bottles, or a total of 5 bottles to be purchased

24. (4 tablets $\times$ 2/day) + (3 tablets $\times$ 2/day) + (1 tablet $\times$ 1/day) = 15 tablets

25. 24 hr/day $\times$ 1 dose/3 hr = 8 doses/day; 8 doses/day $\times$ 10 days = 80 doses; 80 doses $\times$ (1 mL/dose $\times$ 2 cheeks) = 160 mL

26. a. 12 fl oz/bottle = 360 mL/bottle, 1 tsp/dose = 5 mL/dose; 360 mL/bottle $\times$ 25 mg/5 mL = 1800 mg/bottle

    b. 9 g = 9000 mg; 9000 mg/therapy $\times$ 1 bottle/1800 mg = 5 bottles; 5 bottles − 1 initial bottle = 4 refills

27. 2 tsp/dose = 10 mL/dose; 3 doses/day $\times$ 10 mL/dose = 30 mL/day; 30 mL/ day $\times$ 15 days/treatment = 450 mL/ treatment; 450 mL/treatment $\times$ 1 fl oz/30 mL = 15 fl oz/treatment

28. 2 tbsp/dose = 30 mL/dose; 3 doses/day $\times$ 30 mL/dose = 90 mL/day; 20 days/treatment $\times$ 90 mL/day = 1800 mL/treatment

29. 1 tsp = 5 mL
Child 1: 5 mL/dose × 3 doses/day =
15 mL/day; 15 mL/day × 4 days = 60 mL
Child 2: 10 mL/dose × 3 doses/day =
30 mL/day; 30 mL/day × 4 days = 120 mL
60 mL + 120 mL = 180 mL
Since 1 bottle = 4 fl oz, 4 fl oz/bottle ×
30 mL/1 fl oz = 120 mL/bottle
The mother will need 2 bottles, or 240 mL.

30. Child 1: 5 mL × 25 mg/5 mL; x mg = 25 mg
Child 2: 10 mL × 25 mg/5 mL; x mg = 50 mg

31. ¾ tsp = 0.75 tsp; 0.75 tsp × 5 mL/tsp =
3.75 mL; 3.75 mL × 187 mg/5 mL = 140.25 mg

32. 1½ tsp = 1.5 tsp; 1.5 tsp × 5 mL/tsp =
7.5 mL; 7.5 mL × 187 mg/5 mL = 280.5 mg

33. 125 mg × 5 mL/187 mg = 3.3422 mL,
rounded to 3.34 mL

34. 500 mg × 5 mL/187 mg = 13.3689 mL,
rounded to 13.37 mL

35. a. 180 g/3 equal parts = 60 g of each

    b. 180 g × 1 oz/30 g = 6 oz; use a 6 oz jar

    c. 1/3/201X + 6 months = 7/3/201X

36. 12 fl oz bottle × 30 mL/1 fl oz = 360 mL;
360 mL × 1 syringe/60 mL = 6 syringes

5.3 Problem Set

1. (0° − 32°) ÷ 1.8 = -17.777 °C, rounded to
-17.8 °C

2. (23° − 32°) ÷ 1.8 = -5 °C

3. (36° − 32°) ÷ 1.8 = 2.222 °C, rounded to
2.2 °C

4. (40° − 32°) ÷ 1.8 = 4.444 °C, rounded to
4.4 °C

5. (64° − 32°) ÷ 1.8 = 17.777 °C, rounded to
17.8 °C

6. (72° − 32°) ÷ 1.8 = 22.222 °C, rounded to
22.2 °C

7. (98.6° − 32°) ÷ 1.8 = 37 °C

8. (100.5° − 32°) ÷ 1.8 = 38.055 °C, rounded
to 38.1 °C

9. (102.8° − 32°) ÷ 1.8 = 39.333 °C, rounded
to 39.3 °C

10. (105° − 32°) ÷ ÷ 1.8 = 40.555 °C, rounded to
40.6 °C

11. (1.8 × -15°) + 32 = 5 °F

12. (1.8 × 18°) + 32 = 64.4 °F

13. (1.8 × 27°) + 32 = 80.6 °F

14. (1.8 × 31°) + 32 = 87.8 °F

15. (1.8 × 38°) + 32 = 100.4 °F

16. (1.8 × 40°) + 32 = 104 °F

17. (1.8 × 49°) + 32 = 120.2 °F

18. (1.8 × 63°) + 32 = 145.4 °F

19. (1.8 × 99.8°) + 32 = 211.64 °F, rounded to
211.6 °F

20. (1.8 × 101.4°) + 32 = 214.52 °F, rounded to
214.5 °F

21. (1.8 × 130°) + 32 = 266 °F

22. a. (1.8 × -20°) + 32 = -4 °F

    b. 2/1/15 + 6 months = August 1, 2015

23. (300° − 32°) ÷ 1.8 = 148.888 °C, rounded to
148.9 °C

24. a. 2.3 °C

    b. 3.2 °C

    c. 3.9 °C

    d. 2.1 °C

    e. 2.7 °C

    f. 1.6 °C; too cold

    g. 2.4 °C

    h. 2.7 °C

    i. 1.9 °C; too cold

    j. 3.8 °C

5.3 Problem Set, chart for question 24

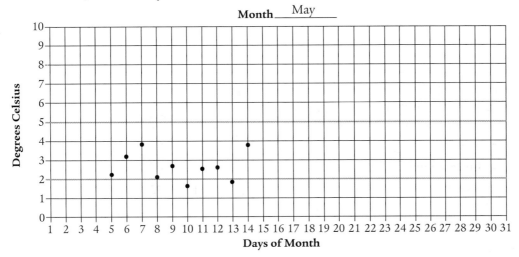

25. a. 35.2 °F; too cold   f. 37.8 °F

    b. 37.6 °F   g. 39 °F

    c. 37 °F   h. 36.5 °F

    d. 37.4 °F   i. 39.4 °F

    e. 40.1 °F   j. 40.5 °F

5.3 Problem Set, chart for question 25

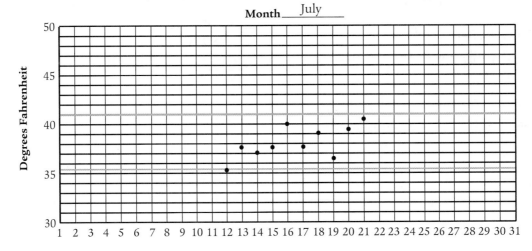

Chapter 6

6.1 Problem Set

1. x mL/50 mg = 1 mL/10 mg; x mL = 5 mL (5 mL syringe filled to 5 mL)

2. x mL/60 mg = 4 mL/40 mg; x = 6 mL; (10 mL syringe filled to 6 mL)

3. x mL/80 mg = 10 mL/100 mg; x mL = 8 mL ; (10 mL syringe filled to 8 mL)

4. x mL/0.75 mg = 1 mL/1 mg; x mL = 0.75 mL (1 mL syringe filled to 0.75 mL)

5. x mL/100 mg = 1 mL/50 mg; x mL = 2 mL ; (3 mL syringe filled to 2 mL)

6. x mL/30 mg = 2 mL/20 mg; x mL = 3 mL ; (3 mL syringe filled to 3 mL)

7. x mL/40 mg = 2 mL/20 mg; x mL = 4 mL (5 mL syringe filled to 4 mL)

8. Reconstitute to 100 mg/mL; x mL/250 mg = 1 mL/100 mg; x mL = 2.5 mL ; (3 mL syringe filled to 2.5 mL)

9. Reconstitute to 100 mg/mL; x mL/400 mg = 1 mL/100 mg; x mL = 4 mL ; (5 mL syringe filled to 4 mL)

10. x mL/50 mg = 100 mL/100 mg; x mL = 50 mL (60 mL syringe filled to 50 mL)

11. x mg/0.5 mL = 15 mg/1 mL; x mg = 7.5 mL

12. x mg/1.75 mL = 60 mg/2 mL; x mg = 52.5 mg

13. x mg/3.75 mL = 20 mg/1 mL; x mg = 75 mg

14. x mg/1.3 mL = 2 mg/2 mL; x mg = 1.3 mg

15. x mg/5 mL = 50 mg/10 mL; x mg = 25 mg

16. x mg/5 mL = 25 mg/5 mL; x mg = 25 mg

17. x mg/5 mL = 10 mg/10 mL; x mg = 5 mg

18. x mg/8 mL = 4 mg/1 mL; x mg = 32 mg

19. x mg/1.5 mL = 4 mg/2 mL; x mg = 3 mg

20. x mg/2.5 mL = 50 mg/1 mL; x mg = 125 mg

21. x g/2 mL = 1 g/1000 mL; x g = 0.002 g = 2 mg

22. x g/1 mL = 1 g/5000 mL; x g = 0.0002 g = 0.2 mg = 200 mcg

23. x g/1.5 mL = 1 g/10,000 mL; x g = 0.00015 g = 0.15 mg = 150 mcg

24. x g/1.4 mL = 1 g/2000 mL; x g = 0.0007 g = 0.7 mg = 700 mcg

25. x mg/2.5 mL = 1 g/10,000 mL; x mg = 0.00025 g = 0.25 mg = 250 mcg

26. Convert 500 mg to 0.5 g; x mL/0.5 g = 1000 mL/1 g; x mL = 500 mL

27. Convert 50 mg to 0.05 g; x mL/0.05 g = 10,000 mL/1 g; x mL = 500 mL

28. Convert 600 mg to 0.6 g; x mL/0.6 g = 300 mL/1 g; x mL = 180 mL

29. Convert 250 mg to 0.25 g; x mL/0.25 g = 500 mL/1 g; x mL = 125 mL

30. x mL/0.01 g = 750 mL/1 g; x mL = 7.5 mL

6.2 Problem Set

1. x mL/30 mEq = 1 mL/4.4 mEq; x mL = 6.81818 mL, rounded to 6.82 mL (10 mL syringe filled to 6.82 mL graduation mark)

2. x mL/45 mEq = 1 mL/4.4 mEq; x mL = 10.22727 mL, rounded to 10.23 mL (10 mL syringe filled to 10 mL graduation mark; 1 mL syringe filled to .23 mL graduation mark)

3. x tablets/32 mEq = 1 tablet/8 mEq; x tablets = 4 tablets

4. x mL/30 mEq = 15 mL/40 mEq; x mL = 11.25 mL; 11.25 mL/ 2 doses = 5.625 mL, rounded to 5.63 mL (10 mL syringe filled to 5.63 mL graduation mark)

5. x mEq/15 mL = 20 mEq/10 mL; x mEq = 30 mEq

6. x mL/30 mEq = 15 mL/20 mEq; x mL = 5.63 mL (10 mL syringe filled to 5.63 mL graduation mark)

7. Select the 20 mEq vial; x mL/14 mEq = 1 mL/2 mEq; x mL = 7 mL (10 mL syringe filled to 7 mL graduation mark)

8. Select the 20 mEq vial; x mL/19 mEq = 1 mL/2 mEq; x mL = 9.5 mL (10 mL syringe filled to 9.5 mL graduation mark)

9. Select the 40 mEq vial ; x mL/27 mEq = 1 mL/2 mEq; x mL = 13.5 mL

10. Select the 10 mEq vial; x mL/50 mEq = 1 mL/2 mEq; x mL = 25 mL

11. x mEq/8 mL = 30 mEq/15 mL; x mEq = 16 mEq or x mEq/8 mL = 2 mEq/1 mL; x mEq = 16 mEq

12. x mEq/15 mL = 40 mEq/20 mL; x mEq = 30 mEq or x mEq/15 mL = 2 mEq/1 mL; x mEq = 30 mEq

13. x mL/132 mEq = 1 mL/4 mEq; x mL = 33 mL (60 mL syringe filled to 33 mL graduation mark)

14. x mL/120 mEq = 1 mL/4 mEq; x mL = 30 mL (60 mL syringe filled to 30 mL graduation mark)

15. x mL/4 units = 1 mL/10 units; x mL = 0.4 mL

16. x units/2.8 mL = 10 units/1 mL; x units = 28 units (30 unit syringe filled to 28 units graduation mark)

17. x mL/3500 units = 1 mL/1000 units; x mL = 3.5 mL

18. x units/0.43 mL = 20,000 units/0.8 mL; x units = 10,750 units

19. x mL/24,000 units = 1 mL/10,000 units; x mL = 2.4 mL

20. x mL/24,000 units = 1 mL/10,000units; x = 2.4 mL

21. x mL/30 mg = 0.8 mL/80 mg; x mL = 0.3 mL

22. x mL/175,000 units = 1 mL/500,000 units; x mL = 0.35 mL

23. x mL/1,500,000 units = 1 mL/600,000 units; x mL = 2.5 mL

24. x mL/385,000 units = 1 mL/50,000 units; x mL = 7.7 mL

25. x mL/45 units = 1 mL/100 units; x mL = 0.45 mL

26. Calculate morning dose: x mL/18 units = 1 mL/100 units; x mL = 0.18 mL
Calculate evening dose: x mL/10 units = 1 mL/100 units; x mL = 0.1 mL
Add morning and evening doses: 0.18 mL/morning + 0.1 mL/evening = 0.28 mL/day
Since the vial shown on the label contains 10 mL, calculate time for 10 mL vial to last: x days/10 mL vial = 1 day/0.28 mL; x days = 35.714 days, rounded to 35 days

27. a. Add morning and evening units: 20 units + 18 units = 38 units/day

b. x mL/38 units = 1 mL/100 units; x mL = 0.38 mL. Calculate the number of days of therapy in a 10 mL vial: 10 mL / 0.38 mL = 26.3 days, rounded down to 26 days for 1 vial. Therefore, 2 vials will be needed for 30 days of therapy.

28. Humulin R: 10 units/dose × 1 dose/day × 30 days = 300 units for month; 300 units × 1mL/100 units = 3mL; 1 vial will be needed
Humulin 70/30 Mix: 15 units/dose × 2 doses/day × 30 days = 900 units for month ; 900 units × 1mL/100 units = 9mL; 1 vial will be needed

29. x units/0.5 mL = 100 units/1 mL; x units = 50 units

30. 20 units/dose x 2 doses/day = 40 units/day; x days/40 units = 1 mL/100 units; x mL = 0.4 mL are used daily
x days/20 mL = 1 day/0.4 mL; x days = 50 days

6.3 Problem Set

1. Convert 375 mg to 0.375 g.
x mL/1.5 g = 1 mL/0.375 g; x mL = 4 mL
4 mL final volume − 3.3 mL diluent volume = 0.7 mL powder volume

2. Convert 250 mg to 0.25 g, and note that 1 tsp = 5 mL.
x mL/5 g = 5 mL/0.25 g; x mL = 100 mL final volume
100 mL final volume − 8.6 mL powder volume = 91.4 mL diluent volume

3. Convert 1 g to 1000 mg.
x mL/1000 mg = 2 mL/125 mg; x mL = 16 mL final volume
16 mL final volume − 14.4 mL diluent = 1.6 mL powder volume

4. Convert 250 mg to 0.25 g.
x mL/2 g = 1 mL/0.25 g; x mL = 8 mL final volume
8 mL final volume − 6.8 mL diluent = 1.2 mL powder volume

5. Convert 125 mg to 0.125 g.
x mL/2 g = 1 mL/0.125 g; x mL = 16 mL final volume
Using the powder volume calculated in #4, 16 mL final volume − 1.2 mL powder volume = 14.8 mL diluent volume

6. Convert 250 mg to 0.25 g.
   x mL/4 g = 1 mL/0.25 g; x mL = 16 mL final volume
   16 mL final volume − 11.7 mL diluent = 4.3 powder volume

7. a. x mL/6 g = 2.5 mL/1 g; x mL = 15 mL final volume; 15 mL final volume − 12.5 mL diluent volume = 2.5 mL powder volume

   b. 2.5 mL powder volume + 2.5 mL diluent volume = 5 mL final volume; 6 g/5mL = 1.2 g/mL = 1200 mg/mL

8. 4 mL final volume − 3.3 mL diluent = 0.7 mL powder volume

9. Using the information from #8, 1 g/4 mL, and converting 1 g to 1000 mg: x mL/100 mg = 4 mL/1000 mg; x mL = 0.4 mL

10. x mL/2 g = 1 mL/0.2 g, x mL = 10 mL final volume; 10 mL final volume − 8.8 mL diluent = 1.2 mL powder volume

11. Convert 10 g to 10,000 mg; 45 mL DV + 5 mL PV = 50 mL FV; x mg/1 mL = 10,000 mg/50 mL; x mg = 200 mg, so there will be 200 mg/mL

12. Convert 8 g to 8000 mg, and remember 1 tsp = 5 mL. x mg/5 mL = 8000 mg/200 mL; x mg = 200 mg, so there are 200 mg/5 mL or 200 mg/tsp

13. a. x mL/20 g = 6 mL/1 g, x mL = 120 mL FV; 120 mL FV − 106 mL DV = 14 mL PV

    b. x mL/20 g = 3 mL/1 g, x mL = 60 mL FV; 60 mL FV − 14 mL PV = 46 mL DV

14. Convert 2 g to 2000 mg; x mL/2000 mg = 1 mL/375 mg, x mL = 5.3 mL FV; 5.3 mL FV − 3.5 mL DV = 1.8 mL PV

15. Convert 2.5 g to 2500 mg; x mL/2500 mg = 5 mL/300 mg, x mL = 41.7 mL FV; 41.7 mL FV − 9.6 mL PV = 32.1 mL DV

16. Convert 5 g to 5000 mg; x mL/5000 mg = 1 mL/250 mg, x mL = 20 mL FV; 20 mL FV − 8.6 mL DV = 11.4 mL PV

17. x mg/10 g = 2.5 mL/1 g, x mL = 25 mL FV; 25 mL FV − 20 mL DV = 5 mL PV; 5 mL PV + 35 mL new DV = 40 mL FV; 10 g/40 mL = 0.25 g/mL or 250 mg/mL

18. 5 mL FV − 4.3 mL DV = 0.7 mL PV

19. 25 mL DV + 5 mL PV = 30 mL FV; x mg = 167 mg, so 167 mg/mL

20. 90 mL DV + 10 mL PV = 100 mL FV; convert 20 g to 20,000 mg; x mg/1 mL = 20,000 mg/100 mL; x mg = 200 mg, so 200 mg/mL

21. 20 mL DV + 5 mL PV = 25 mL FV; convert 3 g to 3000 mg; x mg/1 mL = 3000 mg/25 mL; x mg = 120 mg, so 120 mg/mL

22. 100 mL FV − 67 mL DV = 33 mL PV

23. Convert 35 g to 35,000 mg; x mg/1 mL = 35,000 mg/100 mL, x mg = 350 mg, so 350 mg/mL

24. (1) 15 mL − 9 mL = 6 mL in bottle; (2) 10 mL + 0.2 mL = 10.2 mL vancomycin; (3) 10.2 mL vancomycin + 6 mL bottle = 16.2 mL FV; x mg/1 mL = 500 mg/16.2 mL; x mg = 30.8641 mg, rounded to 31 mg, so 31 mg/mL

25. a. x mg/1 mL = 1000 mg/4.4 mL; x mg = 227 mg, so 227 mg/mL; 1 mL + 9 mL = 10 mL, so 227 mg/10 mL, which is simplified to 22.7 mg/mL

    b. x mg /0.1 mL = 22.7 mg/1 mL = 2.27 mg

Chapter 7

7.1 Problem Set

1. w/v = 10 g/100 mL

2. w/v = 0.45 g/100 mL

3. v/v = 0.25 mL/100 mL

4. v/v = 7 mL/100 mL

5. 10 % = 10 g/100 mL; 10 g /100 mL = x mL/500 mL; 10 × 500 = 5000; 500/100 = 50 g

6. 2% = 2 g/100 mL= x g/1.3 mL; 2 × 1.3 = 2.6; 2.6/100 = 0.026 g; 1.026 × 1000 = 26 mg

7. 15 g/100 mL = 15%

8. 20 g/500 mL × 100; 20/5000 = 0.04; 0.04 × 100 = 4%

9. 0.15 g/1 mL × 100; 0.15/1 = 0.15; 0.15 × 100 = 15%

10. 0.03 g/ 1 mL × 100; 0.03/1 = 0.03; 0.03 × 100 = 3%

11. 0.005 g/1 mL $\times$ 100; 0.005/1 = 0.005; 0.005 $\times$ 100 = 0.5%

12. 0.002 g/1 mL $\times$ 100; 0.002/1 = 0.002; 0.002 $\times$ 100 = 0.2%

13. 0.01 g/1 mL $\times$ 100; 0.01/1 = 0.01. 0.01 $\times$ 100 = 1%

14. 0.002 g/1 mL $\times$ 100; 0.02/1 = 0.02; 0.02 $\times$ 100 = 2%

15. 3.5% = 3.5 g/100 mL = x g/2500 mL; 3.5 $\times$ 2500 = 8750; 8750/100 = 87.5 g

16. 10% = 10 g/100 mL = x g/ 1000 mL; 10 $\times$ 1000 = 10,000; 10,000/100 = 100 g

17. 0.25% = 0.25 g/100 mL = x g/1000 mL; 0.25 $\times$ 1000 = 250; 250/100 = 2.5 g

18. 0.9% = 0.9 g per 100 mL; 0.9 g

19. 4% = 4 g/100 mL = x g/500 mL; 4 $\times$ 500 = 2000; 2000/100 = 20 g

20. 0.45% = 0.45 g/100 mL = x g/1000 mL; 0.45 $\times$ 1000 = 450; 450/100 = 4.5 g

21. 5% = 5 g/100 mL = x g/1000 mL; 5 $\times$ 1000 = 5000; 5000/100 = 50 g

22. 0.4% = 0.4 g/100 mL = x g/500 mL; 0.4 $\times$ 500 = 200; 200/100 = 2 g

23. 4% = 4 g/100 mL = x g/500 mL; 4 $\times$ 500 = 2000; 2000/100 = 20 g

24. 2% = 2 g/100 mL = x g/250 mL; 2 $\times$ 250 = 500; 500/100 = 5 g

25. 7.5% = 7.5 g/100 mL = x g/5 mL; 7.5 $\times$ 5 = 37.5; 37.5/100 = 0.375 g; 0.375 $\times$ 1000 = 375 mg

26. 0.5 % = 0.5 g/100 mL = x g/5 mL; 0.5 $\times$ 50 = 25; 25/100 = 0.25 g; 0.25 $\times$ 1000 = 250 mg

27. 1% = 1 g/100 mL = x g/ 5 mL; 1 $\times$ 5 = 5; 5/100 = 0.05 g; 0.05 $\times$ 1000 = 5 mg

28. 1:1000 = 1000 mg/1000 mL = x mg/1 mL; 1000 $\times$ 1 = 1000; 1000/1000 = 1 mg

29. 1:5000 = 1000 mg/5000 mL = x mg/5 mL; 1000 $\times$ 5 = 5000; 5000/5000 = 1 mg

30. 100 g/ 1000 mL = x g/100 mL; 100 $\times$ 100 = 10,000; 10,000/1000 = 10 g; 10 g/100 mL = 10%

31. 10 g/100 mL = x g/3000 mL; 10 $\times$ 3000 = 30,000; 30,000/100 = 300 g

32. NS = 0.9%

33. Rate = 150 mL per hr; 150 $\times$ 24 = 3600 mL in 24 hr period; 0.9% = 0.9 g/100 mL = x g/3600 mL; 0.9 $\times$ 3600 = 3240; 3240/100 = 32.4 g

34. 0.9 g/100 mL = x g/250 mL; 0.9 $\times$ 250 = 225; 225/100 = 2.25 g

35. 0.9 g/100 mL = x g/500 mL; 0.9 $\times$ 500 = 450; 450/100 = 4.5 g

36. 0.9 g/100 mL = x g/1000 mL; 0.9 $\times$ 1000 = 900; 900/100 = 9 g

37. 0.9 g/100 mL = x g/2225 mL; 0.9 $\times$ 2225 = 2002.5; 2002.5/100 = 20.02 g

38. 0.45 g/100 mL = x g/125 mL; 0.45 $\times$ 125 = 56.25; 56.25/100 = 0.563, rounded to 0.56 g

39. 0.45 g/100 mL = x g/250 mL; 0.45 $\times$ 250 = 112.5/100 = 1.125, rounded to 1.13 g

40. 0.45 g/100 mL = x g/750 mL; 0.45 $\times$ 750 = 337.5; 337.5/100 = 3.375, rounded to 3.38 g

41. 0.45 g/100 mL = x g/1800 mL; 0.45 $\times$ 1800 = 810; 810/100 = 8.1 g

42. 0.45 g/100 mL = x g/2600 mL; 0.45 $\times$ 2600 = 1170; 1170/100 = 11.7 g

43. 5 g/100 mL = x g/75 mL; 5 $\times$ 75 = 375; 375/100 = 3.75 g

44. 5 g/100 mL = x g/385 mL; 5 $\times$ 385 = 1925; 1925/100 = 19.25 g

45. 5 g/100 mL = x g/525 mL; 5 $\times$ 525 = 2625; 2625/100 = 26.25 g

46. 5 g/100 mL = x g/1350 mL; 5 $\times$ 1350 = 6750; 6750/100 = 67.5 g

47. 10 g/100 mL = x g/100 mL; 10 $\times$ 100 = 1000; 1000/100 = 10 g

48. 10 g/100 mL = x g/325 mL; 10 $\times$ 325 = 3250; 3250/100 = 32.5 g

49. 10 g/100 mL = x g/450 mL; 10 $\times$ 450 = 4500; 4500/100 = 45 g

50. 10 g/100 mL = x g/875 mL; 10 $\times$ 875 = 8750; 8750/100 = 87.5 g

7.2 Problem Set

1. $1000/50 = 20$ hr

2. $1000/100 = 10$ hr; 10 hr from 7 PM is 5 AM

3. $500/30 = 16.666$ rounded to 16.67 hr; or approximately 16 hr and 40 min

4. 75 mL/45 min = x mL/60 min; $75 \times 60 = 4500$; $4500/45 = 100$ mL/hr

5. 100 mL/45 min = x mL/60 min; $100 \times 60 = 6000$; $6000/45 = 133.33$ mL/hr

6. $250/5 = 50$ mL/hr

7. $1500/5 = 300$ mg/hr

8. Rate is 50 mL over 60 min or 50 mL/hr

9. Rate is 500 mg over 60 min or 500 mg/hr

10. 100 mL/hr

11. $1000/100 = 10$ hr

12. 1 bag = 10 hr; $24/10 = 2.4$; 2.4, rounded up to 3 IV bags

13. $20/10 = 2$ mEq/hr

14. $D_5 = 5$ g/100 mL = x g/1000 mL; $5 \times 1000 = 5000$; $5000/100 = 50$; $x = 50$ g

15. NS = 0.9 g/100 mL = x g/1000 mL; $0.9 \times 1000 = 900$; $900/100 = 9$; $x = 9$ g

16. $1000/50 = 20$ hr; $24/20 = 1.2$, rounded up to 2 IV bags

17. $1000/75 = 13.33$ hr; $24/13.33 = 1.8$, rounded up to 2 IV bags

18. $1000/100 = 10$ hr; $24/10 = 2.4$, rounded up to 3 IV bags

19. $1000/120 = 8.33$ hr; $24/8.33 = 2.88$, rounded up to 3 IV bags

20. $1000/125 = 8$ hr; $24/8 = 3$ IV bags

21. $1000/130 = 7.69$ hr; $24/7.69 = 3.12$, rounded up to 4 IV bags

22. $1000/150 = 6.66$ hr; $24/6.66 = 3.6$, rounded up to 4 IV bags

23. $1000/175 = 5.71$ hr; $24/5.71 = 4.2$, rounded up to 5 IV bags

24. $1000/200 = 5$ hr; $24/5 = 4.8$, rounded up to 5 IV bags

25. $1000/225 = 4.44$ hr; $24/4.44 = 5.41$, rounded up to 6 IV bags

26. a. $250/4 = 62.5$ mL/hr

    b. $250/4 = 62.5$ mg/hr

27. a. $500/12 = 41.666$, rounded to 41.67 mL/hr

    b. $12,000,000/12 = 1,000,000$ units/hr

28. a. 4% = 4 g/100 mL = x g/500 mL; $4 \times 500 = 2000$; $2000/100 = 20$ g; 20 g = 20,000 mg; $20,000/500 = 40$; 40 mg/1 mL = 800 mg/x mL; $1 \times 800 = 800$; $800/40 = 20$ mL/hr

    b. $500/20 = 25$ hr

29. a. 250 mg/500 mL = 20 mg/x mL; $x = 40$ mL/hr

    b. 20 mg/1 hr = 250 mg/x hr; $x = 12.5$ hr

30. a. 1600 mcg/500 mL = x mcg/1 mL; $1600 \times 1 = 1600$; $1600/500 = 75$ mL/hr

    b. 4 mcg/1 min = x mcg/60 min $4 \times 60 = 240$; $240/1 = 240$; 240 mcg/hr

31. a. 200 mg/5 mL = 800 mg/x mL; $5 \times 800 = 4000$; $4000/200 = 20$; $x = 20$ mL

    b. $800/250 = 3.2$ mg/hr; 3.2 mg/1 mL = 5 mg/x mL; $x = 1.56$ mL/hr

32. a. 3.977, rounded to 3.98 mL

    b. 1.666, rounded to 1.67 mL/hr

7.3 Problem Set

1. 10 mL/60 min × 10; $10/60 = 0.166$; $0.166 \times 10 = 1.67$, rounded down to 1 gtt/min

2. 35 mL/60 min × 60; $35/60 = 0.58$; $0.58 \times 60 = 34.99$, rounded down to = 34 gtts/min

3. 100 mL/60 min × 10; $100/60 = 1.66$; $1.66 \times 10 = 16.66$, rounded down to 16 gtts/min

4. 50 mL/30 min × 60; $50/30 = 1.67$; $1.67 \times 60 = 99.99$, rounded down to 99 gtts/min

5. $500/24 = 20.83$; 20.83/60 min × 15; $20.83/60 = 0.347 \times 15 = 5.21$, rounded down to 5 gtts/min

6. 250 mL/60 min × 15; $250/60 = 4.17$; $4.17 \times 15 = 62.55$, rounded down to 62 gtts/min

7. 50 mL/60 min × 15; $50/60 = 0.83 \times 15 = 12.45$, rounded down to 12 gtts/min

8. 95 mL/60 min × 20; 95/60 = 1.58; 1.58 × 20 = 31.67, rounded down to 31 gtts/min

9. 100 × 10 = 1000 (i.e., 1000 drops in 100 mL); 40/1000 = 0.04 mEq/gtt

10. 25 mL/60 min × 15; 25/60 = 0.42; 0.42 × 15 = 6.3, rounded down to 6 gtts/min

11. 50 mL/60 min × 60; 50/60 = 0.83; 0.83 × 60 = 49.8, rounded down to 49 gtts/min

12. 10 mL/60 min × 20; 10/60 = 0.167; 0.167 × 20 = 3.33, rounded to 3 gtts/min

13. mg/gtt = 450 mg/250 mL × 1 mL/60 gtts = 450 mg/15,000 gtts = 0.03 mg/gtt

14. 250/24 = 10.42 mL/hr; 10.42 mL/60 min × 10; 10.42/60 = 0.174; 0.174 × 10 = 1.74; (8mg/250 mL) ÷ 1.74; 8/250 = 0.032; 0.032/1.74 = 0.018, rounded to 0.02 mg/gtt

15. 25 mL/60 min × 10; 25/60 = 0.417; 0.417 × 10 = 4.17, rounded down to 4 gtts/min

16. 5 mL/60 min × 60; 5/60 = 0.083; 0.083 × 60 = 4.99 gtts/min; (10 mEq/500 mL) ÷ 4.99; 10/500 = 0.02; 0.02/4.99 = 0.004 mEq/gtt

Chapter 8

8.1 Problem Set

1. 30 g/120 g = 30/120 = ¼ ratio
Coal tar 4 g = 4/4 = 1 g
Salicylic acid 1 g = ¼ = 0.25 g
Triamcinolone 0.1% ung 15 g = 15/4 = 3.75 g
Aqua-base ointment 100 g = 100/4 = 25 g

Therefore, you will need 1 g of coal tar, 0.25 g of salicylic acid, 3.75 g of triamcinolone 0.1% ung, and 25 g of aqua-base ointment.

2. 150/30 = 5/1 ratio
Progesterone 2.4 g × 5 = 12 g
Polyethylene glycol 3350 30 g ×5 = 150 g
Polyethylene glycol 1000 90 g × 5 = 450 g

Therefore, you will need 12 g of progesterone, 150 g of polyethylene glycol 3350, and 450 g of polyethylene glycol 1000.

3. 120/20 = 6/1 ratio
Podophyllum resin 25%; 25% = 25 mL/100 mL = x mL/20 mL = 5 mL; 5 × 6 = 30 mL
Benzoin tincture QSAD 120 mL

Therefore, you will need 30 mL of podophyllum resin and QSAD 120 mL of benzoin tincture. *Note:* You could also do this by multiplying 120 × 0.25 = 30 mL; 120-30 = 90 mL.

4. 8 oz = 240 mL
120/240 = ½ ratio
Tetracycline 500 mg capsules; 16/2 = 8
Hydrocortisone suspension 15 mL; 15/2 = 7.5
Lidocaine oral suspension 30 mL; 30/2 = 15
Mylanta suspension QSAD 240 mL; 240/2 = QSAD 120

Therefore, you will need 8 capsules of tetracycline 500 mg, 7.5 mL of hydrocortisone suspension, 15 mL of lidocaine oral suspension, and QSAD 120 mL of Mylanta suspension.

5. 4 × 15 = 60 mL
60/30 = 2/1 ratio
Antipyrine 1.8 g × 2 = 3.6 g
Benzocaine 0.5 g × 2 = 1 g
Glycerin QSAD 30 mL × 2 = QSAD 60 mL

Therefore, you will need 3.6 g of antipyrine, 1 g of benzocaine, and QSAD 60 mL of glycerin.

8.2 Problem Set

1.

10		2.5 parts of 10%
	7.5	
5		2.5 parts of 5%

2.5 + 2.5 = 5 parts total

2.5/5 = x/200 = 100; x = 100 mL of 10% dextrose

2.5/5 = x/200 = 100; x = 100 mL of 5% dextrose

2.

20		3 parts of 20%
	8	
5		12 parts of 5%

$3 + 12 = 15$ parts total

$3/15 = x/400 = 80; x = 80$ mL of 20%

$12/15 = x/400 = 320; x = 320$ mL of 5%

3.

70		7.5 parts of 70%
	12.5	
5		57.5 parts of 5%

$7.5 + 57.5 \ 5 \ 65$ parts total

$7.5/65 = x/500 = 57.69; x = 57.69$ mL of 70%

$57.5/65 = x/500 = 442.31; x = 442.31$ mL of 5%

4.

10		4 parts of 10%
	6	
5		1 part of 5%

$4 + 1 = 5$ parts total

$4/5 = x/250 = 200; x = 200$ mL of 10%

$1/5 = x/250 = 50; x = 50$ mL of 5%

5.

50		2.5 parts of 50%
	7.5	
5		42.5 parts of 5%

$2.5 + 42.5 = 45$ parts total

$2.5/45 = x/500 = 27.78; x = 27.78$ mL of 50%

$42.5/45 = x/500 = 472.22; x = 472.22$ mL of 5%

6.

20		3 parts of 20%
	8	
5		12 parts of 5%

$3 + 12 = 15$ parts total

$3/15 = x/250 = 50; x = 50$ mL of 20%

$12/15 = x/250 = 200; x = 200$ mL of 5%

7.

20		2.5 parts of 20%
	7.5	
5		12.5 parts of 5%

$2.5 + 12.5 = 15$ parts total

$2.5/15 = x/300 = 50; x = 50$ mL of 20%

$12.5/15 = x/300 = 250; x = 250$ mL of 5%

8.

20		2.5 parts of 20%
	12.5	
10		7.5 parts of 10%

$2.5 + 7.5 = 10$ parts total

$2.5/10 = x/500 = 125; x = 125$ mL of 20%

$7.5/10 = x/500 = 375; x = 375$ mL of 10%

9.

10		2.5 parts of 10%
	7.5	
5		2.5 parts of 5%

2.5 + 2.5 = 5 parts total

$2.5/5 = x/150 = 75; x = 75$ mL of 10%

$2.5/5 = x/150 = 75; x = 75$ mL of 5%

10.

20		2.5 parts of 20%
	12.5	
10		7.5 parts of 10%

2.5 + 7.5 = 10 parts total

$2.5/10 = x/250 = 62.5; x = 62.5$ mL of 20%

$7.5/10 = x/250 = 187.5; x = 187.5$ mL of 10%

11.

10		2 parts of 10%
	3	
1		7 parts of 1%

2 + 7 = 9 parts total

$2/9 = x/60 = 13.33; x = 13.33$ g of 10%

$7/9 = x/60 = 46.66; x = 46.66$ g of 1%

12.

15		2.5 parts of 15%
	7.5	
5		7.5 parts of 5%

7.5 + 2.5 = 10 parts total

$2.5/10 = x/30 = 7.5; x = 7.5$ g of 15%

$7.5/10 = x/30 = 22.5; x = 22.5$ g of 5%

13. $4 \times 30 = 120$ g

5		2 parts of 5%
	3	
1		2 parts of 1%

2 + 2 = 4 parts total

$2/4 = x/120 = 60; x = 60$ g of 5%

$2/4 = x/120 = 60; x = 60$ g of 1%

14.

20		5 parts of 20%
	10	
5		10 parts of 5%

10 + 5 = 15 parts total

$5/15 = x/45 = 15; x = 15$ g of 20%

$10/15 = x/45 = 30; x = 30$ g of 5%

15.

10		3 parts of 10%
	8	
5		2 parts of 5%

3 + 2 = 5 parts total

$3/5 = x/100 = 60; x = 60$ g of 10%

$2/5 = x/100 = 40; x = 40$ g of 5%

8.3 Problem Set

1. 2% = 2 g/100 g; 2 g/100 g = x g/75 g; 2 × 75 = 150; 150/100 = 1.5; x = 1.5 g

   Therefore, there are 1.5 g of hydrocortisone in 75 g of the cream.

2. 8 g/ 454 g = x g/100 g; 8 × 100 = 800; 800/454 = 1.76; x = 1.76

   Therefore, the percentage strength of the compound is 1.76%.

3. 2.5% = 2.5 g/100 g

   Therefore, 2.5 g of acyclovir will be needed for this preparation.

4. 10 g + 50 g = 60 g; 10 g/60 g = x g/100 g; 10 × 100 = 1000; 1000/60 = 16.66; x = 16.7

   Therefore, the percentage strength of the compound is 16.7%.

5. 2% = 2 g/100 g; 2g/100 g = x g/30 g; 2 × 30 = 60; 60/100 = 0.6; x = 0.6

   Therefore, 0.6 g of triamcinolone will be needed for this prescription.

6. 0.1% = 0.1 g/100 g; 0.1 g/100 = x g/15 g; 0.1 × 15 = 1.5; 1.5/100 = 0.015

   Therefore, 0.015 g of mometasone fumarate will be needed to prepare the prescription.

7. a. 100 × 200 = 20,000 mg needed for batch

   b. 20000 mg/100 = x mg/1; x = 200 mg; 200 mg = 0.2 g; 0.2/1 = x/100; x = 20%

8. 0.75% = 0.75 g/100 g; 0.75 g/100 g = x g/30 g; 0.75 × 30 = 22.5; 22.5/100 = 0.225 g of metronidazole needed for this prescription.

9. 1% = 1 g/100 g
   1g/100g = x g/30 g
   1 × 30 = 30; 30/100 = 0.3

   0.3 g of clindamycin is needed to prepare this prescription.

10. a. 10% = 10 g/100 g
    10 g/100 g = x g/50 g
    10 × 50 = 500; 500/100 = 5

    5 g of acyclovir are needed to prepare this prescription.

    b. 1 dose = 1 g
    1 g/1 dose = 50g /x doses
    50 × 1 = 50; 50/1 = 50

    There are 50 doses.

8.4 Problem Set

1. a. 10 mg/1 mL = x mg/10 mL; 10 × 10 = 100; 100/1 = 100; x = 100 mg

   b. 100 mg/mL = 1 mL

   c. 10 − 1 = 9 mL

2. a. 10 mg/1 mL = x mg/5 mL; 10 × 5 = 50; 50/1 = 50; x = 50 mg

   b. 40 mg/1 mL = 50 mg/x mL; 1 × 50 = 50; 50/40 = 1. 25; x = 1.25 mL

   c. 5 − 1.25 = 3.75 mL

3. a. 10 mg/1 mL = x mg/10 mL; 10 × 10 = 100; 100/1 = 100; x = 100 mg

   b. 500 mg/5 mL = 100 mg/x mL; 5 × 100 = 500; 500/500 = 1; x = 1 mL

   c. 10 − 1 = 9 mL

4. a. 1 mg/1 mL = x mg/5 mL; 1 × 5 = 5; 5/1 = 5; x = 5 mg

   b. 4 mg/1 mL = 5 mg/x mL; 1 × 5 = 5; 5/4 = 1.25; x = 1.25 mL

   c. 5 − 1.25 = 3.75 mL

5. a. 1 mg/1 mL = x mg/10 mL; 1 × 10 = 10; 10/1 = 10; x = 10 mg

b. 20 mg/2 mL = 10 mg/x mL; 2 × 10 = 20; 20/20 = 1; x = 1 mL

c. 10 − 1 = 9 mL

6. a. 500 × 15 = 7500; 7500/70 = 107.14 mL of 70% dextrose

b. 500 − 107.14 = 392.86 mL of sterile water

7. a. 2000 × 10 = 20,000; 20,000/50 = 400 mL of 50% dextrose

b. 2000 − 400 = 1600 mL of sterile water

8. a. 1000 × 10 = 10,000; 10,000/50 = 200 mL of 50% dextrose

b. 1000 − 200 = 800 mL of sterile water

9. a. 750 × 8 = 6000; 6000/50 = 120 mL of 50% dextrose

b. 750 − 120 = 630 mL of sterile water

10. a. 250 × 7.5 = 1875; 1875/70 = 26.79 mL of 70% dextrose

b. 250 − 26.79 = 223.21 mL of sterile water

11. 1500/70 × 17; 1500/70 = 21.43; 21.43 × 17 = 364.29 mL of $D_{70}W$
1500/10 × 3; 1500/10 = 150; 150 × 3 = 450 mL of Aminosyn 10%
1500/20 × 2.5; 1500/20 = 75; 75 × 2.5 = 187.5 mL of Liposyn 20%

20 × 1.5 = 30; 30/4 = 7.5 mL of sodium chloride
15 × 1.5 = 22.5; 22.5/2 = 11.25 mL of potassium chloride
10 × 1.5 = 15; 15/3 = 5 mL of potassium phosphate
3 × 1.5 = 4.5; 4.5/3 = 1.5 mL of sodium phosphate
10 × 1.5 = 15; 15/4.06 = 3.695 rounded to 3.7 mL of magnesium sulfate
10 mL of MVI

364.29 + 450 + 187.5 + 7.5 + 11.25 + 5 + 1.5 + 3.7 + 10 = 1040.74

1500 − 1040.74 = 459.26 mL of sterile water QSAD to 1500 mL

Chapter 9

9.1 Problem Set

1. $135,000.00 + $52,000.00 + $23,000.00 + $6,000.00 + $4,000.00 + $2,000.00 + $4,000.00 + $4,000.00 + $750,000.00 = $980,000.00; $980,000.00 × 0.18 = $176,400.00; $980,000.00 + $176,400.00 = $1,156,400.00; desired income goal for 18% profit is $1,156,400.00

2. $1,401,489.00 − $980,000.00 = $421,489.00; $421,480.00/$1,401,490.00 = 0.30; 0.3 × 100 = 30%; percentage profit is 30%

3. $1,191,692.00 − $980,000.00 = $211,692.00; $211,692.00/$1,191,692.00 = 0.178; 0.178 × 100 = 17.8%; percentage profit is 17.8%

4. $72,000.00 + $52,000.00 + $13,000.00 + $5,500.00 + $2,000.00 + $1,500.00 + $4,000.00 + $3,500.00 + $50,000.00 = $203,500.00; $203,500.00 × 0.2 = $40,700.00; $203,500.00 + $40,700.00 = $244,200.00; Desired income goal for 20% profit is $244,200.00

5. $991,982.00 − $203,500.00 = $788,482.00; $788,482.00/$991,982.00 = 0.79; 0.79 × 100 = 79%; Percentage profit is 79%

6. $1,248,301.00 − $203,500.00 = $1,044,801.00; $1,044,801.00/$1,248,301.00 = 0.837; 0.837 × 100 = 83.7%; percentage profit is 83.7%

7. $54,617.53 − $3700.83 = $50,916.70; the overhead for the week was $50,916.70

8. $13,033.06 × 0.22 = $2867.27; $2867.27 + $13,033.06 = $15,900.33; weekly sales of $15,900.33 are required for a 22% profit

9. $3.96/100 tablets = $0.0396 per tablet, rounded to $0.04 per tablet; $0.04 × 50 tablets = $2; $8.59 − $2 = $6.59 net profit

$8.59 − $4.25 = $4.34; $4.34 − $2 = $2.34; $2.34/$2 = 1.17 or 117% markup rate

10. $8.50/500 capsules = $0.017 per capsule, rounded to $0.02; $0.02 × 30 capsules = $0.60; $14.80 − $0.60 = $14.20 net profit

$14.80 − $4.25 = $10.55; $10.55 − $0.60 = $9.95; $9.95/$0.60 = 16.58 or 1658% markup rate

11. $118.50/100 tablets = $1.185 per tablet, rounded to $1.19; $1.19 × 30 tablets = $35.70; $45.50 - $35.70 = $9.80 net profit

$45.50 − $4.25 = $41.25; $41.25 − $35.70 = $5.55; $5.55/$35.70 = 0.1554 or 15.5% markup rate

12. $83.50/500 tablets = $0.167 per tablet, rounded to $0.17; $0.17 × 100 tablets = $17.00; $23.16 − $17.00 = $6.16 net profit

$23.16 − $4.25 = $18.91; $18.91 − $17.00 = $1.91; $1.91/$17.00 = 0.1123 or 11.2% markup rate

13. $41.20/100 tablets = $0.412 per tablet, rounded to $0.41; $0.41 × 90 tablets = $36.90; $41.70 − $36.90 = $4.8 net profit

$41.70 − $4.25 = $37.45; $37.45 − $36.90 = $0.55; $0.55/$36.90 = 0.015, or 1.5% markup rate

14. $37.50/16 oz = $2.34 per ounce; $2.34 × 8 oz = $18.75; $25.34 − $18.75 = $6.59 net profit

$25.34 − $4.25 = $21.09; $21.09 − $18.75 = $2.34; $2.34/$18.75 = 0.124, or 12.4% markup rate

15. $62.30/6 packs = $10.38 per pack; $10.38 × 1 pack = $10.38; $17.90 - $10.38 = $7.52 net profit

$17.90 − $4.25 = $13.65; $13.65 − $10.38 = $3.27; $3.27/$10.38 = 0.315, or 31.5% markup rate

16. $5.89 × 0.2 = $1.18; $5.89 − $1.18 = $4.71; discounted selling price is $4.71

17. $1.19 × 0.15 = $0.18; $1.19 − $0.18 = $1.01; discounted selling price is $1.01

18. $7.29 × 0.30 = $2.19; $7.29 − $2.19 = $5.10; discounted selling price is $5.10

19. $5.69 × 0.15 = $0.85; $5.69 − $0.85 = $4.84; discounted selling price is $4.84

20. $3.89 × 0.25 = $0.9725, rounded to 0.97; $3.89 − $0.97 = $2.92; discounted selling price is $2.92

21. $4.26 × 0.30 = $1.28; $4.26 − $1.28 = $2.98; discounted selling price is $2.98

22. $8.70 × 0.5 = $4.35; $8.70 − $4.35 = $4.35; discounted selling price is $4.35

23. $2.99 × 0.40 = $1.20; $2.99 − $1.20 = $1.79; discounted selling price is $1.79

24. $12.50 × 0.3 = $3.75; $12.50 + $3.50 = $16.00; $16.00 × 12 tubes = $195.00; the total selling price is $195.00

25. $111.60/36 = $3.10 (purchase price per bottle); $3.10 + $1.75 = $4.85; selling price is $4.85 per bottle

26. $15.60 × 0.25 = $3.9; the markup amount is $3.90; $15.60 + $3.90 = $19.50; the selling price is $19.50

27. $30.75 − $24.80 = $5.95; $5.95/$24.80 × 100; $5.95/$24.80 = 0.2399; 0.2399 × 100 = 23.99, rounded to 24%; markup rate is 24%

28. $650.00 − $520.00 = $130.00; gross profit is $130.00

29. $2.05/1000 × 100 = $20.50; $130.00 − $20.50 = $109.50; $109.50/1000 = 0.11; net profit is $0.11 per tablet

30. $120.50 × 0.25 = $30.13; markup amount is $30.13; $120.50 + $30.13 = $150.63; selling price is $150.63

31. $24.00 × 0.15 = $3.60; markup amount is $3.60; $24.00 + $3.60 = $27.60; selling price is $27.60

32. $200.00 × 0.27 = $54.00; markup amount is $54.00; $200.00 + $54.00 = $254.00; selling price is $254.00

33. $27.50 × 0.21 = $5.78; markup amount is $5.78; $27.50 + $5.78 = $33.28; selling price is $33.28

34. $67.50 × 0.18 = $12.15; markup amount is $12.15; $67.50 + $12.15 = $79.65; selling price is $79.65

35. $840.00 × 0.32 = $268.80; markup amount is $268.80; $840.00 + $268.80 = $1108.80; selling price is $1108.80

36. $550.00 × 0.30 = $165.00; markup amount is $165.00; $550.00 + $165.00 = $715.00; selling price is $715.00

37. $120.50 + $24.00 + $200.00 + $27.50 + $67.50 + $840.00 + $550.00 = $1829.50; the total amount that the pharmacy spent on the shipment was $1829.50; $150.63 + $27.60 + $254.00 + $33.28 + $79.65 + 1108.80 + $715.00 = $2368.96; $2368.96 − $1829.50 = $539.46; the total amount made by the pharmacy was $539.46; $549.46/$1829.50 × 100; $549.46/$1829.50 = 0.3003; 0.3003 × 100 = 30.03 rounded to 30; the total markup rate was 30%

9.2 Problem Set

1. $48.90 × 0.13 = $6.36; $48.90 − $6.36 = $42.54; $42.54/60 tablets × 20 tablets; $42.54/60 tablets = $0.71 per tablet; $0.71 × 20 tablets = $14.20 for the prescription; the pharmacy will submit for $14.20 reimbursement

2. $84.07 × 0.13 = $10.93; $84.07 − $10.93 = $73.14; $73.14/100 tablets × 30 tablets; $73.14/100 tablets = $0.73 per tablet; 0.73 × 30 tablets = $21.90 for the prescription; the pharmacy will submit for $21.90 reimbursement

3. $30.25 × 0.13 = $3.93; $30.25 − $3.93 = $26.32; $26.32/1000 tablets × 100 tablets; $26.32/1000 tablets = $0.02632 per tablet, rounded to 0.03; 0.03 × 100 tablets = $3.00 for the prescription; the pharmacy will submit for $3.00 reimbursement

4. $120.68 × 0.04 = $4.83; $120.68 + $4.83 = $125.51; $125.51/500 tablets × 30 tablets; $125.51/500 = $0.25 × 30 = $7.50; $7.50 + $6.25 = $13.75; the pharmacy will submit for $13.75 reimbursement

5. $39.78 × 0.04 = $1.59; $39.78 + $1.59 = $$41.37; $41.37/100 tablets × 60 tablets; $41.37/100 = $0.4137 × 60 = $24.82; $24.82 + $6.25 = $31.07; the pharmacy will submit for $31.07 reimbursement

6. $317.50 × 0.04 = $12.70; $317.50 + $12.70 = $330.20; $330.20/30 tablets × 20 tablets; $330.20/30 = $11.01; $11.01 × 20 = $220.20; $220.20 + $6.25 = $226.45; the pharmacy will submit for $226.45 reimbursement

7a. $71.35/100 × 50; $71.35/100 = $0.7135; $0.7135 × 50 = $35.675, rounded to $35.68; the pharmacy cost is $35.68

7b. $71.35 × 0.035 = $2.50; $71.35 + $2.50 = $73.85; $73.85/100 tablets × 50 tablets; $73.85/100 = $0.7385 × 50 = $36.925; $36.925 + $4.50 = $41.425, rounded to $41.43; the pharmacy will submit for $41.43 reimbursement

7c. $41.43 − $35.68 = $5.75; the pharmacy will make a profit of $5.75 on this prescription

8. a. $36.35 × 0.03 = $1.091; $36.35 − $1.091 = $35.259; $35.259 × 2 = $70.518, rounded to $70.52; the pharmacy cost is $70.52

   b. $36.35 × 0.05 = $1.82; $36.35 + $1.82 = $38.17 per inhaler × 2 = $76.34; the pharmacy will submit this for $76.34 reimbursement

   c. $76.34 − $70.52 = $5.82; the pharmacy will make $5.82 on this prescription

9. a. $302.35/30 × 10; $302.35/30 = $10.08; $10.08 × 10 = $100.80; the pharmacy cost is $100.80

   b. $100.80 × 0.03 = $3.024; $100.80 − $3.024 = $97.776; $97.776 + $7.00 = $104.776, rounded to $104.78; the pharmacy will submit this for $104.78 reimbursement

   c. $104.78 − $100.80 = $3.98; the pharmacy will make $3.98 on this prescription

10. a. $117.35/50 × 30; $117.35/50 = $2.35; $2.35 × 30 = $70.5; the pharmacy cost is $70.50

   b. $70.50 × 0.03 = $2.115; $70.50 + $2.115 = $72.615; $72.615 + $4.00 = $76.615, rounded to $76.62; the pharmacy will submit this for $76.62 reimbursement

   c. $76.62 − $70.50 = $6.12; the pharmacy will make $6.12 on this prescription

11. a. $85.35/80 × 15; $85.35/80 = $1.07; $1.07 × 15 = $16.05; the pharmacy cost is $16.05

   b. $16.05 × 0.045 = $0.72; $16.05 + $0.72 = $16.77; the pharmacy will submit this for $16.77 reimbursement

c. $16.77 − $16.05 = $0.72; the pharmacy will make $0.72 on this prescription

12. a. $310.00 × 6 = $1860.00; the pharmacy will be reimbursed $1860.00 for the capitation fee

b. $15.75 + $106.50 + $27.80 + $210.00 + $47.50 + $105.25 + $160.00 + $52.00 + $150.00 + $210.00 + $76.00 + $10.50 + $28.00 + $62.50 + $210.00 + $210.00 + $17.00 = $1698.80; the pharmacy cost is $1698.80

c. The pharmacy made a profit

d. $1860.00 – $1698.80 = $161.20

13. a. $15.75 + $106.50 + $27.80 + 210.00 + 47.50 + 105.25 + 160.00 + $52.00 + $150.00 + $210.00 + $76.00 + $10.50 + $28.00 + $62.50 + $210.00 + $210.00 + $17.00 = $1698.80; the pharmacy cost is $1698.80

b. $1698.80 × 0.03 = $50.96; $1698.80 + $50.96 = $1749.76; $2.00 per prescription × 17 = $34.00; $1749.76 + $34.00 = $1783.76; the pharmacy will submit this for $1783.76 reimbursement

c. The pharmacy made a profit

d. $1783.76 − $1698.80 = $84.96; the pharmacy made a profit of $84.96

e. The pharmacy made more money under Mountain HMO's capitation plan

f. $161.20 − $84.96 = $76.24; the pharmacy made $76.24 more under the capitation plan

14. a. $275.00 × 10 = $2750.00; the total amount that the HMO reimbursed for capitation fees is $2750.00

b. $89.63 + $126.54 + $420.45 + $117.50 + $46.75 = $729.87; the total pharmacy cost is $800.87

c. The pharmacy made a profit

d. $2750.00 − $800.87 = $1949.13; the pharmacy made a profit of $1949.13

15. a. $275.00 × 12 = $3300.00; the total amount that the HMO reimbursed for capitation fees is $3300.00

b. $78.26 + $75.23 + $25.48 + $128.46 + $21.86 + $61.89 + $41.20 + $16.59 + $5.80 + $3.87 + $21.67 + $58.24 = $538.55; the total pharmacy cost is $538.55

c. the pharmacy made a profit

d. $3300.00 − $538.55 = $2761.45; the pharmacy made a profit of $2761.45

16. a. $225.00 × 40 = $9000.00; $9000.00 + $60.00 = $9060.00; the total amount the HMO will reimburse the pharmacy is $9060.00

b. the pharmacy made money

c. $9060.00 − $1867.50 = $7192.50; the pharmacy made a profit of $7192.50

17. a. $210.00 × 42 = $8820.00; $4.25 × 31 = $131.75; $8820.00 + $131.75 = $8951.75; the total amount that the insurance company reimbursed is $8951.75

b. The pharmacy lost money

c. $8951.75 2 $9634.73 5 –$682.98; the pharmacy lost $682.98

9.3 Problem Set

1. 1 bottle of 500

2. 2 bottles of 100

3. 1 bottle of 500

4. 1 bottle of 60

5. 1 bottle of 100

6. no purchase necessary

7. 1 bottle of 50

8. no purchase necessary

9. no purchase necessary

10. 3 of the 15 g; 4 of the 80 g

11. 1 of the 15 g; 1 of the 60 g; 2 of the 80 g

12. 1 of the 60 mL

13. 1 of the 15 g; 1 of the 60 g

14. 3 of the 60 g;

15. 2 of the 15 g; 2 of the 60 g; 1 of the 4 oz

16. 2 of the 15 g; 1 of the 60 g

17. 1 of the 15 g; 1 of the 45 g

18. 1 of the 15 g; 3 of the 30 g; 2 of the 60 g; 2 of the 120 g

19. zero of the 15 g; 1 of the 30 g; 3 of the 60 g

20. 1 of the 15 g; 1 of the 30 g; Could be either 1 or 2 of the 60 g; 1 of the 120 g

21. 1 of the 20 mL; 2 or 3 of the 60 mL

22. 2 bottles of 100

23. 2 bottles of 100

24. 4 bottles of 100

25. 4 bottles of 60

26. 3 bottles of 100

27. 2 bottles of 1000

28. 2 bottles of 100

29. 2 bottles of 1000

30. 2 bottles of 100

31. 2 bottles of 300

32. 3 bottles of 100

33. 2 bottles of 100

34. 2 bottles of 1000

35. 2 bottles of 100

36. 1 bottle of 100

37. a. 7 jars

    b. 3 bottles of 1000

    c. 20 bottles

    d. 3 bottles

    e. 11 bottles

38. a. $38,207.00/7 = $5458.14, rounded to $5458.00; $183,445.00/$5458.00 = 33.61, rounded to 34; they have approximately a 34 day supply

    b. 34 − 28 = 6; they are 6 days over their goal; $5458.00 × 6 = $32,748.00; they are $32,748.00 over their goal

39. a. $26,504.00/7 = $3786.29, rounded to $3786.00; $123,490.00/$3786.00 = 32.62, rounded to 33; they have approximately a 33 day supply

b. 33 − 26 = 7; they are 7 days over their goal; $3786.00 × 7 = $26,502.00; they are $26,502.00 over their goal

40. $147,210.00/24 = $6133.75; the approximate cost of goods sold was $6133.75

41. $51,280.00 + $5000.00 = $56,280.00; $56,280.00/7 = they must average $8,040.00 per day

42. $63,910.00 − $48,891.00 = $15,019.00; $15,019.00/$63,910.00 = 0.2350; 0.2350 × 100 = 23.5%, rounded to 24%; their percentage of profit last week was approximately 24%

43. a. $58,223.00 × 0.21 = $12,226.83; $58,223.00 − $12,226.83 = $45,996.17; the pharmacy cost for last week was $45,996.17

    b. $45,996.00/7 = $6570.57, rounded to $6571.00; $164,590.00/$6571.00 = 25.05, rounded to 25; they have approximately a 25 day supply

    c. 31 − 20 = 6; they are 6 days under their goal; $6571.00 × 6 = $39,426.00; they are $39,426.00 under their goal

44. a. $28,223.00 × 0.26 = $7337.98; $28,223.00 + $7337.98 = $35,560.98; the total amount sold last week was $35,560.98

    b. $28,223.00/7 = $4031.86, rounded to $4032.00; $184,520.00/$4032.00 = 45.76, rounded to 46; they have approximately a 46 day supply

    c. 46 − 34 = 12; $4032.00 × 12 = $48,384.00; they are $48,384.00 over their goal

45. $1,612,00.00/$132,936.00 = 12.123, rounded to 12.13; their turnover rate was 12.13

46. $1,768,000.00/$156,200.00 = 11.318, rounded to 11.32; their turnover rate was 11.32

47. $20,800.00/$520.00 = 40; turnover rate is 40

48. $5760.00/$178.00 = 32.36; turnover rate is 32.36

49. $7213.00/$360.00 = 20.04; turnover rate is 20.04

50. $5060.00/$320.00 = 15.81; turnover rate is 15.81

51. $6000.00/$385.00 = 14.58$; turnover rate is 15.58

52. $52,500.00/$5,000.00 = 10.5$; turnover rate is 10.5

53. $8294.00 - $2138.00 = 6156.00; $6156.00/6 = 1026.00; the annual depreciation is $1026.00

54. $18,350.00 \times 2 = $36,700.00$; $1567.00 \times 2 = 3134.00; $36,700.00 - $3134.00 = $33,566.00$; $33,566.00/12 = 2797.17; the annual depreciation is $2797.17

Appendix B

Additional Practice with Fractions and Percents

B.1 Working with Fractions

Change each of the mixed numbers to improper fractions.

1. $3\frac{1}{4}$

2. $5\frac{1}{2}$

3. $6\frac{1}{8}$

4. $5\frac{3}{4}$

5. $6\frac{7}{8}$

6. $8\frac{11}{12}$

7. $9\frac{13}{16}$

8. $12\frac{1}{4}$

9. $13\frac{2}{3}$

10. $14\frac{5}{6}$

Change each of the improper fractions to mixed numbers.

11. $\frac{55}{7}$

12. $\frac{75}{8}$

13. $\frac{95}{3}$

14. $\frac{89}{12}$

15. $\frac{125}{9}$

16. $\frac{139}{3}$

17. $\frac{147}{5}$

18. $\frac{269}{6}$

19. $\frac{409}{8}$

20. $\frac{293}{5}$

Reduce the following fractions to their lowest terms.

21. $\frac{2}{6}$

22. $\frac{2}{10}$

23. $\frac{4}{10}$

24. $\frac{8}{12}$

25. $\frac{9}{15}$

26. $\frac{8}{18}$

27. $\frac{8}{26}$

28. $\frac{48}{64}$

29. $\frac{52}{76}$

30. $\frac{75}{180}$

31. $\frac{60}{380}$

32. $\dfrac{85}{120}$

33. $\dfrac{96}{128}$

34. $\dfrac{72}{108}$

35. $\dfrac{75}{195}$

36. $\dfrac{88}{220}$

37. $\dfrac{81}{135}$

38. $\dfrac{156}{252}$

39. $\dfrac{85}{135}$

40. $\dfrac{270}{285}$

Add the following fractions.

41. $\dfrac{1}{2} + \dfrac{2}{3} =$

42. $\dfrac{3}{4} + \dfrac{7}{8} =$

43. $\dfrac{1}{3} + \dfrac{2}{7} =$

44. $\dfrac{5}{6} + \dfrac{7}{8} + \dfrac{2}{3} =$

45. $\dfrac{5}{7} + \dfrac{1}{5} + \dfrac{3}{10} =$

46. $\dfrac{1}{4} + \dfrac{7}{12} + \dfrac{1}{2} + \dfrac{7}{8} =$

47. $\dfrac{5}{16} + \dfrac{1}{4} + \dfrac{9}{24} =$

48. $4\dfrac{1}{2} + 2\dfrac{2}{3} =$

49. $9\dfrac{3}{4} + 7\dfrac{7}{8} =$

50. $5\dfrac{7}{8} + 2\dfrac{1}{3} =$

51. $12\dfrac{1}{6} + 13\dfrac{1}{4} =$

52. $8\dfrac{1}{3} + 5\dfrac{5}{6} + 13\dfrac{5}{8} + 19\dfrac{9}{16} =$

Subtract the following fractions.

53. $\dfrac{1}{2} - \dfrac{1}{4} =$

54. $\dfrac{3}{4} - \dfrac{1}{8} =$

55. $\dfrac{4}{9} - \dfrac{1}{3} =$

56. $\dfrac{5}{8} - \dfrac{1}{3} =$

57. $\dfrac{5}{12} - \dfrac{1}{8} =$

58. $\dfrac{2}{3} - \dfrac{1}{16} =$

59. $\dfrac{6}{7} - \dfrac{2}{3} =$

60. $\dfrac{11}{16} - \dfrac{5}{12} =$

61. $8\dfrac{3}{4} - 2\dfrac{1}{4} =$

62. $7\dfrac{1}{2} - 2\dfrac{1}{4} =$

63. $15\dfrac{2}{3} - 7\dfrac{1}{8} =$

64. $32\dfrac{3}{5} - 7\dfrac{3}{8} =$

65. $63\dfrac{5}{6} - 17\dfrac{7}{16} =$

66. $13\dfrac{1}{2} - 8\dfrac{3}{4} =$

67. $29\dfrac{1}{3} - 13\dfrac{3}{8} =$

68. $37\dfrac{2}{9} - 21\dfrac{1}{3} =$

Multiply the following fractions and reduce to lowest terms. Rewrite as a mixed number if necessary.

69. $\dfrac{2}{3} \times \dfrac{5}{12} =$

70. $\dfrac{5}{9} \times \dfrac{4}{8} =$

71. $\dfrac{3}{16} \times \dfrac{4}{5} =$

72. $\dfrac{7}{8} \times \dfrac{2}{3} =$

73. $\dfrac{7}{12} \times 18 =$

74. $\dfrac{5}{9} \times 21 =$

Multiply the following mixed numbers.

75. $3\dfrac{1}{2} \times 8\dfrac{1}{4} =$

76. $9\dfrac{3}{8} \times 11\dfrac{5}{6} =$

77. $15\dfrac{4}{7} \times 6\dfrac{5}{14} =$

78. $2\dfrac{1}{2} \times 3\dfrac{2}{3} \times 2\dfrac{5}{6} =$

79. $6\dfrac{1}{8} \times 5\dfrac{1}{4} \times 3\dfrac{3}{16} =$

80. $5\dfrac{2}{3} \times 3\dfrac{1}{4} \times 8\dfrac{7}{12} =$

Solve the following story problems using fractions.

81. A man pays $3000.00 for a microcomputer with an annual maintenance fee that is ⅕ of the purchase price. How much is the annual maintenance fee for this microcomputer?

82. There were 10,240 persons attending a rock concert, and ⅖ of the audience was female. How many girls and women attended the concert?

83. A jigsaw puzzle contains 5240 pieces. Ralph estimates that the puzzle is ⅝ completed. How many pieces have been put in place?

84. A jigsaw puzzle contains 905 pieces. Sue estimates the puzzle is ⅔ completed. How may pieces are not yet placed in the puzzle?

Divide the following mixed numbers and fractions.

85. $3\dfrac{1}{2} \div \dfrac{3}{4} =$

86. $2\dfrac{1}{3} \div \dfrac{5}{6} =$

87. $5\dfrac{1}{4} \div \dfrac{3}{8} =$

88. $6\dfrac{7}{8} \div \dfrac{5}{16} =$

89. $5\dfrac{1}{2} \div 2 =$

90. $16\dfrac{5}{9} \div 3 =$

91. $3\dfrac{1}{2} \div 1\dfrac{3}{4} =$

92. $15\dfrac{7}{8} \div 5\dfrac{9}{16} =$

Calculate the following.

93. $\dfrac{9}{10}$ of 650

94. $\dfrac{4}{5}$ of 785

95. $\dfrac{3}{8}$ of 248

96. $\dfrac{5}{6}$ of 66

97. $\dfrac{3}{4}$ of 76

98. $\dfrac{5}{7}$ of 56

99. $\dfrac{2}{3}$ of 780

100. $\dfrac{1}{12}$ of 144

Solve the following story problems.

101. An automobile travels 240 miles in $5\frac{1}{2}$ hours. How many miles/hour does the automobile travel?

102. An automobile travels $210^6/_{10}$ miles and uses $16^2/_{10}$ gallons of gasoline. What is the mileage in miles/gallon?

103. A student is able to transfer $84\frac{3}{4}$ credits and $271\frac{1}{5}$ quality points into another school. The student's grade point average is the number of quality points divided by the number of credits received. What is the student's grade point average based on the transfer of credits into the new school?

104. An auditorium has 31,437 square feet of seating space. Each seat will take $3\frac{1}{2}$ square feet. How many seats will fill the seating space?

B.2 Working with Percents

Convert each of the following percents to a decimal and a reduced fraction. The first problem is completed as an example.

Percent	Decimal Equivalent	Fractional Equivalent
20%	0.2	$\frac{20}{100} = \frac{1}{5}$
105. 30%		
106. 5%		
107. 8%		
108. 15%		

Compute the amount for each of the following problems, rounding to two decimal places.

109. 52% of $520.00

110. 3% of $1640.00

111. 20% of $1840.00

112. $\frac{1}{2}$% of $3640.00

113. $4\frac{1}{2}$% of $764.00

114. 8% of $514.85

115. 7% of $316.38

116. $17\frac{3}{4}$% of $42.00

Solve the following story problems.

117. Last year, a musical production was attended by 15,500 persons. This year's attendance was 92% of last year's attendance. How many attended this year?

118. The Monroe City Council voted to impose a 2% tax on personal incomes. If the average income in Monroe is $14,514.00, what is the average tax levied on each taxpayer?

119. Binford Peeples makes $820.00/week. If he receives a raise of 8%, find the amount of (a) his raise and (b) his new salary.

120. Bert Brown and Clara Johansson are partners in a business that has an annual profit of $64,500.00. Mr. Brown receives 47% of the net profit, and Ms. Johansson receives 53%. How much did (a) Mr. Brown and (b) Ms. Johansson receive?

121. Randy Schwartz purchased a condominium for $85,500.00. The depreciation allowance, for tax purposes, is 5% per year. How much is the annual depreciation allowance for the condominium?

122. Roxanne Adams owned a bond worth $2000.00 that paid interest at $8\frac{1}{2}\%$ per year. How much interest did she earn the first year?

The salaries and merit raise indexes for six employees are shown below. Multiply each salary amount by its raise index rate to get the new salary amount.

123. Salary $1500.00
     Raise Index   108%
     New Salary $ _____

124. Salary $1450.00
     Raise Index   109%
     New Salary $ _____

125. Salary $1670.00
     Raise Index $110\frac{1}{2}\%$
     New Salary $ _____

126. Salary $1548.00
     Raise Index $112\frac{1}{2}\%$
     New Salary $ _____

127. Salary $1476.00
     Raise Index $104\frac{3}{4}\%$
     New Salary $ _____

128. Salary $1950.00
     Raise Index   111%
     New Salary $ _____

Solve the following story problems.

129. Dr. Ernest Bishop has a gross earned income of $120,000.00. Of this amount, 42% represents income from patients who paid cash for their medical services, and 58% represents income from patients who charged their medical services. How much of his gross earned income is from (a) cash patients and (b) charge patients?

130. The building owned by Brodnex Jewelry Store has an assessed value of $220,000.00 for property tax purposes. Tax rates are as follows: city, 3.6%; county, 5.3%; and special business, 2.5%. How much tax is owed on the building for (a) city, (b) county, and (c) special business taxes?

131. Mitsumi Takeda owns a house valued at $120,000.00 and furniture worth $25,000.00. The house is insured at 80% of its value, and the furniture at 65% of its value. For how much are (a) the house and (b) the furniture insured? Assuming that the above amounts represent realistic values, (c) how much would Ms. Takeda lose if the house and furniture were completely destroyed by fire?

132. Canty Importers' sales during the first year of operation came to $250,000.00. Second-year sales have been projected to be 125% of first-year sales, and third-year sales have been projected to be 130% of second-year sales. What are the projected sales for (a) the second year and (b) the third year?

133. The delivery truck owned by Bellissimo Floral Shoppe used 2600 L of gasoline last year. By purchasing a more fuel-efficient truck, the store would realize an estimated 7% savings in gasoline. Assuming this is true, (a) how much gasoline would be saved next year, and (b) how much gasoline would be used next year?

134. Yasmin Nwosu gets a monthly salary of $2,400.00. Deductions are made as follows: payroll taxes, 28%; credit union, 8%; and savings account, $12\frac{1}{2}\%$. How much is deducted from her check for (a) payroll taxes, (b) credit union, and (c) savings account?

Appendix C
Common Pharmacy Abbreviations and Acronyms

Abbreviation	Meaning
A-B-C	
ac; a.c.; AC	before meals
ad; a.d.; AD	right ear
AM; a.m.	morning
amp	ampule
APAP	acetaminophen; Tylenol
as; a.s.; AS	left ear
ASA	aspirin
au; a.u.; AU	both ears; each ear
AZT; ZDV	azidothymidine; zidovudine
b.i.d.; BID	twice daily
BSA	body surface area
Ca	calcium
Cap	capsule
D-E-F	
DAW	dispense as written
DC; d/c	discontinue
disp	dispense
EC	enteric-coated
Elix	elixir
E-mycin; Emycin; E.E.S.	erythromycin
epi	epinephrine
ER; XR; XL	extended-release
°F	degrees Fahrenheit; temperature in degrees Fahrenheit
FDA	Food and Drug Administration
fl	fluid
fl oz	fluid ounce
G-H-I	
g, G	gram
gr	grain
gtt; gtts	drop; drops
h; hr	hour
HCTZ	hydrochlorothiazide
h.s.; HS	bedtime
i; ī	one

Abbreviation	Meaning
ii; ĩi	two
iii; ĩĩ	three
IBU	ibuprofen; Motrin
IM	intramuscular
Inj	injection
IV	intravenous
J-K-L	
K; K+	potassium
KCl	potassium chloride
kg	kilogram
L	liter
lb	pound
LR; RL	lactated Ringer's solution; Ringer's lactate
M-N-O	
mcg; μg*	microgram
MDI	metered-dose inhaler
Med; MED; med; meds	medication; medications
mEq	milliequivalent
mg	milligram
mL	milliliter
Na	sodium
NaCl	sodium chloride; salt
NDC	National Drug Code
NPO	nothing by mouth
NS	normal saline; 0.9% sodium chloride
NSAID	nonsteroidal anti-inflammatory drug
NTG	nitroglycerin
od; o.d.; OD	right eye
os; o.s.; OS	left eye
OTC	over the counter; no prescription required
ou; o.u.; OU	both eyes; each eye
oz	ounce

Abbreviation	Meaning
P-Q-R	
p.c.; PC	after meals
PCN	penicillin
PDR	Physicians' Desk Reference
Per	by
PM; p.m.	afternoon; evening
PO	orally; by mouth
PPI	proton pump inhibitor
PRN; p.r.n.	as needed; as occasion requires
q	every
q.h.; qhour	every hour
q2h	every 2 hours
q4h	every 4 hours
q6h	every 6 hours
q8h	every 8 hours
q12h	every 12 hours
q24h	every 24 hours
q48h	every 48 hours
QAM; qam	every morning
qDay; QD†	every day
q.i.d.; QID	four times daily
QOD; Q other day; Q.O. Day	every other day
QPM; qpm	every evening
qs; qsad	quantity sufficient; a sufficient quantity to make
QTY; qty	quantity
Rx	prescription; pharmacy; medication; drug; recipe; take
S-T	
sig	write on label; signa; directions
SL; sub-L	sublingual
SMZ-TMP	sulfamethoxazole and trimethoprim; Bactrim
sol	solution

Abbreviation	Meaning
SR	sustained-release
SS; ss	one-half
SSRI	selective serotonin reuptake inhibitor
Stat	immediately; now
Sub-Q; SC; SQ; sq	subcutaneous
SUPP; Supp	suppository
susp	suspension
SW	sterile water
SWFI	sterile water for injection
Tab	tablet
TBSP; tbsp	tablespoon; tablespoonful; 15 mL
TCN	tetracycline
t.i.d.; TID	three times daily
TPN	total parenteral nutrition
TSP; tsp	teaspoon; teaspoonful; 5 mL
U-V-W	
U	unit
ung	ointment
ut dict	as directed
VAG; vag	vagina; vaginally
w/	with
wk; WK	week
w/o	without
X-Y-Z	
ZnO; ZNO	zinc oxide

† Please note that this abbreviation is on the Joint Commission's Official "Do Not Use" List of Abbreviations. However, you may occasionally encounter its use in your practice. If you see this abbreviation on a prescription or medication order, alert the pharmacist who will, in turn, clarify the order with the prescriber.

* Please note that this abbreviation is being considered for possible future inclusion in the Joint Commission's Official "Do Not Use" List of Abbreviations.

Appendix D
Measures and Conversions

Metric

Volume
1 L = 1000 mL
1 mL = 1 cc

Weight
1 g = 1000 mg
1 mg = 1000 mcg

Household

Volume
1 gal = 4 qt
1 qt = 2 pt
1 pt = 2 cups = 16 fl oz
1 fl oz = 2 tbsp = 6 tsp

Weight
1 lb = 16 oz

Length
1 yd = 3 ft
1 ft = 12 in

Conversions

	Household	Apothecary	Metric
Volume	1 qt = 32 fl oz		0.96 L
	1 pint = 16 fl oz		480 mL *
	1 cup = 8 fl oz		240 mL
	2 tbsp = 1 fl oz	6 f℥ = 1 f℥	30 mL *
	1 tbsp	3 f℥	15 mL
	1 tsp	1 f℥	5 mL †
		1 ♏	0.0625 mL
Weight	2.2 lb		1 kg
	1 lb		454 g
	1 oz	8 ℥	30 g
Length	1 in		2.5 cm

* There are actually 29.57 mL in 1 fl oz, but 30 mL is usually used. When packaging a pint, companies will typically include 473 mL, rather than the full 480 mL, thus saving money over time.

† There are actually 3.75 mL in an apothecary f℥. However, convention dictates that 1 f℥ = 5 mL = 1 tsp.

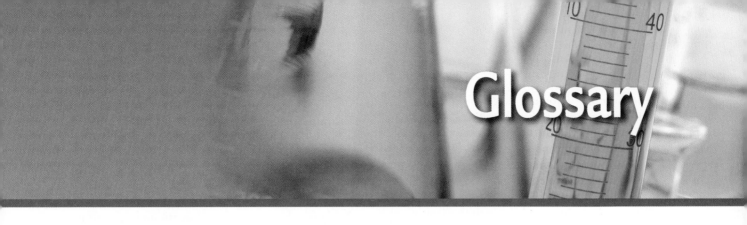

Glossary

A

accuracy the correctness of a number in its representation of a given value

active ingredient the component of a pharmaceutical preparation or medication that exerts pharmacological activity designed to treat or prevent disease

additive a pharmaceutical substance, such as a medication, electrolyte, or other ingredient, that is added to another product, such as a compounded sterile preparation, to be easily administered to a patient

alligation method the mathematical calculation used to determine the amounts of two or more dilutions of differing strengths that will be mixed to prepare a product of a desired strength and quantity

Arabic numbers a numbering system that uses numeric symbols to indicate numbers, fractions, and decimals; uses the numerals 0, 1, 2, 3, 4, 5, 6, 7, 8, 9

assets properties, furnishings, inventory, supplies, and equipment owned by the pharmacy; may be put into two categories: current, or short-term, assets and long-term assets

atomic weight the weight of a single atom of an element compared with the weight of a single atom of hydrogen

average wholesale price (AWP) an average price at which drugs are purchased at the wholesale level, or the average value at which wholesalers sell a particular drug to pharmacies

B

base profit the amount of profit determined by subtracting the total pharmacy overhead amount from the pharmacy's income

body surface area (BSA) a measurement related to a patient's weight and height, expressed in meters squared (m²), and used to calculate patient-specific doses of medications

brand name the name under which the manufacturer markets a drug; a registered trademark of the manufacturer; also known as the *trade name*

C

capitation fee a monthly fee paid by some insurance plans to a pharmacy under a specific prescription reimbursement plan

Celsius a thermometric scale in which 100° is the boiling point of water and 0° is the freezing point of water

Clark's Rule a formula used to determine an appropriate pediatric dose by using the child's weight in pounds and the normal adult dose; weight in lb/150 lb × adult dose = pediatric dose

common denominator a number into which each of the unlike denominators of two or more fractions can be divided evenly

complex fraction a fraction in which both the numerator and the denominator are fractions

compounded sterile preparation (CSP) the mixing of one or more sterile parenteral products using aseptic technique

compounded stock preparation a solution that is prepared in a large amount and kept in stock in the pharmacy to be divided for individual prescriptions

compounding the process of using raw ingredients and/or other prepared ingredients to create a drug product for a patient

conversion factor an equivalency equal to 1 that can be used when converting units of measure using the ratio-proportion method

current formula a standard pharmaceutical recipe that is commonly used in pharmacy compounding; a recipe often used to prepare compounded stock preparations

current percentage of profit the amount of profit that is determined by dividing the base profit by income and then multiplying that quotient by 100; often used to determine the desired percentage of profit

D

days' supply the number of days that a prescription or medication order will last a patient when taken as directed by the prescriber

DEA number a number issued by the Drug Enforcement Administration (DEA) to signify the authority of the holder to prescribe or handle controlled substances; made up of two letters followed by seven digits, the last of which is a checksum digit used to check the validity of the DEA number

decimal a fraction value in which the denominator is 10 or some power of 10

denominator the number in the bottom part of a fraction

depreciation an allowance made to account for the decreasing value of a fixed asset; properties, furnishings, and equipment owned by the pharmacy are called *fixed assets*, or simply *assets*

desired formula a specialized pharmaceutical recipe that may be ordered by the prescriber and that results from altering various components of the current formula

desired percentage of profit the percentage of profit the pharmacy intends to make on the product after the overall cost is subtracted from the selling price

dimensional analysis method a conversion method in which the given number and unit are multiplied by the ratio of the desired unit to the given unit, which is equivalent to 1

discount a price that is reduced from what is typically charged

discount rate the percent that the discounted price is reduced from the regular selling price

dispensing fee the amount that is charged over and above the pharmacy's purchase price for a medication; this amount is meant to cover all costs related to filling a prescription, beyond the purchase price of the drug

disposal value the value of an item should it be sold or otherwise disposed of at the end of its useful life

dose on a prescription, the indication of how much medication the patient will take at each administration

dosing schedule on a prescription, the indication of how often the drug is to be taken

dosing table a table providing dose recommendations based on the age and/or the weight of the patient; often used to determine the safe dose for a pediatric patient

drop factor the number of drops an IV set takes to make 1 mL; also called *drip set*

E

electrolytes substances such as mineral salts that conduct an electrical charge when dissolved in a solution

F

Fahrenheit a thermometric scale in which 212° is the boiling point of water and 32° is the freezing point of water

flat rate a low pharmacy selling price for a certain amount of medication, a supply designed to last a specific number of days

flow rate the rate, expressed in milliliters per hour or drops per minute, at which medication is flowing through an IV line; also called *infusion rate* and *rate of infusion*

formula a written document listing the ingredients and instructions needed to prepare a compound

fraction a portion of a whole that is represented as a ratio

G

generic name the name under which a drug is approved by the Food and Drug Administration; sometimes denotes a drug that is not protected by a trademark; also referred to as a *USAN (United States Adopted Name)*

gram the basic unit for measuring weight in the metric system

gross profit the difference between the pharmacy's selling price and purchase price

H

household measure a system of measure used in homes, particularly in kitchens, in the United States; units of measure for volume include teaspoonful, tablespoonful, cup, pint, quart, and gallon; units for weight are pound and ounce

I

improper fraction a fraction with a value greater than 1 (the value of the numerator is larger than the value of the denominator)

inactive ingredient an inert ingredient that is used as a base, or vehicle, to deliver the active ingredient in a compounded preparation; for example, petrolatum is used as a base in many topical preparations

income the money or equivalent received from the sale of medications, supply items, or equipment

infusion the administration of a large volume of liquid medication given parenterally over a long period of time

injection a method of administering medications in which a syringe with a needle or cannula is used to penetrate through the skin or membrane into the tissue below

intramuscular (IM) injection an injection given into the aqueous muscle tissue

intravenous (IV) infusion the injection of fluid into the veins

inventory a listing of all of the items that are available for sale in a business

inventory value the total value of all of the drugs and merchandise in stock on a given day

L

leading zero a zero that is placed to the left of the decimal point, in the ones place, in a number that is less than 1 and is being represented by a decimal value

liter the basic unit for measuring volume in the metric system

lowest known place value the last digit on the right of a written numeral

M

markup rate a percentage amount that is determined by subtracting the pharmacy's purchase price for an item from the pharmacy's selling price for that item

meter the basic unit for measuring length in the metric system

metric system a measurement system based on subdivisions and multiples of 10; made up of three basic units: meter, gram, and liter

military time a system of time based on a 24-hour format

milliequivalent (mEq) the ratio of the weight of a molecule to its valence, used to measure the concentration of electrolytes in a volume of solution; also an amount of medication that will provide the patient with a specific amount (equivalent amount) of an electrolyte

millimole (mM) molecular weight expressed in milligrams

mini-drip set a drop set at a rate of 60 gtts/mL

mixed number a whole number and a fraction

molecular weight the sum of the atomic weights of all atoms in one molecule of a compound

N

net profit the difference between the selling price and the overall cost

numerator the number in the top part of a fraction

O

overall cost the sum of the cost to purchase the drug from the manufacturer (known as the pharmacy's purchase price) and the cost to dispense the drug

overhead the pharmacy's cost of doing business; this cost includes personnel salaries, equipment, and operating expenses such as rent, taxes, and utilities

P

par level an average inventory range for an item, which generally includes the minimum and maximum stock levels for the item

parenteral administered by injection or infusion and not by way of the GI system

percent the number of parts per 100; can be written as a fraction, a decimal, or a ratio

percentage of error the percentage by which a measurement is inaccurate

percentage strength a mathematical formula or expression used to identify the number of grams of active ingredient per 100 mL of solution (or per 100 g of solid); may be referred to as *percent strength*

pharmacy benefits manager (PBM) a large prescription processing service that contracts with insurance companies and pharmacies to process insurance reimbursement

place value the location of a numeral in a string of numbers that describes the numeral's relationship to the decimal point

powder volume (PV) the space occupied by dry pharmaceuticals, calculated as the difference between the final volume and the volume of the diluting ingredient, or the diluent volume; the amount of space occupied by lyophilized (freeze-dried) medication in a sterile vial, used for reconstitution

prescription an order for medication for a patient that is written by a physician or a qualified licensed practitioner to be filled by a pharmacist

product the result of multiplying one number by another

profit the financial gain made when the amount earned is greater than the amount spent during a specified period

profit margin the difference between the cost of doing business (the pharmacy's purchase price, overhead, and preparation costs) and the selling price of a drug or product

proper fraction a fraction with a value of less than 1 (the value of the numerator is smaller than the value of the denominator)

proportion an expression of equality between two ratios

purchase price the cost to purchase the drug from the wholesaler or manufacturer

Q

quotient the result of dividing one number by another

R

ratio a numerical representation of the relationship between two parts of the whole or between one part and the whole

ratio strength a means of describing the concentration of a liquid medication based on a ratio such as *a* grams:*b* milliliters

ratio-proportion method a conversion method based on comparing a complete ratio to a ratio with a missing component

Roman numerals a numbering system that uses alphabetic symbols to indicate a quantity; uses the letters I, V, and X to represent 1, 5, and 10, respectively

route of administration on a prescription, the indication of how the medication is to be given

S

scientific notation a method used to write numbers that have a very large or very small numerical value; uses "× 10" with an exponent

selling price the amount that the pharmacy charges for a particular drug or product

signa (sig) from the Latin word for "write"; the part of the prescription that provides instructions for proper use of the medication, including the dose, route of administration, and dosing schedule

significant figures the figures in a numeral that are known values and have not been rounded or estimated in the process of mathematical calculation, plus the digit in the lowest place value, which is approximate

solute the substance dissolved in the liquid solvent in a solution

solution a mixture of two or more substances

solvent the liquid that dissolves the solute in a solution

special dilution a custom-made CSP that provides accurate dosage of a medication prepared according to a desired recipe or formula; a term often associated with certain neonatal or pediatric CSPs

standard time a system of time that relates to the natural day and is based on a 12-hour format

subcutaneous (SC) injection an injection given into the vascular, fatty layer of tissue under the skin

sum the result of adding two or more numbers together

T

total parenteral nutrition (TPN) IV administration of total nutrient requirements to patients who require a long-term alternative to enteral feeding

TPN base solution components of the TPN solution that provide the primary volumetric source of hydration and calories, often composed of a combination of dextrose, amino acids, fat emulsion, and sterile water

trailing zero a zero that appears at the end of a decimal string and is not needed except when considered significant

turnover rate the number of times the amount of goods in inventory was sold during the year

U

unit the amount of activity associated with a medication that has a biological impact on a patient

V

valence the ability of a molecule to bond, as indicated by its positive or negative charge; represented by a superscript plus or minus sign next to an element's chemical symbol

vehicle an inert medium, such as a syrup, in which a drug is administered

volume in volume (v/v) the number of milliliters of a drug (solute) in 100 mL of the final product (solution)

W

weight in volume (w/v) the number of grams of a drug (solute) in 100 mL of the final product (solution)

weight-in-weight (w/w) formula the number of grams of a drug (solid) in 100 g of the final product (solid)

wholesaler a company that sells and distributes a large number of goods such as medications and supply items to a pharmacy; a company that acts as a go-between for pharmacies and manufacturing companies such as drug manufacturers

Y

Young's Rule a formula used to determine an appropriate pediatric dose by using the child's age in years and the normal adult dose; age in years/(age in years + 12 years) × adult dose = pediatric dose

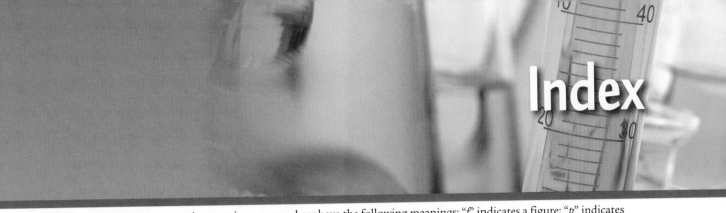

Index

Note: The letters accompanying certain page numbers have the following meanings: "*f*" indicates a figure; "*p*" indicates a photo; "*t*" indicates a table.

Photo and Art Credits

1 © Paradigm Publishing; **2** © Paradigm Publishing; **8** Reprinted with permission of Mylan Pharmaceuticals Inc. All rights reserved; **9** Reprinted with permission of Mylan Pharmaceuticals Inc. All rights reserved; **13** © Paradigm Publishing; **17** © Paradigm Publishing; **44** © Paradigm Publishing (illustration and photo); **46** © Copyright Eli Lilly and Company. All Rights Reserved. Used with Permission. Cymbalta is a trademark of Eli Lilly and Company; Copyright Pfizer Inc. Used with permission; **47** Image courtesy of American Regent, Inc.; © Paradigm Publishing; **49** Images used with permission from Fresenius Kabi USA, LLC; **51** © Paradigm Publishing; **53** © Paradigm Publishing; **55** Images used with permission from Fresenius Kabi USA, LLC; **59** Images used with permission from Fresenius Kabi USA, LLC; **60** Images used with permission from Fresenius Kabi USA, LLC; **61** Images used with permission from Fresenius Kabi USA, LLC; Courtesy of Apothecary Products, Inc.; **62** Courtesy of Apothecary Products, Inc.; **74** © Paradigm Publishing; **75** © Paradigm Publishing; **77** Copyright Pfizer Inc. Used with permission; **78** Reprinted with permission of Mylan Pharmaceuticals Inc. All rights reserved; Images used with permission from Fresenius Kabi USA, LLC; **79** Image courtesy of American Regent, Inc.; Courtesy of Apothecary Products, Inc. (2); Courtesy of Tova Wiegand-Green; **80** Image courtesy of Optimer; **83** Macrobid container label used with permission. Macrobid is a registered trademark of Almatica Pharma, Inc.; © Copyright Eli Lilly and Company. All Rights Reserved. Used with Permission. Prozac is a trademark of Eli Lilly and Company (2); Reprinted with permission of Mylan Pharmaceuticals Inc. All rights reserved; **84** Copyright Pfizer Inc. Used with permission; Mallinckrodt LLC; **93** Reprinted with permission of Mylan Pharmaceuticals Inc. All rights reserved; Image courtesy of Salix; **99** © Paradigm Publishing (5 photos); **107** Images used with permission from Fresenius Kabi USA, LLC; **112** Mallinckrodt LLC; **113** Images used with permission from Fresenius Kabi USA, LLC; Copyright Pfizer Inc. Used with permission; **114** Images used with permission from Fresenius Kabi USA, LLC; **118** Copyright © Novartis Pharmaceuticals Corp. Used with permission; **119** Copyright © Novartis Pharmaceuticals Corp. Used with permission; **134** © Paradigm Publishing; **135** © Paradigm Publishing; **139** © Paradigm Publishing; **140** © Paradigm Publishing; **140** Mallinckrodt LLC; **145** © Paradigm Publishing; **147** Mallinckrodt LLC; **150** © Paradigm Publishing; **161** © iStockphoto/malerapaso; **164** © Paradigm Publishing (2); **176** Images used with permission from Fresenius Kabi USA, LLC; **177** © Paradigm Publishing (2); Images used with permission from Fresenius Kabi USA, LLC; **178** Images used with permission from Fresenius